POLYMER DRUGS IN THE CLINICAL STAGE

ADVANTAGES AND PROSPECTS

ADVANCES IN EXPERIMENTAL MEDICINE AND BIOLOGY

Recent Volumes in this Series

Volume 510
OXYGEN TRANSPORT TO TISSUE XXIII: Oxygen Measurements in the 21st Century: Basic Techniques and Clinical Relevance
Edited by David F. Wilson, Sydney M. Evans, John Biaglow, and Anna Pastuszko

Volume 511
PEDIATRIC GENDER ASSIGNMENT: A Critical Reappraisal
Edited by Stephen A. Zderic, Douglas A. Canning, Michael C. Carr, and Howard McC. Snyder, III.

Volume 512
LYMPHOCYTE ACTIVATION AND IMMUNE REGULATION IX: Homeostasis and Lymphocyte Traffic
Edited by Sudhir Gupta, Eugene Butcher, and William Paul

Volume 513
MOLECULAR AND CELLULAR BIOLOGY OF NEUROPROTECTION IN THE CNS
Edited by Christian Alzheimer

Volume 514
PHOTORECEPTORS AND CALCIUM
Edited by Wolfgang Baehr

Volume 515
NEUROPILIN: From Nervous System to Vascular and Tumor Biology
Edited by Dominique Bagnard

Volume 516
TRIPLE REPEAT DISEASES OF THE NERVOUS SYSTEM
Edited by Lubov T. Timchenko

Volume 517
DOPAMINERGIC NEURON TRANSPLANTATION IN THE WEAVER MOUSE MODEL OF PARKINSON'S DISEASE
Edited by Lazaros C. Triarhou

Volume 518
ADVANCES IN MALE MEDIATED DEVELOPMENTAL TOXICITY
Edited by Bernard Robaire and Barbara F. Hales

Volume 519
POLYMER DRUGS IN THE CLINICAL STAGE: Advantages and Prospects
Edited by Hiroshi Maeda, Alexander Kabanov, Kazurori Kataoka, and Teruo Okano

POLYMER DRUGS IN THE CLINICAL STAGE

ADVANTAGES AND PROSPECTS

Edited by

Hiroshi Maeda
Kumamoto University School of Medicine
Kumamoto, Japan

Alexander Kabanov
University of Nebraska Medical Center
Omaha, Nebraska

Kazurori Kataoka
University of Tokyo
Tokyo, Japan

and

Teruo Okano
Tokyo Women's Medical College
Tokyo, Japan

Springer Science+Business Media, LLC

Proceedings of the International Symposium on Polymer Therapeutics—Recent Progress in Clinics and Future Prospects, held July 13–14, 2001, in Nara, Japan.

ISSN 0065-2598

DOI 10.1007/978-0-306-47932-8

Originally published by Kluwer Academic/Plenum Publishers, New York in 2003
MyCopy version of the original edition 2003

http://www.wkap.nl/

10 9 8 7 6 5 4 3 2 1

A C.I.P. record for this book is available from the Library of Congress

Preface

Progress in research on polymeric-drugs has been remarkable in the past few decades, whereas development of clinical applications of these drugs has been slow. The oldest and most widely used polymer-based drug is an antiseptic agent, povidone-iodine, which consists of a complex of poly (1-vinyl-2-pyrrolidone) and iodine. Used since the 1950s, it is still the best antiseptic agent available. True polymer-based drugs that can be administered by injection did not become practical until the 1990s, although the numbers of polymeric drugs such as SMANCS and interferon that are now being used in clinics is still limited. As will be apparent in this volume, however, the great potential of these drugs is now clear, especially in view of their prolonged plasma half-life and enhanced targeting to sites of either cancerous or inflammatory lesions. Use of these drugs will result in great benefits for patients in terms of compliance and quality of life, as well as improved therapeutic efficacy and cost effectiveness of the drugs. Realization of such advantages becomes a strong incentive for research scientists and entrepreneurs, and there are probably more than three-dozen candidate drugs with polymer conjugates currently under development.

The technology of polymer science has developed considerably during the past half-century, and in this volume, we describe some of the aspects of this technology that will have a great impact in the future. Among these advances, for example, are gene delivery to specific disease sites and carrier polymers that respond to a stimulus or particular environment. We include discussions of as many examples as possible of polymer drugs that have achieved, or are close to clinical use. We have limited our concept of "Polymer drugs" here to primarily injectable and water-soluble agents, although we have also covered some drugs in micellar form or liposomes.

This book is intended for students and researchers in the field of pharmacology who have particular interests in drug delivery, targeting, and formulation, as well as for clinicians such as oncologists who are interested in the field. People who work at regulatory agencies should also be aware such that drugs with great potential are being developed and will be beneficial to many patients, as well as to health insurance agencies because of improved cost effectiveness. Thus, a great impact on society at large is anticipated.

Finally, we want to acknowledge that this book was initiated as a result of the enthusiasm generated during the "*International Symposium of Polymer Therapeutics – Recent Progress in Clinic and Future Prospects*", which was held in Nara, July 13 and 14, 2001. Most of the chapters treated in this monograph are thus based on the symposium, with a few new additions.

The Editors,

Hiroshi Maeda
Alexander Kabanov
Kazurori Kataoka
Teruo Okano

June, 2002

Contents

Challenges in Polymer Therapeutics

State of the Art and Prospects of Polymer Drugs

ALEXANDER V. KABANOV* AND TERUO OKANO#

College of Pharmacy, Department of Pharmaceutical Sciences, University of Nebraska Medical Center, 986025 Nebraska Medical Center, Omaha, NE 68198-6025, USA; akabanov@unmc.edu; *# Institute of Biomedical Engineering, Tokyo Women's Medical University, 8-1 Kawadacho, Shinjuku, Tokyo 162, Japan;* tokano@lab.twmu.ac.j

1. INTRODUCTION

The field of drug delivery has attracted tremendous attention during the last two decades. The principal reason for this attention, and the resulting impact on the advance of the field, is the awareness that substantial improvements over current therapies will likely occur primarily through improved delivery of current and yet to be discovered drugs. This realization arises primarily due to the existence of the many barriers that must be circumvented before a drug molecule will reach its target site within the body. In addition, delivery systems can address and correct problems related to the physical characteristic of a drug, including solubility and stability. Consequently, the technologies currently under development for drug delivery and drug targeting systems will have a tremendous impact on the improvement of novel drug therapies.

One particular subset of drug delivery systems, those that are based on synthetic polymers, appears particularly promising [1]. This has lead to the emergence of new field, coined "*polymer therapeutics*". Generally speaking, polymer therapeutics refers to the use of a polymer as a component of a pharmaceutical formulation for the purpose of improving drug or gene performance. The array of polymers enlisted for this task is quite broad, and includes polymers, exhibiting inherent biological activity, as well as polymers that can exist in the form of polymer-drug conjugates, polymeric micelles, nanoparticles and polymer-coated liposomes. A growing number of polymer therapeutic agents have been approved by the regulatory authorities in the

Polymer Drugs in the Clinical Stage, Edited by Maeda et al.
Kluwer Academic/Plenum Publishers, New York, 2003

North America, Europe and Asia for clinical use in treatment of cancer, infectious and genetic diseases.

There are several fundamental properties of polymers that are useful in solving drug delivery problems. First, polymers can be designed to be intrinsically multifunctional and can, for example, be combined either covalently or non-covalently with drugs to overcome multiple problems such as solubility, stability, permeability, etc. Second, polymers can be easily modified with various targeting vectors to direct drugs to specific sites in the body. Third, polymers can be designed to be environmentally responsive materials, allowing for the controlled and sustained release of a drug at its site of action. And finally, polymers themselves can be biologically active, and this property can be exploited in order to modify the activity of various endogenous drug transport systems within the body to improve delivery and, therefore, to improve drug performance.

The field of polymer therapeutics has advanced significantly over the past two decades, resulting in the current state of the field, which is marked by initiated, ongoing, and even several completed clinical trials. A landmark symposium, "*The International Symposium on Polymer Therapeutics: Recent Progress in Clinic and Future Prospects*" was held in Nara, Japan in July 2001, to overview the current state of the field and the future prospects of polymer-based drugs. This symposium was striking in that the entire program of lectures was devoted to reports on the clinical aspects of polymer therapeutics. The symposium ended with a very dynamic podium-organized discussion that focused specifically on the challenges and future prospects of polymer therapeutics. This discussion evolved into a prolific 'think tank', fueled by the knowledge, experience and thought processes of each and every meeting attendee. The result was the successful identification the key issues of highest priority to the further development of this field of research. The present chapter serves to briefly summarize this discussion. This short summary is not intended to serve as an in-depth critical review of the field, but rather to present some of the identified key issues that should be focal to researchers within this field.

2. DISCOVERY AND DEVELOPMENT OF NEW POLYMER MATERIALS

There appears to be a consensus in literature that new polymer materials for applications in drug and gene delivery are needed. However, the process of material development for pharmaceutical applications requires a significant commitment of both time and money, including the daunting requirement to address regulatory issues. Therefore, the prospect of development of new, novel polymer materials cannot be taken lightly. As a result, it is imperative that the goals and requirements for any new material development be precisely outlined.

Identification of the goals and requirements for new material development could only occur following critical evaluation of currently existing polymer therapeutics. At the present time, only a relatively small number of polymer materials have been administered in the human body. Of those materials, only an even smaller subset, including examples of amphiphilic, hydrophobic and hydrophilic molecules, has been clinically validated as safe for the systemic administration in the body. Each of the validated materials represents a tremendous advancement in therapy from both clinical and commercial viewpoints.

Examples of approved water-soluble or amphiphilic neutral polymers include polyethyleneglycol (PEG) [2], poly(vinylpyrolidone) (PVP) [3], copolymers of N-(2-hydroxypropyl)methacrylamide (pHPMA) [4], and poly(ethylene oxide)-*b*-poly(propylene oxide)-*b*-poly(ethylene oxide) block copolymers (poloxamers or Pluronic®) [5, 6]. These polymers have been utilized in a broad range of applications including, but not limited to, the preparation of soluble polymer-drug conjugates (pHPMA), the surface modification of proteins, liposomes and nanoparticles (PEG, pHPMA, Pluronic®), the preparation of micellar drug formulations (Pluronic®), as well as the employment of these polymers as biological response modifying agents (PVP, Pluronic®).

Examples of clinically validated water-insoluble, biodegradable polymers include material such as poly(D,L,lactide-*co*-glycolide (PLGA) [7], poly(ortho esters) (POE) [8], and polyisohexylcyanoacrylate (PIHCA) [9]. These materials have been used for the preparation of nanoparticles, biodegradable implants and viscous injectable materials. In addition, one amphiphilic material, poly(styrene-co-maleic acid) copolymer conjugated with neocarzinostatin (SMANCS) dissolved in lipid contrast medium Lipiodol, has proven efficacious in several clinical trials for the treatment of cancer [10, 11].

Charged polymers are also present within the inventory of successful polymer therapeutics. For example, high molecular mass polyanions, such as polyacrylic resins and copolymers of acrylic acid have been utilized in various oral dosage forms, however, there is less clinical data regarding their use in systemic drug delivery formulations [12]. The few well-known examples of systemically administered anionic polymers, include heparin and its synthetic analogs, e.g. highly sulfated glycosaminoglycans [13]. However these are biologically active compounds that are used as drugs rather than components of drug delivery formulations. One example of a synthetic polyanion administered in the body is poly(dicarboxylato-phenoxyphosphazene) (PCPP) that was evaluated in clinical trials as immunoadjuvant in a number of preventive vaccines, such as influenza [14, 15]. This is a biodegradable polymer which slowly degrades producing low molecular weight compounds – ammonium phosphate and hydroxybenzoic acid. This polymer is interesting not only because of its unique immunoajuvants properties, but also because it can be used as a polyanionic component of constructs for drug delivery and drug release in the body [16, 17].

In this context, it is important to point out that polycations, as a rule, are substantially more toxic than water-soluble nonionic polymers and polyanions. Therefore, the development of cationic polymer therapeutics, such as is currently under way for gene delivery applications, obviously represents a substantial challenge to the field. Nonetheless some polycation-based therapeutics have indeed been developed and tested in clinical applications. For instance, chitosan, has been incorporated in a number of oral, topical and injectable drug therapeutics and vaccines [18, 19]. Another example of a successful polycation-based polymer therapeutic is "polyoxidonium", a partially N-alkylated, partially N-oxidized copolymer of poly(1,4-ethylenepiperaside) [20]. Polyoxidonium is biodegradable polymer that serves as an immunomodulating component of artificial polymer-antigen conjugated vaccines. The most notable of which is an anti-influenza vaccine "Grippol", which has been approved by Russian regulatory authorities and has been administered in over 15 million human subjects [21].

The studies using polymeric micelles, block ionomer complexes and other similar materials for drug and gene delivery have been very promising [22-47]. These materials form as result of self-assembly of block- or graft copolymers containing polymer segments of different structure and functionality, for example, ionic and nonionic block, or hydrophilic and hydrophobic block, etc. The use of such materials in pharmaceutics is contingent upon successful development of various block or graft copolymers. This leads to a whole lot of issues of synthesis, characterization and pharmacological evaluation of block copolymers, as well as other polymers of different architecture. The characterization of such polymers both *in vitro* and *in vivo* is quite complex and further studies in this area are needed.

Overall, one should expect, based on the already available clinical data, including the identification of short fallings and limitations of the current polymer therapeutics that further validation of existing polymers and the appearance of several new and novel materials appropriate for a diverse array of therapeutic applications will rapidly progress.

3. ARE BIODEGRADABLE POLYMERS NEEDED?

The successful application of a particular polymer in polymer therapeutics cannot be predicted based on that polymer's characteristic of biodegradability or non-biodegradability. For example, PLGA and PEG are both highly successful materials, however, PLGA is biodegradable, while PEG is not. This points out one of the most quintessential questions in polymer therapeutics today: are new biodegradable polymer materials needed and, if they are, what are the likely situations requiring their use? In order to properly address this question, the multitude of unique drug delivery situations, as well as the classes of materials to be employed, require consideration.

Water-soluble nonionic polymers are usually characterized by relatively low toxicity. While some of these water-soluble polymers can be degradable, they arguably do not have to be degradable if their administration in therapeutically needed amounts is not associated with toxic effects. Furthermore, frequently the degradation of such polymers in the organism should be avoided, because it might complicate the analytical procedures and obscure the approval of the formulation by the regulatory authorities. When administered systemically these polymers are often removed from the body without degradation within an acceptable time frame. The rates and mechanisms of clearance of the polymers are dependent on their molecular mass. Polymers (both nonionic and ionic) with a molecular mass below the renal threshold barrier are usually cleared quickly from the blood and are eliminated from the body primarily by renal excretion. For example, the upper molecular mass limit for renal excretion of intravenously injected hyaluronic acid is about 25 000 [48]. Similar values for the renal threshold barrier are displayed by pHPMA copolymers, which are cleared from blood circulation in a molecular-mass dependent manner [49]. Poloxamer 188 (Pluronic® F68) a hydrophilic block copolymer, m.w. 8,400, which is also under the above threshold, is excreted mainly through the renal clearance [50]. The use of polymers displaying a molecular mass above the renal threshold limit permits the polymers to escape renal clearance, shifting the primary route of blood clearance to elimination through extravasation into tissues [49, 51, 52]. If very large polymer molecules are needed for drug delivery, one can produce such molecules by cross-linking several smaller nondegradable polymers via biodegradable links. The cleavage of those linkages in the body will result in the release of the smaller polymers, which can be eventually removed through the renal clearance route.

Insoluble polymers are used in the preparation of implants, micro- and nanoparticles, particularly among those that are administered locally [53-55]. Generally speaking, these polymers cannot be removed from the body unless they are degraded. Furthermore, the mechanism of drug release from such materials is generally anchored on the principles of erosion and polymer degradation in the biological milieu, allowing the rate of the polymer degradation to be one factor that controls the rate of drug release [56]. Therefore, for this particular application, it is quite apparent that the development of such biodegradable polymers was a clear necessity to advance the research in this area over the last two decades.

In contrast, research in the area of biodegradable polyelectrolytes is much less advanced. Polyelectrolytes are generally significantly more toxic than water-soluble nonionic polymers. This problem is particularly severe in the case of polycations, which exhibit toxic effects through interactions with various charged species present in the body. At the same time, the advancement of novel technologies, such as gene delivery and stimulus-sensitive drug carrier systems, has underscored the increasing need for the development of polyelectrolyte materials that can be safely administered in the body. This toxicity can, to an extent, be alleviated simply by making those materials biodegradable. One of the early examples of successful use of this approach is polyoxidonium, developed in early 80's as immunomodulating agent by the groups of V. Kabanov, R. Petrov and R. Khaitov [57], which is now widely used in many vaccines administered in humans. A more recent example is poly[alpha-(4-aminobutyl)-l-glycolic acid] (PAGA), a biodegradable nontoxic polymer, developed by the group of S.-W. Kim for the delivery of plasmid DNA [58]. In contrast to the majority of polycations used for gene delivery, this polymer has remarkably low toxicity while maintaining the ability to deliver therapeutic genes *in vivo* [59, 60]. One should expect significant new developments in the area of biodegradable nontoxic polyelectrolytes in the near future.

4. IS SPECIFIC TARGETING OF POLYMER THERAPEUTICS USEFUL?

On first sight, the question posed in the title of this section might appear irrelevant in view of the successful clinical development of immunotoxins [61] and targeted radioimaging agents [62]. However, the situation is actually far more complex that it might appear. First of all, poor extravasation within interstitial spaces of macromolecular objects with sizes exceeding 5-10 nm severely limits the ability of these objects to reach their precise cellular targets within a normal tissue or organ [63]. As a result, specific targeting of such objects to those sites is difficult, if not impossible. Therefore, with rare exceptions, targeting of polymer therapeutics will be mainly limited to those sites readily accessible to the circulatory system, such as blood components, endothelial cells, subendothelial structures and ischemic regions of the heart [63, 64]. Selected polymer therapeutics display elevated circulation times, which may, to some extent, mitigate the effect of the poor extravasation of the therapeutics in the tissues. However, some existing examples, such as PEGylated liposomes also suggest that increased circulation times may come at a cost of deposition of liposomes to skin resulting in the skin toxicity effects [65].

The second set of problems is associated with situations when there is a need to deliver a drug or biomacromolecule into a cell or across a cellular barrier. Such situations are realized, for example, during the delivery of DNA into cells, the transport of drug across the blood brain barrier (BBB), or the delivery of a drug *via* the oral route, when the delivery vehicle is required to cross the intestinal epithelium. One way to enhance delivery in these cases is to target appropriate receptors expressed at the cell surface that would allow for endocytosis (into cell) or transcytosis (across cell) of the drug carrier. For example, several studies have used antibodies to transferrin receptor to deliver macromolecular constructs across the BBB [66]. The questions that arise with respect to such studies are as follows: First, are there enough receptor molecules displayed at the cell surface to allow for the transport of a therapeutic dose of targeted materials to its site of action? Second, is the endocytosis machinery in those cells efficient enough to deliver the therapeutic dose to the appropriate target within the cell or to deliver it across cellular barriers? Another question arises with respect to the fact that moieties designed to target cell receptors often display biological activity of their own and, as a result of their administration to the body, some harmful and unexpected side effects may be displayed.

The concept of using polymeric drug carriers in combination with the targeting moieties is, generally speaking, very attractive [67]. A single unit of a given polymeric drug carrier can incorporate many molecules of drug, resulting in high "payloads" per one targeting moiety and/or receptor engaged. Furthermore, by increasing the payload of the carrier, one might improve the efficacy of the delivery while maintaining a relatively low level of involvement of numbers of targeted moieties and receptors. However, there might be an additional problem here. Specifically, an increase in the cargo space of the pharmaceutical carrier is usually associated with an increase in the volume and surface area of this carrier. As a result, nonspecific molecular interactions of the carrier with biological objects present in the body (cell surfaces, biomacromolecules, etc.) might elevate to the extent that the net contribution of such interactions becomes comparable with or greater than the contribution of the specific binding of the targeting moieties with the receptors. At this point the advantages of specific targeting should drop drastically due to the high levels of nonspecific binding of carrier with cells and tissues, such as macrophages or reticuloendothelial cells. One obvious remedy could be, firstly, to modify the surface of the carrier with "inert" moieties such as PEG chains that would have minimal interactions with the cells and, secondly, to attach the specific targeting moieties at the surface or above the inert layer to allow for specific binding of the targeting moiety with its receptor. This approach has been used, for example, with various PEG-modified species including block copolymer micelles, polyelectrolyte complexes and liposomes (hence, "stealth" liposomes) [42, 68-70].

Overall, targeting strategies employing specific "vector" molecules are being actively pursued in many laboratories. Success with this approach has already been demonstrated *in vivo* with a variety of pharmaceutical carriers, including soluble polymers, microcapsules, microparticles, cells, cell ghosts, liposomes, and micelles, for a review see [67]. However, the actual usefulness of this approach for drug delivery in human trials remains to be seen.

5. DRUG TARGETING IN THE ABSENCE OF SPECIFIC TARGETING MOIETIES

One potential disadvantage of the specific targeting approach discussed in the previous section involves the increase in the complexity and the cost of the manufacture of the pharmaceutical carrier as a result of conjugation of this carrier with the specific targeting groups. Therefore alternative approaches that will allow for site-specific drug delivery without the use of targeting moieties, are of significant interest. Currently, such approaches include direct local application of a drug to the site of action, magnetic targeting of drugs immobilized on paramagnetic materials, "passive" drug targeting (a technique that exploits local variations in vascular permeability based on so-called "*enhanced permeability and retention*" (EPR) effect, and finally, "physical" drug targeting (a technique that exploits local variations in pH and/or temperature including arterial infusion method using catheter)[67].

Administration of a drug delivery system directly to the site of action would be the most straightforward and cost effective approach to drug targeting. However, there are many drug delivery situations in which that approach is not feasible. In such situations, the other targeting techniques mentioned, passive, physical and magnetic targeting, may provide viable alternatives. For example, magnetically targeted carriers (MTCs), micro- or nanoparticles made from paramagnetic material, can be localized and retained at the target site, such as a tumor using an externally positioned permanent dipole magnet [71, 72]. Several of these MTC systems have been evaluated in clinical trials, including a delivery vehicle for doxorubicin (MTC-DOX). It is reasonable to expect substantial further development of MTCs in the future [71].

Passive physical targeting, such as techniques that exploit the presence of leaky vasculature, are of particular interest from the standpoint of the current discussion (see the following chapter). The spontaneous accumulation of drug within areas of leaky vasculature is referred to as the "EPR effect". The EPR effect is responsible for a significant enhancement in the accumulation of polymeric drugs in tumor tissue compared to normal tissue [73-77]. This is an intrinsic effect of polymer therapeutics, and is displayed for a broad assortment of polymers of different molecular composition and structure. Recent studies using HPMA copolymers with different molecular masses illustrate the EPR effect very well [49, 76]. In these studies, it was observed that intravenously administered pHPMA copolymers of various sizes accumulated in the tumor, regardless of molecular mass (up to 1.0-1.5% of injected dose per g of tumor). However, those copolymers exhibiting higher molecular masses (> 50 K) were still retaining within the tumor after 6 h, while the lower molecular mass copolymers (< 40 K) had been rapidly removed from the tumor tissue and subsequently excreted in the urine. The elevated level of polymer extravasation into the tumors compared the level of polymer extravasation observed in other tissues is clearly the result of the 'leakiness' of the tumor vasculature, a phenomena referred to as "enhanced permeability". The enhanced retention of the larger molecules within the tumor is due to the much slower rate of diffusion of those molecules out of the tumor and into the blood compared to the diffusion rate of the smaller molecules, a phenomena referred to as "retention". Furthermore, the differences between large and small molecules are amplified by the rapid renal excretion of small molecules, while the larger molecules, which surpass the renal barrier limit, remain in circulation longer, thereby increasing the duration of exposure to the tumor tissue.

Low molecular mass drugs will, after an initial extravasation into tumors, rapidly diffuse back into the circulating blood and then be rapidly removed from the body via renal excretion. However, if the same drugs are linked to a polymer, diffusion following extravasation will be significantly retarded, effectively resulting in drug targeting to the tumor. Importantly the EPR effect is applicable not only to soluble polymers such as pHPMA but also to micelles, liposomes, nanoparticles and other nanoscale supramolecular species as well lipid vehicle (such as Lipidol as discussed later), which can carry low molecular mass drug to the tumor matter.

Thus far, the EPR effect has been credited for the clinical development of SMANCS [11] and the pHPMA-doxorubicin conjugate (PK1) [4]. For example, arterially administered SMANCS in patients with primary hepatoma displayed tumor/blood ratios as great as 2000 when combined with Lipidol as carrier [11]. Furthermore, the clinical trials of PK1 suggested that this drug displayed antitumour activity in chemotherapy-refractory patients, considerably reduced toxicity compared with doxorubicin, and provided evidence of tumor-selective targeting [4].

As the clinical evidence for the EPR effect continues to mount, it appears that this phenomenon be beneficial to the development of many polymer therapeutics, including those for targeted delivery of genes, antisense oligonucleotides, proteins and peptides to tumors [4]. In this respect, it is vital that the various factors that could impact the EPR effect in the clinical setting need to be thoroughly studied. This includes the possible effects of the tissue origin, localization, type and morphology of the tumors, as well as the route and the rate of drug administration. Furthermore, the pharmacological and clinical criteria for successful induction of the EPR effect need to be defined and applied in clinical trials of novel polymer therapeutics.

6. TRIGGERED DRUG RELEASE AT THE SITE OF ACTION

Poor aqueous solubility is a major problem faced by about 80 % of newly discovered drug candidates [78]. Furthermore, many currently employed drugs are insoluble and must be administered in either solid or liquid drug formulations, this frequently results in poor bioavailability, often accompanied by side effects induced by various toxic components (surfactants, organic solvents etc.) present in the formulations. It is not surprising, therefore, that a major effort is underway in many industrial and academic laboratories to improve the formulation of existing drugs and to develop formulations for novel agents by incorporating those agents into dispersed pharmaceutical carriers, including liposomes, micelles and nanoparticles. Although this may seem, at first, to be a simple strategy, the problem of solubilization of many insoluble compounds is in fact quite formidable and does not provide for a universal solution, i.e. there is no single drug carrier that allows for incorporation of various structurally distinct compounds [79]. The problem of drug solubilization in a pharmaceutical carrier is fundamentally related to another issue of drug delivery, namely, effective retention of drug delivered to the body [5]. One widespread concept in drug delivery is that the effect of the pharmaceutical carrier on the behavior of the drug is maximized when the highest stability of the drug-carrier complex is achieved. For instance, effective retention of the drug in the carrier is essential to the use of the carrier in order to achieve efficient drug delivery to a specific site in the body. Several studies have demonstrated that stable liposomes and block copolymer micelle systems, characterized by strong drug retention in the carrier particles, enable extended circulation times for drugs in the blood stream, as well as high metabolic stability of those drugs in the body [24]. However, increased drug solubilization and retention in the pharmaceutical carrier usually comes at a cost of decreased efficacy of drug release form this carrier. As a result, an increase in the circulation time through stabilization of the drug-carrier complex is not necessarily sufficient to improve the therapeutic index of the drug. Indeed, if the attachment of a drug to the carrier is too strong, the release of drug will be decreased, which may result in lower concentrations of the released drug in the body.

Therefore recent studies have focused on controlling drug release from the carrier by triggering changes in environmental parameters, or through the localized application of a physical field such as temperature or acoustic waves at the desired sites in the body. For instance, certain tumors are characterized by low pH values, which could be used to induce structural transitions in the carriers resulting in the drug release within the tumor [80]. Similarly, acidification of the environment within endosomes can trigger drug release within the cells. For example, polyelectrolyte complexes formed by weak polyacids or polybases can undergo pH-induced transitions displaying high cooperativity. This property is currently being investigated as a potential trigger mechanism for pH-induced drug release from the block ionomer complexes [81]. Another example, pH-sensitive liposomes, has been successfully used to deliver various biological agents into tumor cells *in vitro* and *in vivo* [82, 83]. Various techniques to prepare pH-sensitive liposomes have been developed, including the use of pH-sensitive lipid formulations [84-86], incorporation of pH-sensitive peptides in lipid bilayers [87], steric stabilization of liposomes by PEG linked to the lipids though cleavable groups [88], anchoring of pH sensitive polymers in the lipid bilayers [89, 90]. Each of these approaches involve structural transitions in the liposome-forming material triggered by acidification of the external environment and resulting in liposome destabilization. In principle, similar strategies can be applied in the design of various other pH-sensitive polymer drug carriers such as micelles, nanoparticles and nanogels.

Okano's group has been exploring another approach involving triggered drug release at the site of action by altering the temperature [91]. These studies employ block copolymer micelles with a corona of poly(*N*-isopropylacrylamide-*co*-*N*,*N*'-diethylacrylamide) (pNIPAAM) and a core of poly(D,L-lactide), as the temperature-responsive drug delivery systems. The corona of these micelles reveals lower critical solution temperature (LCST) behavior, resulting in micelle precipitation and drug release upon elevation of temperature (from 37°C to 42.5°C) [91]. The temperature responsive micelles can potentially be used for the delivery and controlled release of drugs within specific sites in the body. In another study, Rapoport *et al.* [92-94] have explored drug release from micelles triggered by application of ultrasound. In these studies, anticancer drugs were first delivered to cancer cells using Pluronic® micelles and then ultrasound was applied to promote drug release [92, 93]. The application of acoustic treatment at a desired time resulted in induced controlled release of the drug inside the cells. Overall, the design of environmentally responsive pharmaceutical carriers for controlled drug delivery and release is an area of research with great potential, in which new and important developments are expected in the near future.

7. INTRACELLULAR DRUG AND GENE DELIVERY

Many drugs enter cells through endocytosis; therefore, one common problem is how to increase drug release from the endocytic vesicles. Specifically, how to ensure that a protein, plasmid DNA or antisense oligonucleotide molecule delivered into a cell with a pharmaceutical carrier is then effectively released in the cytoplasm? To address this problem several groups are developing pH-responsive polymers that mimic the membrane disruptive properties of viruses and toxins, enabling endosomal escape of the delivered material [95, 96]. One such material is based on a copolymer of poly(2-propylacrylic acid) (pPAAc), which displays pH-dependent hemolytic properties and disrupts lipid membranes after a decrease of pH from 7.4 to 5.0 [97, 98]. Gene delivery using cationic liposomes mixed with pPAAc resulted in an enhancement of DNA delivery and transfection in cell culture [99]. Furthermore, co-administration of pPAAc with plasmid DNA in healing wounds demonstrated successful enhancement of transgene expression *in vivo* [100].

Following escape from endocytic vesicles, a drug must be delivered into the target intracellular compartment(s). A recent study examined a strategy for targeting macromolecules to the nucleus via the endocytic pathway [101]. For this purpose a model compound, bovine serum albumin (BSA), was encapsulated into pH-sensitive liposomes (dioleoyl phosphatidyl ethanolamine: cholesterylhemisuccinate) in order to direct endosomal escape of the BSA under conditions of low pH. Selective targeting to the nucleus was achieved by adding the nuclear localization signal (NLS) of SV-40 directly to the BSA. Thus, by combining polymer therapeutics with localization signals derived from toxins, viruses or endogenous intracellular proteins, one might be able to target drugs to selected locations within the cells.

One approach to increase cellular transport of macromolecules and their complexes is to make the species more hydrophobic. For example, point modification of water-soluble proteins with fatty acid residues was used successfully to render these proteins membrane-active and to enhance delivery of these proteins into a cell [102-104]. This approach has been particularly successful in two general situations. First, when the fatty acid binding receptors were expressed at the cell surface the fatty acylation of the proteins drastically enhanced binding and uptake of these proteins allowing their targeting to cells expressing the receptor, such as hepatocytes [105]. Second, when the protein had a specific receptor at the cell surface the fatty acylation provided for an additionall point of attachment with the membrane resulting in a drastically enhanced binding of the modified protein through two points - protein receptor and a fatty residue "anchor". This in turn led to an increased cellular uptake of protein through its receptor-mediated pathway and/or enhanced affect of the protein on the cells (such as anti-viral and anti-proliferative affect of interferons) [104, 106].

Modification of hydrophilic proteins with hydrophobic polymers has been also explored as a way to enhance protein transport into a cell. For example, conjugation of a small water-soluble peptide neocarzinostatin, with poly(styrene-co-maleic acid) copolymer (SMANCS) resulted in a 20 to 30 fold enhancement of the transport of the peptide into a cell. This polymer conjugate also displayed facilitated uptake into cells at acidic pH, which may be due to protonation of carboxylic groups of the polymer chain rendering it even more hydrophobic [107, 108]. Since more acidic environment is characteristic of many tumors compared to normal tissue this property of SMANCS may have an additional benefit by potentiating the anticancer effects of the conjugate in the tumors [108].

In early 90's, during the graduate studies under supervision of one of the co-authors of this manuscript, Slepnev has examined effects of covalent modification of proteins with Pluronic® block copolymers [109]. In particular, these studies used horseradish peroxidase (HRP) as a probe to examine transport and localization of various modified proteins into a cell. Non-modified HRP enters cell via endocytosis and remains entrapped in the intracellular vesicles without any substantial cytoplasmic release. Slepnev synthesized a conjugate of HRP with Pluronic® P85 and studied transport and localization of this conjugate in MDCK cell line. While the extent of accumulation of this conjugate into the cell was practically the same as that on non-modified HRP, the internalized protein conjugate was released from the vesicles into the cytoplasm displaying a characteristic cytoplasmic staining. Therefore, modification of a protein with an amphiphilic block copolymer allowed for an effective escape of this protein from the endocytic vesicles. Recently, Pluronic® block copolymers were used to enhance intracellular delivery of DNA/polycation complexes ("polyplxes") [46, 47, 110]. In this work molecules Pluronic® molecules were grafted to polyethyleneimine chains. The resulting graft copolymers were subsequently reacted with the DNA to form polyplexes. These studies demonstrated that incorporation of Pluronic® into the complexes resulted in significant enhancement of DNA delivery into and cell increase in the transfection activity of the polyplexes. The mechanism of Pluronic® effects observed in these studies is not completely understood. However, it is likely that it includes enhanced interaction of the complexes with the cell membranes due to the presence of the hydrophobic poly(propylene oxide) segments in Pluronic® molecules. It is noteworthy that Pluronic® molecules proper display an ability to translocate inside a cell [111], and, therefore, they may contribute to enhanced endocytic escape of the polyplexes.

To achieve efficient intracellular drug and DNA delivery, attempts were made to target drug carriers into cytoplasm bypassing the endocytotic pathway [112, 113]. One such promising strategy to facilitate intracellular drug and DNA delivery involves the use of TAT peptides derived from the HIV-1 TAT protein. Attachment of TAT peptide, for example, on the surface of liposomes affords the efficient intracellular delivery of the liposomes even at low temperature and in the presence of metabolic inhibitors [114]. This suggests that the TAT-modified liposomes are in fact transported directly from the external solution to the cell cytoplasm, an unusual trafficking route, which deserves very serious exploration.

Target cells often display and/or adapt survival mechanisms that hinder drug transport into a cell, including the over expression of ATP-dependent drug efflux proteins, such as P-glycoprotein (Pgp). This phenomenon has been observed in both drug resistant cancer as well as normal cells such as brain microvessel endothelial cells that form the BBB and intestinal epithelial cells that form the intestinal barrier [115-118]. Such transport proteins actively pump drug out of the cells, contributing to multiple drug resistance (MDR) phenotype, as well as poor transport of many compounds across the BBB and intestinal barrier. One approach to overcome MDR consists of conjugating drug to a soluble polymer carrier. For example Kopecek's group demonstrated that a conjugate of doxorubicin with pHPMA is equally effective against both MDR and non-MDR cancers [119]. Furthermore, in contrast to the effects of free drug, chronic exposure to pHPMA-doxorubicin conjugates did not induce MDR in cancer cells [120, 121]. The reason for the differential behavior of the pHPMA-doxorubicin is obviously due to differences in the mechanism of its transport into cell compared to that of the free drug. As a result of the conjugation to the polymer chain, doxorubicin is rendered inaccessible to the Pgp efflux pump in MDR. The resulting conjugate most likely enters the cells via endocytosis, a Pgp-independent pathway, while the free drug is transported across membrane through diffusion, a pathway that in MDR cells is affected by Pgp [122]. This study is consistent with the prior observation by Maeda's group that polymer drugs, which are internalized into cells by endocytosis, are not excreted from the cells by active efflux and exhibited a pronounced anticancer effect against MDR cells [123]. Further, a recent study by Minko et al. [124] suggested that HPMA-bound doxorubicin induced additional caspase-dependent apoptosis signaling pathways, which led to more pronounced apoptosis when compared to the free drug. Therefore, the polymer-drug conjugate not only enhanced drug delivery in MDR cells but also acted as a biological response modifier that potentiates the drug cytotoxic effect in a cell.

Another approach to overcome MDR involves the use of polymeric surfactants, such as Pluronic® block copolymers, as chemosensitizing agents [5]. The affect of Pluronic® block copolymers on MDR cells has two components: first, the polymers alter membrane microviscosity and, second, they cause ATP depletion selectively in MDR cells [111, 125]. Both effects combine to result in very efficacious inhibition of drug efflux transporters, which greatly increases drug accumulation in MDR cancer cells as well as drug transport across the BBB and intestinal barriers [126, 127]. Furthermore, Pluronic® abolishes sequestration of drug in cytoplasmic vesicles, an event often observed within the MDR cells, resulting in efficient drug delivery to the nucleus [128]. Phase I clinical trial of a Pluronic®-based formulation of doxorubicin has recently been completed and Phase II trials are currently underway. These copolymers appear quite promising for improving the chemotherapy of tumors as well as for increasing brain and oral bioavailablity of select drugs.

Overall, the studies of the potential use of polymers to improve intracellular trafficking of biologically active agents have intensified during last several years. One should expect that research in this area will remain extremely active throughout the next decade and will result in novel pharmaceutical carriers capable of delivering drugs inside cells with high efficacy and with the precision characteristic of natural trafficking mechanisms.

8. FUNCTIONAL EXCIPIENTS AND BIOLOGICAL RESPONSE MODIFIERS

The concept of pharmaceutical excipients as components of a formulation other than the active substance has undergone recently a substantial evolution [129]. This is because many excipients that have been considered as "inert" in actuality display important and sometimes very useful activities, making them essential constituents of the formulation. As a result, those components are now sometimes termed "functional excipients". Many polymer therapeutic materials can be placed in this category. One example, considered in the previous section, is Pluronic® block copolymers. Pluronic®-based systems clearly belong in this group because they exhibit a variety of useful biological properties. For example, water-in-oil, oil-in-water and water-in-oil-in-water emulsions formulated with select Pluronic® block copolymers have been extensively used as immunoajuvants [130-140]. These studies suggested significant enhancement of both cell-mediated and humoral immune response with respect to a very broad spectrum of antigens induced by addition of block copolymer formulations. Selected block copolymers, such as Pluronic® F127, have been found to significantly enhance the rate of wound and burn healing, and therefore have been included in cream formulations and skin substitutes for the treatment of burns and for other tissue engineering applications [141-148]. Several Pluronic®-based formulations were shown to effectively prevent postoperative adhesions or to at least reduce the adhesion area following surgery [149, 150]. Furthermore, Pluronic® block copolymers can enhance the sealing of cell membranes that have been permeabilized by ionizing radiation and electroporation, thus preventing cellular necrosis. This attribute could be extremely helpful for improving drug and gene delivery in skeletal muscle [151-153]. Furthermore, as discussed above, select Pluronic® block copolymers can interact with multidrug resistant (MDR) cancer cells resulting in chemosensitization of these cells [125, 126, 128, 154, 155]. These examples show that the Pluronic® block copolymers are valuable biological adjuvants exhibiting useful biological properties, which can be of considerable importance for various therapeutic applications.

Polymers like Pluronic® that can change the performance of a biologically active agent without changing the mechanism of the action of this agent are classified as "biological response modifiers". Some other examples of polymers displaying biological response modifying activity include polycation immunomodulators, such as polyoxidonium, that have been shown to greatly enhance the immune response to various antigens [57]. Furthermore, a recent study suggests that the electroneutroneutral polymer, pHPMA, in pHPMA-conjugates, exhibits a biological response modifying activity, namely, the potentiation of the cytotoxic effect of the drug on cells. This is likely the result of alterations in the plasma membrane permeability and disturbances in cellular metabolism caused by the pHPMA [156]. One should expect that there are many, yet unrealized, examples of biological response modifying effects of various polymers. At present we know relatively little about these effects, therefore, studies in this are likely continue. The purpose of such studies should be, on one hand, to discover new polymers with potentially valuable effects and, on the other hand, to characterize the possible effects of existing polymers that need to be either exploited or avoided in various pharmaceutical formulations.

9. REGULATORY ISSUES WITH POLYMER THERAPEUTICS

Just slightly over a decade ago many individuals in the pharmaceutical sector believed that polymer therapeutics would stand little, if any chance, to be approved by regulatory authorities, particularly, as injectable formulations. Today those views are clearly obsolete. However, many questions regarding the regulatory approval of the polymer therapeutics still exist. Investigators working in the field of polymer therapeutics need to focus on addressing those questions in order to provide the regulatory authorities with a comprehensive outlook that will allow the establishment of consistent guidelines and policies regarding polymer therapeutics.

There are well-established analytical procedures and criteria that are applied during the regulatory approval processes for low molecular mass compounds [157, 158]. However, the situation is more complicated in the case of polymers therapeutics. In such cases, the lack of validated analytical procedures is often compounded by difficulties associated with the identification of various possible products of polymer metabolism, which is inherent due to complexity of the polymer systems. These issues create enough problems when establishing criteria for manufacture and storage of polymer therapeutics, since the criteria applied to determine purity, stability and shelf life of those materials are often arbitrary [129]. However, those problems are greatly magnified upon administration of the polymer therapeutics in the body. For example, criteria need to be established in regard to the biodegradation of synthetic polymers in the body. This is particularly important if biodegradation results in the production of the lower molecular mass polymers consisting of the same repeating units, which may potentially differ in their biological effects. One approach could be, since synthetic polymers are generally characterized by molecular mass distribution (i.e. are set of the chains with the same structure but different lengths), to measure the molecular mass distribution in the body in order to derive information regarding the destruction of the polymer chain. However, this approach is currently not exceedingly feasible given the currently available techniques for such measurements. Therefore, the development of novel techniques, such as, for example, mass spectroscopy, that would provide sufficient sensitivity to characterize polymer structure in the presence of the biological milieu, is highly desirable.

There exists an additional set of hurdles to the *in vivo* evaluation of those polymer therapeutics that self-assemble into supramolecular structures, such as block copolymer micelles or interpolyelectrolyte complexes. Evaluation of the stability of such structures and drug retention in these structures following administration into the body is technically difficult, if not impossible. This is because the physicochemical techniques normally employed for supramolecular complex characterization, such as dynamic light scattering, fluorescent probes or ultracentrifugation, are severely limited by the presence of cells, proteins and other macromolecular components in the whole blood. For example, the large size and high concentration of the blood components prevents use of scattering techniques for examination of the block copolymer micelles due to strong light scattering of those components [159]. Likewise, strong auto-fluorescence of blood components and their interference with molecular probes complicate use of the fluorescence probe method. On the other hand, techniques involving isolation of the complexes from blood components, such as chromatography, frequently cannot be used because of the dynamic character of certain pharmaceutical carriers, such as the block copolymers that disassemble into single chains ("unimers") upon dilution.

The issue of the release of the biological agent from its polymer carrier *in vivo* is also of significance, since in many cases, some of the convenient techniques, such as mass spectroscopy or capillary electrophoresis, do not allow for discrimination between free and polymer-bound drug. This is a formidable task, particularly in those situations in which the biological agent is non-covalently incorporated in the polymer carrier, or in the case of macromolecular therapeutics, when the therapeutic agents (i.e. DNA) is incorporated into the carrier through multiple cooperative interactions. Such interactions may drastically change upon transfer of the biologically derived sample to the conditions needed for the analysis. As a result, the actual portions of the biological agent associated with the carrier in the body may differ immensely from those determined in the assay. Therefore, the development of new assays and the improved utilization of already existing assays to measure the amounts of free drug directly in the body fluids are of utmost importance.

ACKNOWLEDGEMENT

The authors thank Dr. Catherine L. Gebhart (University of Nebraska Medical Center) for editing this manuscript.

REFERENCES

1. Langer, R., 1998, Drug delivery and targeting. *Nature* 392:5-10.
2. Northfelt, D. W., B. J. Dezube, J. A. Thommes, B. J. Miller, M. A. Fischl, A. Friedman-Kien, L. D. Kaplan, C. Du Mond, R. D. Mamelok and D. H. Henry, 1998, Pegylated-liposomal doxorubicin versus doxorubicin, bleomycin, and vincristine in the treatment of AIDS-related Kaposi's sarcoma: results of a randomized phase III clinical trial. *J. Clin. Oncol.* 16:2445-2451.
3. Rosenblum, M. G. and G. N. Hortobagyi, 1986, Pharmacokinetics and tissue disposition of the biological response modifier BAY i 7433 (copovithane) in patients with cancer. *Cancer Chemother. Pharmacol.* 18:247-251.
4. Duncan, R., S. Gac-Breton, R. Keane, R. Musila, Y. N. Sat, R. Satchi and F. Searle, 2001, Polymer-drug conjugates, PDEPT and PELT: basic principles for design and transfer from the laboratory to clinic. *J. Control. Release* 74:135-146.
5. Kabanov, A. V. and V. Alakhov, 2002, Pluronic block copolymers in drug delivery: From micellar nanocontainers to biological response modifiers. *Cr Rev Ther Dr Targ* 19:1-73.
6. Maynard, C., R. Swenson, J. A. Paris, J. S. Martin, A. P. Hallstrom, M. D. Cerqueira and W. D. Weaver, 1998, Randomized, controlled trial of RheothRx (poloxamer 188) in patients with suspected acute myocardial infarction. RheothRx in Myocardial Infarction Study Group. *Am Heart J* 135:797-804.
7. Fournier, C., B. Hecquet, P. Bouffard, M. Vert, A. Caty, M. O. Vilain, L. Vanseymortier, S. Merle, A. Krikorian, J. L. Lefebvre and et al., 1991, Experimental studies and preliminary clinical trial of vinorelbine- loaded polymeric bioresorbable implants for the local treatment of solid tumors. *Cancer Res* 51:5384-5391.
8. Einmahl, S., S. Capancioni, K. Schwach-Abdellaoui, M. Moeller, F. Behar-Cohen and R. Gurny, 2001, Therapeutic applications of viscous and injectable poly(ortho esters). *Adv. Drug Deliv. Rev.* 53:45-73.
9. Kattan, J., J. P. Droz, P. Couvreur, J. P. Marino, A. Boutan-Laroze, P. Rougier, P. Brault, H. Vranckx, J. M. Grognet, X. Morge and et al., 1992, Phase I clinical trial and pharmacokinetic evaluation of doxorubicin carried by polyisohexylcyanoacrylate nanoparticles. *Invest New Drugs* 10:191-199.
10. Seymour, L. W., S. P. Olliff, C. J. Poole, P. G. De Takats, R. Orme, D. R. Ferry, H. Maeda, T. Konno and D. J. Kerr, 1998, A novel dosage approach for evaluation of SMANCS [poly-(styrene-co- maleyl-half-n-butylate) - neocarzinostatin] in the treatment of primary hepatocellular carcinoma. *Int. J. Oncol.* 12:1217-1223.
11. Maeda, H., 2001, SMANCS and polymer-conjugated macromolecular drugs: advantages in cancer chemotherapy. *Adv. Drug Deliv. Rev.* 46:169-185.
12. Ardizzone, S., M. Petrillo, P. Molteni, S. Desideri and G. Bianchi Porro, 1995, Coated oral 5-aminosalicylic acid (Claversal) is equivalent to sulfasalazine for remission maintenance in ulcerative colitis. A double- blind study. *J. Clin. Gastroenterol.* 21:287-289.

13. Schenk, J. F., P. Radziwon, S. Morsdorf, P. Eckenberger and H. K. Breddin, 1999, Effects of aprosulate, a novel synthetic glycosaminoglycan, on coagulation and platelet function parameters: a prospective, randomized phase I study. *Clin. Appl. Thromb. Hemost.* 5:192-197.
14. Payne, L. G., S. A. Jenkins, A. L. Woods, E. M. Grund, W. E. Geribo, J. R. Loebelenz, A. K. Andrianov and B. E. Roberts, 1998, Poly[di(carboxylatophenoxy)phosphazene] (PCPP) is a potent immunoadjuvant for an influenza vaccine. *Vaccine* 16:92-98.
15. Payne, L. G., S. A. Jenkins, A. Andrianov and B. E. Roberts, 1995, Water-soluble phosphazene polymers for parenteral and mucosal vaccine delivery. *Pharm Biotechnol* 6:473-493.
16. Andrianov, A. K., J. Chen and L. G. Payne, 1998, Preparation of hydrogel microspheres by coacervation of aqueous polyphosphazene solutions. *Biomaterials* 19:109-115.
17. Payne, L. G. and A. K. Andrianov, 1998, Protein release from polyphosphazene matrices. *Adv Drug Deliv Rev* 31:185-196.
18. Song, J., C. H. Suh, Y. B. Park, S. H. Lee, N. C. Yoo, J. D. Lee, K. H. Kim and S. K. Lee, 2001, A phase I/IIa study on intra-articular injection of holmium-166-chitosan complex for the treatment of knee synovitis of rheumatoid arthritis. *Eur. J. Nucl. Med.* 28:489-497.
19. Pittler, M. H., N. C. Abbot, E. F. Harkness and E. Ernst, 1999, Randomized, double-blind trial of chitosan for body weight reduction. *Eur. J. Clin. Nutr.* 53:379-381.
20. Nekrasov, A. V., N. G. Puchkova, R. I. Attaullakhanov, R. V. Petrov and A. S. Ivanova, 1996, Compounds having immunostimulating activity and methods of use thereof., 5503830
21. El'shina, G. A., M. A. Gorbunov, T. A. Bektimirov, N. I. Lonskaia, L. I. Pavlova, A. A. Nikul'shin, R. M. Khaitov, A. V. Nekrasov, A. S. Ivanova, M. N. Matrosovich and N. G. Puchkova, 2000, [The evaluation of the reactogenicity, harmlessness and prophylactic efficacy of Grippol trivalent polymer-subunit influenza vaccine administered to schoolchildren]. *Zh. Mikrobiol. Epidemiol. Immunobiol.*:50-54.
22. Kataoka, K., A. Harada and Y. Nagasaki, 2001, Block copolymer micelles for drug delivery: design, characterization and biological significance. *Adv Drug Deliv Rev* 47:113-131.
23. Katayose, S. and K. Kataoka, 1997, Water-soluble polyion complex associates of DNA and poly(ethylene glycol)-poly(L-lysine) block copolymer. *Bioconj. Chem.* 8:702-707.
24. Kwon, G. S. and K. Kataoka, 1995, Block copolymer micelles as long-circulating drug vehicles. *Adv. Drug Delivery Rev.* 16:295-309.
25. Yokoyama, M., M. Miyauchi, N. Yamada, T. Okano, Y. Sakurai, K. Kataoka and S. Inoue, 1990, Characterization and anticancer activity of the micelle-forming polymeric anticancer drug adriamycin-conjugated poly(ethylene glycol)-poly(aspartic acid) block copolymer. *Cancer Res.* 50:1693-1700.
26. Seymour, L., K. Kataoka and A. Kabanov, 1998, Cationic block copolymers as self-assembling vectors for gene delivery, In *Self-assembling Complexes for Gene Delivery. From Laboratory to Clinical Trial* (A. Kabanov, P. Felgner and L. Seymour eds), John Wiley & Sons, Chichester, UK pp 219-239.
27. Harada, A. and K. Kataoka, 1997, Formation of stable and monodispersive polyion complex micelles in aqueous medium from poly(L-lysine) and poly(ethylene glycol)-poly(aspartic acid) block copolymer. *J. Macromol. Sci., Pure Appl. Chem.* A34:2119-2133.
28. Harada, A. and K. Kataoka, 1998, Novel polyion complex micelles entrapping enzyme molecules in the core: preparation of narrowly-distributed micelles from lysozyme and poly(ethylene glycol)-poly(aspartic acid) block copolymer in aqueous medium. *Macromolecules* 31:288-294.

29. Harada, A. and K. Kataoka, 1999, Chain length recognition: core-shell supramolecular assembly from oppositely charged block copolymers. *Science* 283:65-67.
30. Harada, A. and K. Kataoka, 1999, On-Off control of enzymatic activity synchronizing with reversible formation of supramolecular assembly from enzyme and charged block copolymers. *J. Am. Chem. Soc.* 121:9241-9242.
31. Harada, A. and K. Kataoka, 1999, Novel polyion complex micelles entrapping enzyme molecules in the core. 2. Characterization of the micelles prepared at nonstoichiometric mixing ratios. *Langmuir* 15:4208-4212.
32. Harada, A., H. Togawa and K. Kataoka, 2001, Physicochemical properties and nuclease resistance of antisense- oligodeoxynucleotides entrapped in the core of polyion complex micelles composed of poly(ethylene glycol)-poly(L-Lysine) block copolymers. *Eur. J. Pharm. Sci.* 13:35-42.
33. Dash, P. R., V. Toncheva, E. Schacht and L. W. Seymour, 1997, Synthetic polymers for vectorial delivery of DNA: characterization of polymer-DNA complexes by photon correlation spectroscopy and stability to nuclease degradation and disruption by polyanions in vitro. *J. Controlled Release* 48:269-276.
34. Dekie, L., V. Toncheva, P. Dubruel, E. H. Schacht, L. Barrett and L. W. Seymour, 2000, Poly-L-glutamic acid derivatives as vectors for gene therapy. *J Control Release* 65:187-202.
35. Oupicky, D., C. Konak, K. Ulbrich, M. A. Wolfert and L. W. Seymour, 2000, DNA delivery systems based on complexes of DNA with synthetic polycations and their copolymers. *J Control Release* 65:149-171.
36. Read, M. L., T. Etrych, K. Ulbrich and L. W. Seymour, 1999, Characterisation of the binding interaction between poly(L-lysine) and DNA using the fluorescamine assay in the preparation of non-viral gene delivery vectors. *FEBS Lett* 461:96-100.
37. Benns, J. M., J. S. Choi, R. I. Mahato, J. S. Park and S. W. Kim, 2000, pH-sensitive cationic polymer gene delivery vehicle: N-Ac-poly(L- histidine)-graft-poly(L-lysine) comb shaped polymer. *Bioconjug. Chem.* 11:637-645.
38. Choi, Y. H., F. Liu, J.-S. Kim, Y. K. Choi, J. S. Park and S. W. Kim, 1998, Polyethylene glycol-grafted poly-L-lysine as polymeric gene carrier. *J. Contr. Release* 54:39-48.
39. Choi, Y. H., F. Liu, J. S. Park and S. W. Kim, 1998, Lactose-poly(ethylene glycol)-grafted poly-L-lysine as hepatoma cell- tapgeted gene carrier. *Bioconjug Chem* 9:708-718.
40. Choi, Y. H., F. Liu, J. S. Choi, S. W. Kim and J. S. Park, 1999, Characterization of a targeted gene carrier, lactose-polyethylene glycol-grafted poly-L-lysine and its complex with plasmid DNA. *Hum Gene Ther* 10:2657-65.
41. Allen, C., D. Maysinger and A. Eisenberg, 1999, Nano-engineering block copolymer aggregates for drug delivery. *Coll. Surfaces, B: Biointerfaces* 16:3-27.
42. Kabanov, A. V., V. P. Chekhonin, V. Y. Alakhov, E. V. Batrakova, A. S. Lebedev, N. S. Melik-Nubarov, S. A. Arzhakov, A. V. Levashov, G. V. Morozov, E. S. Severin and V. A. Kabanov, 1989, The neuroleptic activity of haloperidol increases after its solubilization in surfactant micelles. Micelles as microcontainers for drug targeting. *FEBS Lett.* 258:343-345.
43. Kabanov, A. V., S. V. Vinogradov, Y. G. Suzdaltseva and V. Y. Alakhov, 1995, Water-soluble block polycations as carriers for oligonucleotide delivery. *Bioconjug. Chem.* 6:639-643.
44. Kabanov, A. V., 1999, Taking polycation gene delivery systems from *in vitro* to *in vivo*. *Pharm. Sci. Tech. Today* 2:365-372.
45. Vinogradov, S. V., T. K. Bronich and A. V. Kabanov, 1998, Self-assembly of polyamine-poly(ethylene glycol) copolymers with phosphorothioate oligonucleotides. *Bioconjug. Chem.* 9:805-812.

46. Nguyen, H. K., P. Lemieux, S. V. Vinogradov, C. L. Gebhart, N. Guerin, G. Paradis, T. K. Bronich, V. Y. Alakhov and A. V. Kabanov, 2000, Evaluation of polyether-polyethyleneimine graft copolymers as gene transfer agents. *Gene Ther* 7:126-138.
47. Gebhart, C. L. and A. V. Kabanov, 2001, Evaluation of polyplexes as gene transfer agents. *J. Contr. Release* 73:401-416.
48. Fraser, J. R., T. C. Laurent, H. Pertoft and E. Baxter, 1981, Plasma clearance, tissue distribution and metabolism of hyaluronic acid injected intravenously in the rabbit. *Biochem J* 200:415-424.
49. Kissel, M., P. Peschke, V. Subr, K. Ulbrich, J. Schuhmacher, J. Debus and E. Friedrich, 2001, Synthetic macromolecular drug carriers: biodistribution of poly[(N-2-hydroxypropyl)methacrylamide] copolymers and their accumulation in solid rat tumors. *PDA J Pharm Sci Technol* 55:191-201.
50. Jewell, R. C., S. P. Khor, D. F. Kisor, K. A. LaCroix and W. A. Wargin, 1997, Pharmacokinetics of RheothRx injection in healthy male volunteers. *J. Pharm. Sci.* 86:808-812.
51. Mitra, G., S. Mumtaz and B. K. Bachhawat, 1993, Enhanced stability and therapeutic utility of proteins upon conjugation with hydrophilic polymers. *Hindustan Antibiot Bull* 35:133-156.
52. Hoste, K., E. Schacht and L. Seymour, 2000, New derivatives of polyglutamic acid as drug carrier systems. *J Control Release* 64:53-61.
53. Douglas, S. J., S. S. Davis and L. Illum, 1987, Nanoparticles in drug delivery. *Crit Rev Ther Drug Carrier Syst* 3:233-261.
54. Jung, T., W. Kamm, A. Breitenbach, E. Kaiserling, J. X. Xiao and T. Kissel, 2000, Biodegradable nanoparticles for oral delivery of peptides: is there a role for polymers to affect mucosal uptake? *Eur J Pharm Biopharm* 50:147-160.
55. Darney, P. D., 1994, Hormonal implants: contraception for a new century. *Am J Obstet Gynecol* 170:1536-43.
56. Rothen-Weinhold, A., K. Besseghir, Y. De Zelicourt and R. Gurny, 1998, Development and evaluation in vivo of a long-term delivery system for vapreotide, a somatostatin analogue. *J Control Release* 52:205-213.
57. Petrov, R. V., R. M. Khaitov, A. A. Mikhailova, V. M. Manko and V. A. Kabanov, 1984, *Cell interactions and vaccines of tomorrow*. Mir publishers, Moscow.
58. Maheshwari, A., R. I. Mahato, J. McGregor, S. Han, W. E. Samlowski, J. S. Park and S. W. Kim, 2000, Soluble biodegradable polymer-based cytokine gene delivery for cancer treatment. *Mol. Ther.* 2:121-130.
59. Koh, J. J., K. S. Ko, M. Lee, S. Han, J. S. Park and S. W. Kim, 2000, Degradable polymeric carrier for the delivery of IL-10 plasmid DNA to prevent autoimmune insulitis of NOD mice. *Gene Ther.* 7:2099-2104.
60. Ko, K. S., M. Lee, J. J. Koh and S. W. Kim, 2001, Combined administration of plasmids encoding IL-4 and IL-10 prevents the development of autoimmune diabetes in nonobese diabetic mice. *Mol Ther* 4:313-316.
61. Thorpe, P. E. and F. J. Burrows, 1995, Antibody-directed targeting of the vasculature of solid tumors. *Breast Cancer Res Treat* 36:237-251.
62. Goodwin, D. A. and C. F. Meares, 1999, Pretargeted peptide imaging and therapy. *Cancer Biother Radiopharm* 14:145-152.
63. Torchilin, V. P., 1998, *In vitro* and *in vivo* availability of liposomes, In *Self-assembling complexes for gene delivery: From laboratory to clinical trial* (A. V. Kabanov, P. L. Felgner and L. W. Seymour eds), John Wiley, Chichester, New York, Weinheim, Brisbane, Singapore, Toronto pp 277-293.

64. Poste, G., C. Bucana, A. Raz, P. Bugelski, R. Kirsh and I. J. Fidler, 1983, Site-specific (targeted) drug delivery in cancer therapy. *Biotech* 1:869-868.
65. Judson, I., J. A. Radford, M. Harris, J. Y. Blay, Q. van Hoesel, A. le Cesne, A. T. van Oosterom, M. J. Clemons, C. Kamby, C. Hermans, J. Whittaker, E. Donato di Paola, J. Verweij and S. Nielsen, 2001, Randomised phase II trial of pegylated liposomal doxorubicin (DOXIL/CAELYX) versus doxorubicin in the treatment of advanced or metastatic soft tissue sarcoma: a study by the EORTC Soft Tissue and Bone Sarcoma Group. *Eur J Cancer* 37:870-877.
66. Shi, N. and W. M. Pardridge, 2000, Noninvasive gene targeting to the brain. *Proc Natl Acad Sci U S A* 97:7567-7572.
67. Torchilin, V. P., 2000, Drug targeting. *Eur J Pharm Sci* 11 Suppl 2:S81-S91.
68. Yokoyama, M., T. Okano, Y. Sakurai, K. Kataoka and S. Inoue, 1989, Stabilization of disulfide linkage in drug-polymer-immunoglobulin conjugate by microenvironmental control. *Biochem. Biophys. Res. Commun.* 164:1234-1239.
69. Khaw, B. A., J. daSilva, I. Vural, J. Narula and V. P. Torchilin, 2001, Intracytoplasmic gene delivery for in vitro transfection with cytoskeleton-specific immunoliposomes. *J Control Release* 75:199-210.
70. Vinogradov, S., E. Batrakova, S. Li and A. Kabanov, 1999, Polyion Complex Micelles with Protein-Modified Corona for Receptor-Mediated Delivery of Oligonucleotides into Cells. *Bioconjug. Chem.* 10:851-860.
71. Lubbe, A. S., C. Alexiou and C. Bergemann, 2001, Clinical applications of magnetic drug targeting. *J Surg Res* 95:200-206.
72. Rudge, S., C. Peterson, C. Vessely, J. Koda, S. Stevens and L. Catterall, 2001, Adsorption and desorption of chemotherapeutic drugs from a magnetically targeted carrier (MTC). *J Control Release* 74:335-340.
73. Maeda, H., T. Sawa and T. Konno, 2001, Mechanism of tumor-targeted delivery of macromolecular drugs, including the EPR effect in solid tumor and clinical overview of the prototype polymeric drug SMANCS. *J Control Release* 74:47-61.
74. Maeda, H., 2001, The enhanced permeability and retention (EPR) effect in tumor vasculature: the key role of tumor-selective macromolecular drug targeting. *Adv Enzyme Regul* 41:189-207.
75. Duncan, R., 1999, Polymer conjugates for tumour targeting and intracytoplasmic delivery. The EPR effect as a common gateway? *Pharm. Sci. Technol. Today.* 2:441-449.
76. Noguchi, Y., J. Wu, R. Duncan, J. Strohalm, K. Ulbrich, T. Akaike and H. Maeda, 1998, Early phase tumor accumulation of macromolecules: a great difference in clearance rate between tumor and normal tissues. *Jpn J Cancer Res* 89:307-314.
77. Malik, N., E. G. Evagorou and R. Duncan, 1999, Dendrimer-platinate: a novel approach to cancer chemotherapy. *Anticancer Drugs* 10:767-776.
78. Huuskonen, J., 2001, Estimation of aqueous solubility in drug design. *Comb Chem High Throughput Screen* 4:311-316.
79. Alakhov, V., G. Pietrzynski and A. Kabanov, 2001, Combinatorial approaches to formulation development. *Curr Opin Drug Discov Devel* 4:493-501.
80. Wike-Hooley, J. L., J. Haveman and H. S. Reinhold, 1984, The relevance of tumour pH to the treatment of malignant disease. *Radiother Oncol* 2:343-366.
81. Solomatin, S. V., T. K. Bronich, V. A. Kabanov, A. Eisenberg and A. V. Kabanov, 2001, Block ionomer complexes: novel environmentally responsive materials. *Polym. Prepr.* 42:107-108.
82. Ponnappa, B. C., I. Dey, G. C. Tu, F. Zhou, M. Aini, Q. N. Cao and Y. Israel, 2001, In vivo delivery of antisense oligonucleotides in pH-sensitive liposomes inhibits

lipopolysaccharide-induced production of tumor necrosis factor-alpha in rats. *J Pharmacol Exp Ther* 297:1129-1136.
83. Drummond, D. C., M. Zignani and J. Leroux, 2000, Current status of pH-sensitive liposomes in drug delivery. *Prog Lipid Res* 39:409-460.
84. Straubinger, R. M., N. Duzgunes and D. Papahadjopoulos, 1985, pH-sensitive liposomes mediate cytoplasmic delivery of encapsulated macromolecules. *FEBS Lett* 179:148-154.
85. Liu, D. and L. Huang, 1989, Role of cholesterol in the stability of pH-sensitive, large unilamellar liposomes prepared by the detergent-dialysis method. *Biochim Biophys Acta* 981:254-260.
86. Reddy, J. A. and P. S. Low, 2000, Enhanced folate receptor mediated gene therapy using a novel pH- sensitive lipid formulation. *J Control Release* 64:27-37.
87. Parente, R. A., L. Nadasdi, N. K. Subbarao and F. C. Szoka, Jr., 1990, Association of a pH-sensitive peptide with membrane vesicles: role of amino acid sequence. *Biochemistry* 29:8713-8719.
88. Ishida, T., M. J. Kirchmeier, E. H. Moase, S. Zalipsky and T. M. Allen, 2001, Targeted delivery and triggered release of liposomal doxorubicin enhances cytotoxicity against human B lymphoma cells. *Biochim Biophys Acta* 1515:144-158.
89. Meyer, O., D. Papahadjopoulos and J. C. Leroux, 1998, Copolymers of N-isopropylacrylamide can trigger pH sensitivity to stable liposomes. *FEBS Lett* 421:61-64.
90. Leroux, J., E. Roux, D. Le Garrec, K. Hong and D. C. Drummond, 2001, N-isopropylacrylamide copolymers for the preparation of pH-sensitive liposomes and polymeric micelles. *J Control Release* 72:71-84.
91. Kohori, F., K. Sakai, T. Aoyagi, M. Yokoyama, M. Yamato, Y. Sakurai and T. Okano, 1999, Control of adriamycin cytotoxic activity using thermally responsive polymeric micelles composed of poly(N-isopropylacrylamide-co-N,N-dimethylacrylamide)-b-poly(D,L-lactide). *Colloids Surf., B: Biointerfaces* 16:195-205.
92. Munshi, N., N. Rapoport and W. G. Pitt, 1997, Ultrasonic activated drug delivery from Pluronic P-105 micelles. *Cancer Lett.* 118:13-19.
93. Rapoport, N. Y., J. N. Herron, W. G. Pitt and L. Pitina, 1999, Micellar delivery of doxorubicin and its paramagnetic analog, ruboxyl, to HL-60 cells: effect of micelle structure and ultrasound on the intracellular drug uptake. *J. Controlled Release* 58:153-162.
94. Husseini, G., G. D. Myrup, W. G. Pitt, D. A. Christensen and N. Y. Rapoport, 2000, Factors affecting acoustically triggered release of drugs from polymeric micelles. *J. Controlled Release* 69:43-52.
95. Stayton, P. S., A. S. Hoffman, N. Murthy, C. Lackey, C. Cheung, P. Tan, L. A. Klumb, A. Chilkoti, F. S. Wilbur and O. W. Press, 2000, Molecular engineering of proteins and polymers for targeting and intracellular delivery of therapeutics. *J Control Release* 65:203-220.
96. Hoffman, A. S., P. S. Stayton, V. Bulmus, G. Chen, J. Chen, C. Cheung, A. Chilkoti, Z. Ding, L. Dong, R. Fong, C. A. Lackey, C. J. Long, M. Miura, J. E. Morris, N. Murthy, Y. Nabeshima, T. G. Park, O. W. Press, T. Shimoboji, S. Shoemaker, H. J. Yang, N. Monji, R. C. Nowinski, C. A. Cole, J. H. Priest, J. M. Harris, K. Nakamae, T. Nishino and T. Miyata, 2000, Founder's Award, Society for Biomaterials. Sixth World Biomaterials Congress 2000, Kamuela, HI,May 15-20, 2000. Really smart bioconjugates of smart polymers and receptor proteins. *J Biomed Mater Res* 52:577-586.
97. Lackey, C. A., N. Murthy, O. W. Press, D. A. Tirrell, A. S. Hoffman and P. S. Stayton, 1999, Hemolytic activity of pH-responsive polymer-streptavidin bioconjugates. *Bioconjug Chem* 10:401-405.

98. Murthy, N., J. R. Robichaud, D. A. Tirrell, P. S. Stayton and A. S. Hoffman, 1999, The design and synthesis of polymers for eukaryotic membrane disruption. *J Control Release* 61:137-143.
99. Cheung, C. Y., N. Murthy, P. S. Stayton and A. S. Hoffman, 2001, A pH-sensitive polymer that enhances cationic lipid-mediated gene transfer. *Bioconjug Chem* 12:906-910.
100. Kyriakides, T. R., C. Y. Cheung, N. Murthy, P. Bornstein, P. S. Stayton and A. S. Hoffman, 2002, pH-sensitive polymers that enhance intracellular drug delivery in vivo. *J Control Release* 78:295-303.
101. Tachibana, R., H. Harashima, M. Shono, M. Azumano, M. Niwa, S. Futaki and H. Kiwada, 1998, Intracellular regulation of macromolecules using pH-sensitive liposomes and nuclear localization signal: qualitative and quantitative evaluation of intracellular trafficking. *Biochem Biophys Res Commun* 251:538-544.
102. Kabanov, A. V., A. V. Levashov and V. Y. Alakhov, 1989, Lipid modification of proteins and their membrane transport. *Protein Eng.* 3:39-42.
103. Kabanov, A. V., A. V. Ovcharenko, N. S. Melik-Hubarov, A. I. Bannikov, V. Alakhov, V. I. Kiselev, P. G. Sveshnikov, O. I. Kiselev, A. V. Levashov and E. S. Severin, 1989, Fatty acid acylated antibodies against virus suppress its reproduction in cells. *FEBS Lett.* 250:238-240.
104. Kabanov, A. V., V. Y. Alakhov and V. P. Chekhonin, 1992, Enhancement of macromolecule penetration into cells and nontraditional drug delivery systems, In, Harwood Academic Publishers, Glasgow pp 1-77.
105. Slepnev, V. I., L. Phalente, H. Labrousse, N. S. Melik-Nubarov, V. Mayau, B. Goud, G. Buttin and A. V. Kabanov, 1995, Fatty acid acylated peroxidase as a model for the study of interactions of hydrophobically-modified proteins with mammalian cells. *Bioconjug. Chem.* 6:608-615.
106. Alakhov, V., A. V. Kabanov, E. V. Batrakova, I. A. Koromyslova, A. V. Levashov and E. S. Severin, 1990, Increasing cytostatic effects of ricin A chain and Staphylococcus aureus enterotoxin A through in vitro hydrophobization with fatty acid residues. *Biotechnol. Appl. Biochem.* 12:94-98.
107. Oda, T. and H. Maeda, 1987, Binding to and internalization by cultured cells of neocarzinostatin and enhancement of its actions by conjugation with lipophilic styrene-maleic acid copolymer. *Cancer Res* 47:3206-3211.
108. Oda, T., F. Sato and H. Maeda, 1987, Facilitated internalization of neocarzinostatin and its lipophilic polymer conjugate, SMANCS, into cytosol in acidic pH. *J Natl Cancer Inst* 79:1205-1211.
109. Slepnev, V. P., 1992, Modification of proteins for transport of biologically active compounds within the cell, Dissertation, Moscow State University.
110. Gebhart, C. L., S. Sriadibhatla, S. Vinogradov and A. Kabanov, 2001, Pluronic-polyethyleneimine conjugates for gene delivery. *Polym. Prepr. (Am. Chem. Soc., Div. Polym. Chem.)* 42:119-120.
111. Batrakova, E. V., S. Li, S. V. Vinogradov, V. Y. Alakhov, D. W. Miller and A. V. Kabanov, 2001, Mechanism of pluronic effect on p-glycoprotein efflux system in blood brain barrier: contributions of energy depletion and membrane fluidization. *J. Pharmacol. Exp. Ther.* 299:483-493.
112. Snyder, E. L. and S. F. Dowdy, 2001, Protein/peptide transduction domains: potential to deliver large DNA molecules into cells. *Curr Opin Mol Ther* 3:147-152.
113. Schwartz, J. J. and S. Zhang, 2000, Peptide-mediated cellular delivery. *Curr Opin Mol Ther* 2:162-167.
114. Torchilin, V. P., R. Rammohan, V. Weissig and T. S. Levchenko, 2001, TAT peptide on the surface of liposomes affords their efficient intracellular delivery even at low

temperature and in the presence of metabolic inhibitors. *Proc Natl Acad Sci U S A* 98:8786-8791.
115. Ambudkar, S. V., S. Dey, C. A. Hrycyna, M. Ramachandra, I. Pastan and M. M. Gottesman, 1999, Biochemical, cellular, and pharmacological aspects of the multidrug transporter. *Ann. Rev. Pharmacol. Toxicol.* 39:361-398.
116. Zhang, Y., H. Han, W. F. Elmquist and D. W. Miller, 2000, Expression of various multidrug resistance-associated protein (MRP) homologues in brain microvessel endothelial cells. *Brain Res.* 876:148-153.
117. Naito, S., A. Yokomizo and H. Koga, 1999, Mechanisms of drug resistance in chemotherapy for urogenital carcinoma. *Int. J. Urol.* 6:427-439.
118. Nooter, K. and G. Stoter, 1996, Molecular mechanisms of multidrug resistance in cancer chemotherapy. *Pathol. Res. Pract.* 192:768-780.
119. Minko, T., P. Kopeckova, V. Pozharov and J. Kopecek, 1998, HPMA copolymer bound adriamycin overcomes MDR1 gene encoded resistance in a human ovarian carcinoma cell line. *J Control Release* 54:223-233.
120. Minko, T., P. Kopeckova and J. Kopecek, 1999, Chronic exposure to HPMA copolymer-bound adriamycin does not induce multidrug resistance in a human ovarian carcinoma cell line. *J Control Release* 59:133-148.
121. Tijerina, M., K. D. Fowers, P. Kopeckova and J. Kopecek, 2000, Chronic exposure of human ovarian carcinoma cells to free or HPMA copolymer-bound mesochlorin e6 does not induce P-glycoprotein-mediated multidrug resistance. *Biomaterials* 21:2203-2210.
122. Omelyanenko, V., P. Kopeckova, C. Gentry and J. Kopecek, 1998, Targetable HPMA copolymer-adriamycin conjugates. Recognition, internalization, and subcellular fate. *J Control Release* 53:25-37.
123. Miyamoto, Y., T. Oda and H. Maeda, 1990, Comparison of the cytotoxic effects of the high- and low-molecular- weight anticancer agents on multidrug-resistant Chinese hamster ovary cells in vitro. *Cancer Res* 50:1571-1575.
124. Minko, T., P. Kopeckova and J. Kopecek, 2001, Preliminary evaluation of caspases-dependent apoptosis signaling pathways of free and HPMA copolymer-bound doxorubicin in human ovarian carcinoma cells. *J Control Release* 71:227-237.
125. Batrakova, E. V., S. Li, W. F. Elmquist, D. W. Miller, V. Y. Alakhov and A. V. Kabanov, 2001, Mechanism of sensitization of MDR cancer cells by Pluronic block copolymers: selective energy depletion. *Br. J. Cancer* 85:1987-1997.
126. Alakhov, V. Y., E. Y. Moskaleva, E. V. Batrakova and A. V. Kabanov, 1996, Hypersensitization of multidrug resistant human ovarian carcinoma cells by pluronic P85 block copolymer. *Bioconjug. Chem.* 7:209-216.
127. Batrakova, E. V., S. Li, D. W. Miller and A. V. Kabanov, 1999, Pluronic P85 increases permeability of a broad spectrum of drugs in polarized BBMEC and Caco-2 cell monolayers. *Pharm. Res.* 16:1366-1372.
128. Venne, A., S. Li, R. Mandeville, A. Kabanov and V. Alakhov, 1996, Hypersensitizing effect of pluronic L61 on cytotoxic activity, transport, and subcellular distribution of doxorubicin in multiple drug- resistant cells. *Cancer Res.* 56:3626-3629.
129. Pifferi, G., P. Santoro and M. Pedrani, 1999, Quality and functionality of excipients. *Farmaco* 54:1-14.
130. Bomford, R., 1981, The adjuvant activity of fatty acid esters. The role of acyl chain length and degree of saturation. *Immunology* 44:187-192.
131. Hunter, R., M. Olsen and S. Buynitzky, 1991, Adjuvant activity of non-ionic block copolymers. IV. Effect of molecular weight and formulation on titre and isotype of antibody. *Vaccine* 9:250-256.

132. Hunter, R., F. Strickland and F. Kezdy, 1981, The adjuvant activity of nonionic block polymer surfactants. I. The role of hydrophile-lipophile balance. *J. Immunol.* 127:1244-1250.
133. Hunter, R. L. and B. Bennett, 1984, The adjuvant activity of nonionic block polymer surfactants. II. Antibody formation and inflammation related to the structure of triblock and octablock copolymers. *J. Immunol.* 133:3167-3175.
134. Hunter, R. L. and B. Bennett, 1986, The adjuvant activity of nonionic block polymer surfactants. III. Characterization of selected biologically active surfaces. *Scand. J. Immunol.* 23:287-300.
135. Hunter, R. L., J. McNicholl and A. A. Lal, 1994, Mechanisms of action of nonionic block copolymer adjuvants. *AIDS Res Hum Retroviruses* 10:S95-S98.
136. Allison, A. C. and N. E. Byars, 1986, An adjuvant formulation that selectively elicits the formation of antibodies of protective isotypes and of cell-mediated immunity. *J. Immunol. Methods* 95:157-168.
137. Allison, A. C. and N. E. Byars, 1990, Adjuvant formulations and their mode of action. *Semin. Immunol.* 2:369-374.
138. Ke, Y., C. L. McGraw, R. L. Hunter and J. A. Kapp, 1997, Nonionic triblock copolymers facilitate delivery of exogenous proteins into the MHC class I and class II processing pathways. *Cell Immunol.* 176:113-121.
139. Millet, P., M. L. Kalish, W. E. Collins and R. L. Hunter, 1992, Effect of adjuvant formulations on the selection of B-cell epitopes expressed by a malaria peptide vaccine. *Vaccine* 10:547-550.
140. Takayama, K., M. Olsen, P. Datta and R. L. Hunter, 1991, Adjuvant activity of non-ionic block copolymers. V. Modulation of antibody isotype by lipopolysaccharides, lipid A and precursors. *Vaccine* 9:257-265.
141. Schmolka, I. R., 1972, Artificial skin. I. Preparation and properties of pluronic F-127 gels for treatment of burns. *J. Biomed. Mater. Res.* 6:571-582.
142. Rodeheaver, G., V. Turnbull, M. T. Edgerton, L. Kurtz and R. F. Edlich, 1976, Pharmacokinetics of a new skin wound cleanser. *Am. J. Surg.* 132:67-74.
143. Rodeheaver, G. T., L. Kurtz, B. J. Kircher and R. F. Edlich, 1980, Pluronic F-68: a promising new skin wound cleanser. *Ann. Emerg. Med.* 9:572-576.
144. Nalbandian, R. M., R. L. Henry, K. W. Balko, D. V. Adams and N. R. Neuman, 1987, Pluronic F-127 gel preparation as an artificial skin in the treatment of third-degree burns in pigs. *J. Biomed. Mater. Res.* 21:1135-1148.
145. Gear, A. J., T. B. Hellewell, H. R. Wright, P. M. Mazzarese, P. B. Arnold, G. T. Rodeheaver and R. F. Edlich, 1997, A new silver sulfadiazine water soluble gel. *Burns* 23:387-391.
146. Follis, F., B. Jenson, K. Blisard, E. Hall, R. Wong, R. Kessler, T. Temes and J. Wernly, 1996, Role of poloxamer 188 during recovery from ischemic spinal cord injury: a preliminary study. *J. Invest. Surg.* 9:149-156.
147. Agren, M. S., 1998, An amorphous hydrogel enhances epithelialisation of wounds. *Acta Derm. Venereol.* 78:119-122.
148. Cao, Y. L., E. Lach, T. H. Kim, A. Rodriguez, C. A. Arevalo and C. A. Vacanti, 1998, Tissue-engineered nipple reconstruction. *Plast. Reconstr. Surg.* 102:2293-2298.
149. Vlahos, A., P. Yu, C. E. Lucas and A. M. Ledgerwood, 2001, Effect of a composite membrane of chitosan and poloxamer gel on postoperative adhesive interactions. *Am. Surg.* 67:15-21.
150. Leach, R. E. and R. L. Henry, 1990, Reduction of postoperative adhesions in the rat uterine horn model with poloxamer 407. *Am. J. Obstet. Gynecol.* 162:1317-1319.

151. Hannig, J., D. Zhang, D. J. Canaday, M. A. Beckett, R. D. Astumian, R. R. Weichselbaum and R. C. Lee, 2000, Surfactant sealing of membranes permeabilized by ionizing radiation. *Radiat. Res.* 154:171-177.
152. Lee, R. C., D. J. Canaday and S. M. Hammer, 1993, Transient and stable ionic permeabilization of isolated skeletal muscle cells after electrical shock. *J. Burn. Care Rehabil.* 14:528-540.
153. Lee, R. C., J. Hannig, K. L. Matthews, A. Myerov and C. T. Chen, 1999, Pharmaceutical therapies for sealing of permeabilized cell membranes in electrical injuries. *Ann. NY Acad. Sci.* 888:266-273.
154. Batrakova, E. V., S. Li, V. Y. Alakhov and A. V. Kabanov, 2000, Selective energy depletion and sensitization of multiple drug resistant cancer cells by Pluronic block copolymers. *Polym. Prepr.* 41:1639-1640.
155. Batrakova, E. V., S. Lee, S. Li, A. Venne, V. Alakhov and A. Kabanov, 1999, Fundamental relationships between the composition of pluronic block copolymers and their hypersensitization effect in MDR cancer cells. *Pharm. Res.* 16:1373-1379.
156. Demoy, M., T. Minko, P. Kopeckova and J. Kopecek, 2000, Time- and concentration-dependent apoptosis and necrosis induced by free and HPMA copolymer-bound doxorubicin in human ovarian carcinoma cells. *J Control Release* 69:185-196.
157. Keatley, K. L., 1999, A review of US EPA and FDA requirements for electronic records, electronic signatures, and electronic submissions. *Qual Assur* 7:77-89.
158. Nishi, H., 1999, Capillary electrophoresis of drugs: current status in the analysis of pharmaceuticals. *Electrophoresis* 20:3237-3258.
159. Kabanov, A. V., I. R. Nazarova, I. V. Astafieva, E. V. Batrakova, V. Y. Alakhov, A. A. Yaroslavov and V. A. Kabanov, 1995, Micelle formation and solubilization of fluorescent probes in poly(oxyethylene-b-oxypropylene-b-oxyethylene) solutions. *Macromolecules* 28:2303-2314.

Factors and Mechanism of "EPR" Effect and the Enhanced Antitumor Effects of Macromolecular Drugs Including SMANCS

JUN FANG, TOMOHIRO SAWA and HIROSHI MAEDA
Department of Microbiology, Kumamoto University School of Medicine, Kumamoto 860-0811, Japan, msmaedah@gpo.kumamoto-u.ac.jp

1. INTRODUCTION

Increasing attention has been paid in recent decades for the tumor angiogenesis and its inhibition, resulting in finding of angiogenesis factors and vascular endothelial growth factor (VEGF). The latter was first identified as vascular permeability factor (VPF) by Senger et al.[1]. Inhibition of angiogenesis by various antidotes or inhibitors such as endostatin and angiostatin, and hence controlling cancer growth is the most recent challenge in cancer therapy along this line.

Notwithstanding the importance of angiogenesis, the other side of biological activity of VEGF (VPF), namely, the enhancement of vascular permeability also plays a critically important role in tumor growth by facilitating adequate supply of nutrients, and possibly oxygen, to meet the great demands of rapidly growing tumors. Embolization of tumor vessels with or without anticancer agents results in tumor regression or necrosis, although it is not fully effective in eradicating tumor cells because tumors quickly regenerate lateral neovasculature and nullify the embolization effect. Antibody directed against VEGF also had a limited effect in controlling the tumor growth in rodent models unable to eradicate the tumor [2].

Tumor vascular permeability, i.e., enhanced permeability and retention (EPR) effect, is important not only in tumor biology but more so in selective delivery of macromolecular anti-cancer agents to tumor [3-6]. In this article,

Polymer Drugs in the Clinical Stage, Edited by Maeda et al.
Kluwer Academic/Plenum Publishers, New York, 2003

the issue of vascular permeability is discussed in terms of macromolecular (or polymeric) drug targeting with high selectivity to tumor tissues. In contrast, such selective targeting is not possible with low-molecular-weight drugs. Small molecules, as are many of the drugs being used today for cancer chemotherapy, do not discriminate tumor tissue from normal tissue; they reach to most normal tissues and organs as well as tumor tissues by free diffusion-dependent equilibrium. For example, common drugs such as antihistamine spread throughout the body within a few minutes after intramuscular or subcutaneous injection. Like inflammatory tissues, tumor tissues exhibit extravasation of macromolecules, including plasma proteins and liposomes. However, unlike the situation with tumor tissues, clearance of macromolecules and lipids from the interstitial space of normal and inflammatory tissues proceeds though slowly via the lymphatic system after extravasation from blood vessels. Clearance of macromolecules and lipids from tumor is so impaired that they remain in the tumor interstitium for longer time [3-7]. This phenomenon has been characterized and termed the tumor-selective enhanced permeability and retention (EPR) effect of macromolecules and lipidic particles. The EPR effect is now recognized as a general characteristic of viable and rapidly growing solid tumor, thus regarded as a "gold standard" in drug design for new anti-cancer agents [3, 4, 8]. This article will, therefore, describe the mechanism of vascular permeability effect in tumor tissues, macromolecular drug delivery, and pathophysiology of tumor vessels using SMANCS as the prototype, and also a few other new polymeric anticancer agents will be discussed briefly.

2. MECHANISM OF ENHANCED VASCULAR PERMEABILITY AND RETENTION (EPR) EFFECT OF SOLID TUMOR TISSUE

Blood vessels in most solid tumors possess unique characteristics that are not usually observed in normal blood vessels. Examples of such characteristics are summarized in Table 1:

(i) ***extensive angiogenesis and hence high vascular density*** [9, 10];

(ii) ***extensive extravasation (vascular permeability) induced by various vascular mediators*** such as (a) bradykinin, which is produced via the activated kallikrein-kinin cascade involving various proteolytic steps [3-5, 11-14], (b) nitric oxide (NO) generated by the inducible form of nitric oxide synthase (iNOS) in leukocytes or in tumor cells [14-16], (c) VPF/VEGF and other cytokines [1, 17-20], (d) prostaglandins involving cyclooxygenases [14, 21, and our unpublished data], and (e) matrix metalloproteinases (MMPs/collagenases) [22];

(iii) ***defective vascular architecture*** [23-25];

(iv) **impaired lymphatic clearance from the interstitial space of tumor tissues** [3, 4, 26-30].

Table 1. Factors affecting the EPR effect of macromolecular drugs in solid tumor

1. Active angiogenesis and high vascular density
2. Extensive production of vascular mediators that facilitate extravasation
    a) bradykinin,
    b) nitric oxide,
    c) VPF/VEGF,
    d) prostaglandins,
    e) collagenase (matrix metalloproteinases, MMPs),
    f) peroxynitrite,
   etc.
3. Defective vascular architecture: for example, lack of smooth muscle layer cells, lack of or reduced receptors for angiotensin II, large gap in endothelial cell-cell junctions, anomalous conformation of tumor vasculature (branching or stretching etc.)
4. Impaired lymphatic clearance of macromolecules and lipids from interstitial tissue (→retention)

The characteristics of vascular pathophysiology just enumerated, i.e., enhanced extravasation of macromolecular compounds through blood vessels in tumor tissues and the impaired clearance of the macromolecules and lipidic particles from the interstitial space of tumor tissue contributes to the prolonged retention of these drugs in tumor [3, 4, 27-30]. In normal tissues, however, the lipid contrast medium Lipiodol and lipids as well as plasma proteins and macromolecules are cleared from the reticuloendothelial/ lymphatic system [7, 26-30]. To describe this phenomenon related to the fate of macromolecular drugs and lipids in solid tumor, we coined the term ***EPR (enhanced permeability and retention) effect*** in 1984 [3, 26, 30, 31]. According to the EPR concept, biocompatible macromolecules accumulate at much higher (> 6 fold more) concentrations in tumor tissues than in normal tissues or organs, even higher than those in plasma [26, 27, 30, 31]. This EPR effect can be observed with macromolecules having an apparent molecular size larger than 50 kDa (Figure 1) which have long plasma half-lives [3, 4, 26, 31]. It is also seen with large liposomes and some lipids (edible oils) in various experimental as well as human tumor systems [25-30], such as sarcoma 180, colon 38 adenocarcinama, Walker 256 carcinoma, melanoma B16, AH (Yoshida hepatoma) 109B and 136B, VX-2, in mice, rats, and rabbits respectively; and most of human solid tumors, as described later. It should be noted that non-stealth liposome are, however, cleared from circulation or before delivery to the target by macrophages via phagocytosis as shown in earlier studies in 1970s. Therefore, in general, most stealth biocompatible polymeric drugs accumulate in tumor tissue at concentrations 5-10 times higher than the concentration in plasma 24 hr after intravenous injection, and frequently at levels more than 10 times higher than that in normal tissue such as noncancerous muscle [3, 4, 26, 31]. The concept of EPR effect in tumor tissue is depicted in Figure 1.

A Normal tissue

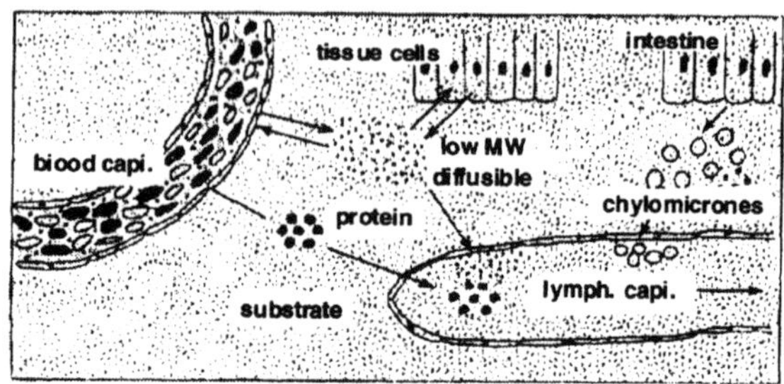

B Tumor tissue

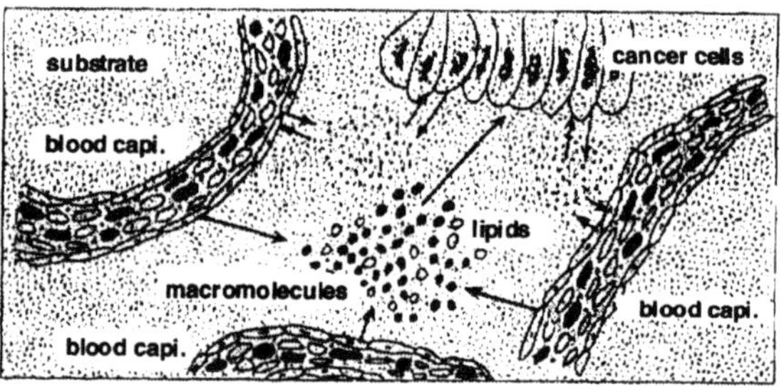

Figure 1. Schematic representation of differences in vascular anatomy of normal tissue (A) and tumor tissue (B). Note the excessive network development of vessels and extravasation of macromolecules and lipid particles in tumor (B). (A from Courtice (7), and B from Maeda (4).)

Most conventional low molecular weight drugs have a plasma half-life of less than 3 min in mouse. However, it takes about 6 hr or longer for drugs in circulation to exert the EPR effect (Figure 2A). This means that any candidate drug must have a large molecular size, above the renal clearance threshold to circulate for a long time. Indeed, as shown in Figure 2B, the plasma AUC (area under the concentration curve) paralleled the accumulation of drug in tumor. Polymer conjugation confers increased residence time of drugs in plasma to a great extent, when compared with the native low molecular drugs. For example, we found that the $t_{1/2}$ of neocarzinostain (12 kDa) in mice is 1.8 min, whereas, the $t_{1/2}$ for its conjugate with poly(styrene-co-maleic acid)half-*n*-butyl ester copolymer (SMA), known as SMANCS becomes about 19 min, i.e., a 10-fold increase.

Native superoxide dismutase (SOD, 30 kDa) had a $t_{1/2}$ of about 3 min in mice, whereas SMA and other polymer conjugates has a $t_{1/2}$ of 25 min or longer. The $t_{1/2}$ of native human interferon-α (approx. 20 kDa) in human plasma was about 8 hr when given intramuscularly, which became 80 hr after PEG conjugation. These data are summarized in Tables 2 and 3.

Table 2. Plasma clearance times of various proteins and their polymer conjugates or modified proteins (from Ref. 4 with permission)

Protein	Type of polymer or modification	Molecular mass (kDa)	$t_{1/2}$	$t_{1/10}$	Test animal
Neocarzinostatin (NCS)	None	12	1.8 min	15 min	Mouse
SMANCS	SMA-NCS[a]	16	19 min	5 hr	Mouse
Ribonuclease	None	13.7	5 min	30 min	Mouse
Ribonuclease dimer	Cross-linked	27	18 min	5 hr	Mouse
Soybean trypsin inhibitor (SBTI[b])	None	20	< 2 min	3 min	Rabbit
Dextran-SBTI	Dextran	127	20 min	> 80 min	Rabbit
Ovomucoid	DTPA/NH_2/^{51}Cr[c]	29	5 min	34 min	Mouse
Cu^{2+}, Zn^{2+} superoxide dismutase (SOD)	None	30	4 min	30 min	Rat
SOD-SMA	SMA conjugate[a]	40	> 300 min	> 10 hr	Rat
Bilirubin oxidase	None	50	< 1 min	1.8 min	Rat
PEG[d]-biliribin oxidase	PEG	70	5 min	48 hr	Rat
Serum albumin, mouse	None	68	3-4 day[e]	-	Mouse
Serum albumin, mouse	Evans blue dye	-	2 hr	30 hr	Mouse
Serum albumin, human	Formaldehyde/^{125}I	-	25 min	4 hr	Rat
L-Asparaginase	None	65 × (2-8)	1.5-3.4 hr	-	Rat
L-Asparaginase-PEG	PEG	-	56 hr	11 day	Mouse
Immunoglobin G, mouse	DTPA	150	60 hr	-	Rat
α_2-Macroglobulin[f]	Iodination/^{125}I	180 × 4	140 hr	22 day	Mouse
α_2-Macroglobulin[f]-plasmin complex	Iodination/^{125}I	180 × 2	2.5 min	20 min	Mouse

[a]binds to albumin; [b] SBTI, Kunitz type; [c] DTPA, diethylenetriaminepentaacetic acid; [d] PEG, polyethylene glycol; [e] Human albumin in humans: 19 days; [f] Human.

Another notion to be emphasized is that polymeric drugs should not be cationic but either neutral or anionic because the luminal surface of blood vessels is highly negatively charged, and thus cationic polymer drugs are adsorbed on the vascular surface and are expected to have a short *in vivo* half-life. In addition, it is obvious that these molecules should not exhibit antigenic or immunogenic characteristics [3-6].

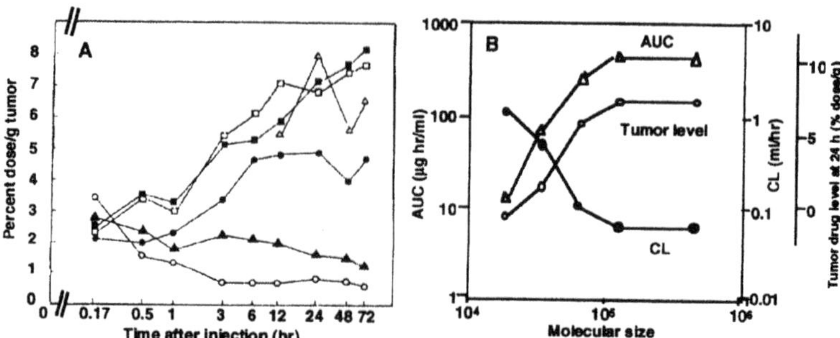

Figure 2. A. Intratumor accumulation of various ^{51}Cr-tagged proteins in solid tumor-bearing mice: ○, neocarzinostatin (NCS) (12 kDa); •, SMANCS (16 kDa, but known to bind to albumin); ▲, ovomucoid (29 kDa); □, bovine serum albumin (69kDa); ■, mouse serum albumin (68 kDa); □, mouse immunoglobulin G (160 kDa). Radiolabeled proteins were injected i.v. at time zero. Values are based on radioactivity (cf. Fig. 2). The tumor model in both A and B was solid sarcoma S-180 in mice. (From ref. 26, with permission). B. Relationship of drug distribution and molecular size to plasma concentration, AUC (area under the concentration curve), renal clearance, and intratumor uptake as expressed by percentage of injected dose. Putative polymer drugs are ^{125}I-Tyr-HPMA-copolymers of various molecular sizes given i.v. at 1.8×10^6 cpm. The tumor model was sarcoma S-180 in mice. (From ref. 28 with permission).

Table 3 Pharmacokinetic parameters of native and polymer conjugated interferon in human, monkey, rat and mice.

Types on conjugates of Interferon	Approximate molecular size (kDa)	$t_{2/1}$ (h) and route of adminisration			
		human, s.c.	monkey, i.v.	rat, i.v.	mice, i.v.
Native IFN-α	18	8	-	-	4
Native IFN-β1a	22.3	-	3.2	1.5	0.92
FMS_7-IFN-α-2	21.4	-	-	-	34
PEG-IFN-β1a	42.27	-	9.5	10.1	9.96
PEG-IFN-α-2b	30	54	-	-	-
PEG-IFN-α-2a	52	80	-	-	-

$t_{1/2}$, plasma half-life; FMS_7-IFN-α2, seven moieties of 2-sulfo-9-fluorenylmethoxycarbonyl conjugate with interferon-α2; PEG-IFN-β1a, 20 kDa straight chain PEG-conjugate with interferon- β1a; PEG-IFN-α2b, 12kDa straight chain PEG-conjugate with interferon-α2b; PEG-IFN-α2a, 40kDa branched chain PEG-conjugate with interferon-α2a.
Data were adapted from reference 32 with permission.

3. MODULATION OF TUMOR BLOOD FLOW AND AUGMENTATION OF THE EPR EFFECT

3.1 Angiotensin II

In 1981, Suzuki et al. found that elevating the systemic blood pressure by infusing angiotensin II in tumor-bearing rats resulted in an increase of tumor blood flow by 2-6 times, in parallel to the blood pressure applied, whereas the blood flow in normal organs and tissues remained constant. In other words, vessels in normal organs, but not in cancerous tissue, show excellent homeostatic autoregulation of blood flow [33].

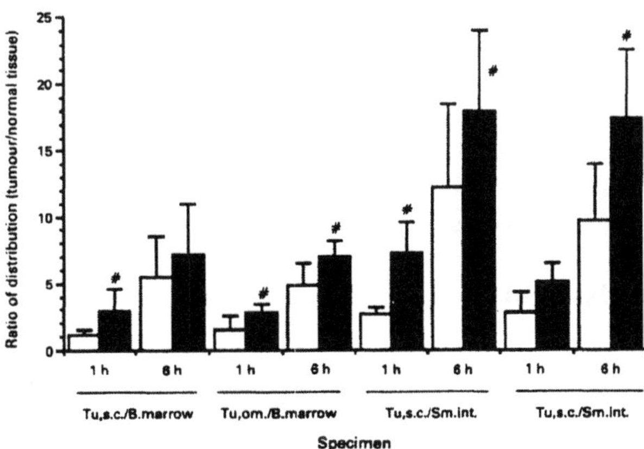

Figure 3. Enhancement of macromolecular drug delivery to tumor (Walker carcinoma 256) in rats given angiotensin II by i.v. infusion. Rats also had the systemic blood pressure elevated for about 15 min from about 100 to 150 mmHg by angiotensin II infusion. To albumin ^{14}C-glycine was attached via amide bond chemically using carbodiimide to a putative macromolecular drug (bovine serum albumin) (From refs. 30, 31). Tu,s.c., tumor implanted subcutaneous location; Tu,om, tumor inoculated peritoneally and metastatic tumor nodule on the omentum; Drug concentration in; Sm. int., small intestine; B. marrow, bone marrow. Tu,sc/sm.int. indicates the ratio of drug concentration between that in tumor subcutaneous over the small intestine, a normal tissue. Solid bars show values obtained after angiotensin II induced hypertension procedure. White bars, normotensive state.

We previously investigated whether this increased tumor blood flow would influence the EPR effect, i.e., if an angiotensin II-induced hypertensive state would improve macromolecular drug delivery. As shown in Figure 3, both radiolabeled bovine serum albumin and SMANCS, which binds to albumin in vivo, thereby becoming an apparent molecular mass of about 80 kDa, accumulated about 1.3 – 3 fold more when arterial blood pressure was elevated from 100 to 150 mmHg by infusion of angiotensin II, and was maintained for 15 min after i.v. injection of [^{51}Cr] labeled SMANCS or the putative macromolecular drug (radiolabeled bovine serum albumin) [34]. Drug delivery to normal organs such as the kidney and the bone marrow was reduced because of the induced vasoconstriction of normal organs, so that the tighter endothelial cell gap suppressed transvascular transfer of macromolecules (Figure 3). Consequently, the side effects such as diarrhea, bone marrow-cellularity, and body weight were decreased to a significant extent [34]. Although the therapeutic dose of an anticancer agent cannot usually be increased 2-3 times more than the recommended dose because of the very narrow safety margin of any conventional anticancer agents, the angiotensin II-induced hypertensive state permits administration of higher dosages for macromolecular drugs. Thus, one may achieve a better therapeutic effect but with fewer and less severe side effects by this method. This therapeutic maneuver is valid only for macromolecular drugs, however.

3.2 Bradykinin

Bradykinin, which has been studied extensively in inflammation, infection [35] and in cancer [11-15, 36], is an important mediator of the EPR effect. It is well known that bradykinin mediates pain and increases vascular permeability and even angiogenesis [37]. We reported previously that the bradykinin-generating cascade is activated in the tumor compartment [11-13], and that bradykinin may be involved in malignant ascitic and pleural fluid accumulation [11, 12, 14, 15].

Enalapril and other similar agents, so-called angiotensin I-converting enzyme (ACE) (E.C. 3.4.15.1) inhibitors, can inhibit the degradation of bradykinin , thus elevating its local level. This is a similar effect to the inhibition of conversion of angiotensin I to II, because of the amino acid sequence homology between bradykinin and angiotensin I near their C-termini. Because bradykinin has a short half-life, inhibition of either kinin-degrading kininase (E.C. 3.4.15.1) or ACE will potentiate the biological activity of kinin in vivo. Indeed, we have shown that inhibition of kallikrein (E.C. 3.4.21.8), which generates bradykinin from high-molecular-weight kininogen (see Figure 4), by soybean trypsin inhibitor (Kunitz type) results in suppression of ascitic fluid accumulation of tumor-bearing mice because the reduced amount of kinin suppresses extravasation [12-14, 38]. In contrast, raising the kinin level in the ascites by administering enarapril, an ACE inhibitor, increased the volume of the ascitic fluid accumulation (Figure 5) [11-14].

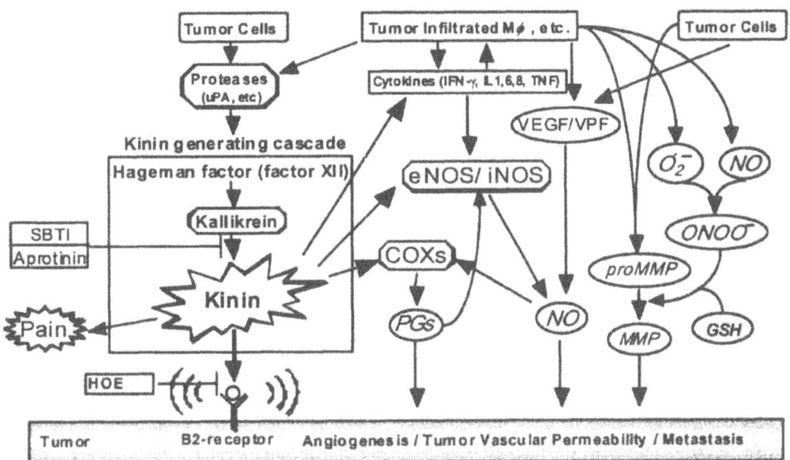

Figure 4. Kinin generating cascade and various vascular mediators in cancer tissues affecting the EPR effect. Mediators, enzymes, and inhibitors are shown. See text for details. Mϕ, macrophage; PMN, polymorphoneuclear cells; COXs, cyclooxygenases; PGs, prostaglandins. SBTI, soybean trypsin inhibitor (Kunitz type); $ONOO^-$, peroxynitrite; NO, nitric oxide; MMP, matrix metalloproteinases.

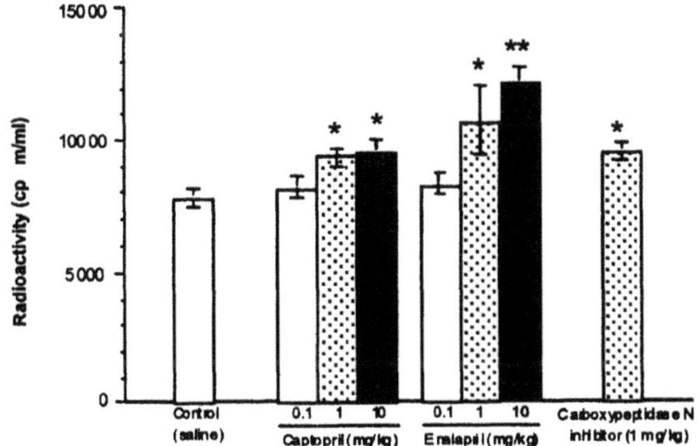

Figure 5. Enhanced extravasation and accumulation of ^{51}Cr-labeled albumin in the peritoneal cavity of mice with ascitic S-180 tumor. Each agent was administrated orally. Data are expressed as means ±S.E., n = 5. See text for details. Adapted from Ref. 12. * $P < 0.05$; ** $P < 0.01$ (versus control).

We recently showed that another ACE inhibitor, temocapril, selectively suppressed blood flow in tumor, whereas blood flow in the kidney, the liver, and the brain was almost unaffected (Figure 6) [39]. A similar effect, i.e., selective suppression (>90%) of tumor blood flow, was observed by using the prostaglandin I_2 (PGI_2) analogue beraprost (our unpublished data). Injection of this PGI_2 analogue, which has much longer in vivo $t_{1/2}$ than PGI_2, resulted in much enhanced EPR effect as that seen with ACE inhibitors in course of several hours: it increased 2-3 times extravasation of Evans blue/albumin. Systemic blood pressure decreased only 10-20%, whereas blood flow in the tumor (AH136B) decreased 90-95%. We believe that this mechanism involves the opening of the tight junction of the endothelium at the postcapillary venule so that plasma components do leak out more effectively into the extravascular space before reaching the postcapillary venous side. As an incidental finding, these vasoactive mediators reduced blood flow downstream to an almost negligible amount (to less than 10%). In this way, we may also achieve more selective accumulation of macromolecular anticancer agents in tumor as well as similar imaging agents though we need to demonstrate in clinical setting.

Therefore, one might improve tumor-selective drug delivery by using macromolecular drugs under angiotensin II-induced hypertensive conditions, together with appropriate vascular mediators such as ACE inhibitors. It should also be mentioned that when [^{14}C]methylglucose, a representative of low-molecular-weight drug mimic, was studied, the EPR effect was only marginal and lasted no longer than 10 min. Such low-molecular-weight drugs seem to be washed out rapidly into the general circulation within 10-min [33] and excreted via the urine.

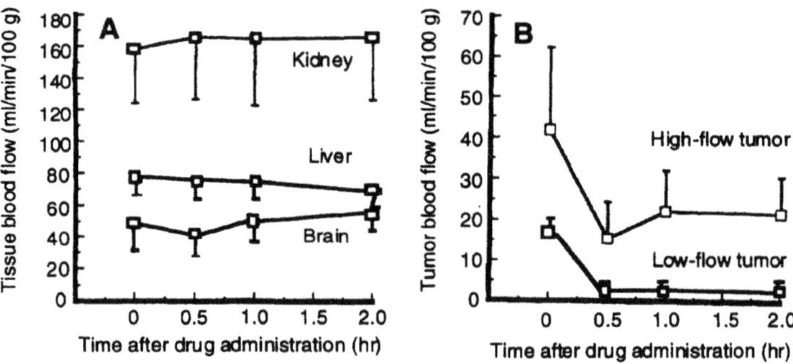

Figure 6. Effect of a second-generation ACE inhibitor, temocapril, on tumor blood flow. Note the great difference in flow rate in normal organs (A) vs that in tumor (B). Tumor blood flow was most affected by elevating blood pressure. The tumor used was LY80 in rats. (Adapted from ref. 39).

3.3 Other inflammatory mediators

Besides VPF (VEGF) and bradykinin system, many other factors involve in the EPR effect in solid tumor. Figure 4 shows various vascular mediators and their interaction for regulating tumor blood flow and vascular permeability.

Prostaglandin biosynthesis by cyclooxygenase (COX-1 and -2), particularly for prostaglandin E2 production, are markedly elevated in human and experimental tumors (40, 41), and many studies have shown that administration of prostaglandin synthesis inhibitors brought about a reduced risk of growth of tumor such as colon cancer, thus that they are beneficial for cancer prevention [42]. In our studies, it was found that prostaglandins are involved in enhanced solid tumor vascular permeability, because the COX inhibitor indomethacin significantly suppressed vascular permeability in S-180 and other solid tumor models [14]. Thus, suppression of COX activity in tumor might be applicable not only to cancer prevention but also to cancer chemotherapy.

We also found that nitric oxide (NO) is involved in tumor vascular permeability. We demonstrated previously that the NO synthase (NOS) inhibitor decreased vascular permeability in solid tumor [14, 15]. Meyer et al. [43] also found that NOS inhibitor N^{ω}-monomethyl-L-arginine irreversibly attenuated blood flow in R3230Ac rat mammary adenocarcinoma. Tozer et al. [44] demonstrated the selective reduction of tumor blood flow with the NOS inhibitor N^{ω}-nitro-L-arginine in rats bearing P22 tumor. Moreover, inhibition of NO synthesis appears to suppress tumor growth, because NO is now known to play a key role in angiogenesis as well as in extravasation, which supply nutrients [14-16, 38, 45-47].

Recently, we found that MMPs, which are known to facilitate cancer metastasis and to enhance angiogenesis to support growth of solid tumors, also facilitated the vascular permeability of solid tumor in mice, and this effect is inhibited by many MMP inhibitors [22].

When one suppresses this enhanced vascular permeability in tumor by using the inhibitors of the kallikrein-kinin system, or cyclooxygenase or NOS in animal models, fluid accumulation in ascitic or pleural carcinomatosis is reduced [12-14, 38]. Thus, suppression of ascitic and pleural fluid accumulation has immediate applications in the clinical setting to support patients inclined to develop cachexia resulting from such fluid (albumin) loss. This application can be accomplished by use of kallikrein inhibitors or bradykinin antagonists (e.g., HOE 140), and most probably also NO scavengers and cyclooxygenase inhibitors [14-16, 38].

Prostaglandins, NO, and bradykinin exert their actions co-dependently, or by cross talking to up-regulate inflammatory mediators [47], so it may be beneficial to simultaneously suppress multiple mediators all together.

4. THERAPEUTIC CHALLENGES OF POLYMER DRUGS: A TUMOR-TARGETING STRATEGY BASED ON THE EPR EFFECT

4.1 SMANCS

We have developed the prototype macromolecular anticancer agent SMANCS (Figure 7) at first 1979 [3, 4, 48-51] as an active principle. SMANCS is more commonly used with Lipiodol®, a carrier vehicle, given by arterial injection using catheter via the tumor-feeding arteries [50-51]. Lipiodol is an iodinated ethylester of poppyseed oil manufactured by Laboratoire Guerbet in France; it can be administered intraarterially upstream from the tumor-feeding artery, i.e., the hepatic artery for hepatoma, and the bronchial artery for lung cancer for example. In an experimental model of metastatic hepatoma in rabbits, the ratio of the drug (lipid) concentration in the tumor (T) to that in blood plasma (B) (T/B) is more than 2000 [27, 29]. Furthermore, the drug remains at high concentration without being cleared from the tumor matrix for up to several weeks, because of its slow clearance as a result of EPR effect [3-6, 8, 14-16, 26, 49-57]; this pronounced retention of lipid contrast agent (Lipiodol) given arterially achieve most remarkable EPR effect, partly by first-pass capture and it is of course much effective than proteins.

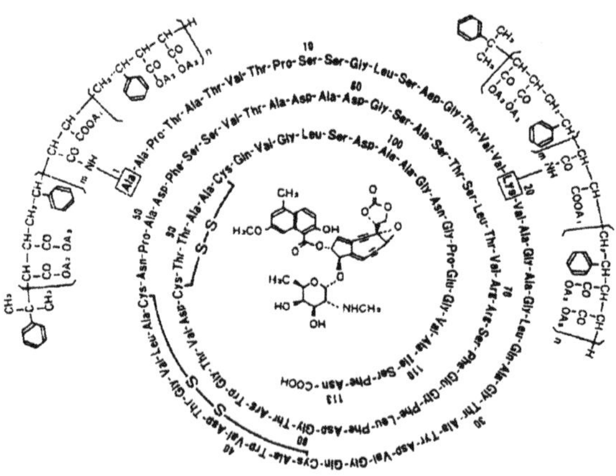

Figure 7. Chemical structure of SMANCS.

Treatment of primary hepatoma by the SMANCS/Lipiodol method has been approved in Japan for more than 6 years, since 1995. When the drug is delivered by intraarterial administration using catheter, this treatment produces definite tumor size reduction (in >90% of cases), improved survival scores, and especially a good quality of life with very little side effect (Table 4)[58]. Furthermore, patients can be out of bed within a few days after the procedure (the Seldinger method is used for arterial infusion under the X-ray system). For all cases of primary hepatoma combined (including Child's criteria of A-C cirrhosis), the 5- to 7- year survival rate is about 30% with this method. With other treatments, no survival would be expected during this time frame. Hepatoma patients with milder liver cirrhosis (such

Table 4. Side effects of intraaterial SMANCS/LPD therapy in hepatoma patients [a]

Symptoms		%	
Dermatological (exanthema)		0.36	
Nausea		5.35	
Vomiting		4.06	b)
Anorexia		3.63	
Abdominal pain (transitory)		5.53	
Liver function			
GOT, increased		2.16	
GPT, increased		2.12	b)
Bilirubin (>1.5 mg/dl)		3.45	
Hypotension		2.22	
Blood counts [c]			
WBCs,	decreased	0.38	
	increased	0.83	
PMNs,	decreased	0.04	
	increased	0.28	b)
Platelets,	decreased	0.83	
Renal function [c], impaired		0.71	
BUN,	increased	0.41	
Anaphylaxis/shock		0.14	
Rigor (transitory)		4.88	
Chest pain (transitory)		0.20	
Fever (low grade, 2-7 days)		27.80	
CRP[c], increased		0.67	
Ascites formation		1.35	

[a] Based on 3956 patients (from PMS data, Yamanoguchi Pharmaceutical Co.).

[b] These results are frequently associated with impaired hepatic functions (e.g., due to liver cirrhosis), and most patients tend to show these effects as liver function deteriorates and disease progresses without the use of SMANCS.

[c] GOT, glutamic-oxaloacetic transaminase; GPT, glutamic-pyruvate transaminase; PMNs, polymorhonuclear neutrophils; WBC, white blood cells; BUN, blood urea nitrogen; CRP, C-reactive proteins

as Child's A grade) and with tumor spread confined to one to two segments of the liver show about 90% survival at 7 years with the SMANCS/Lipiodol treatment.

Side effects of SMANCS/Lipiodol, when used via the intraarterial route for hepatoma patients, are summarized in Table 4. The major side effect is a low-grade fever, which depends on the procedural technique as well as on the individual patient, namely, some of which may also be due to the immunological host response. If the dose is appropriate, there seems to be little liver toxicity, although many, if not all, liver cancer patients have liver cirrhosis and tend to deteriorate progressively. There seems to be no fatal issue with this therapy.

4.2 Poly(ethylene glycol) conjugated xanthine oxidase (PEG-XO)

It has been known that reactive oxidative species (ROS) is potentially cytotoxic, thus can be utilized for treating tumor, which is named oxidation therapy. Xanthine oxidase (XO) is an iron-containing metalloflavoprotien that catalyzes the oxidation of purines, in which ROS including superoxide anion radical (O_2^-) and hydrogen peroxide (H_2O_2) are generated. XO mediates anticancer activity by means of ROS production, however, the high binding affinity of it to blood vessels would cause systemic vascular damage and hence limits the use of native XO in clinical settings. To overcome this drawback, and selectively deliver the drug to tumor by EPR effect, we developed a chemical conjugation of XO with poly(ethylene glycol) (PEG), which hereafter referred to as PEG-XO [58]. To this conjugate, ε-amino groups of lysine residues of XO, which play a crucial role in binding of XO to blood vessels, was conjugated to PEG. PEG-XO injected i.v. showed a 2.8-fold higher accumulation in solid tumor compared with that of native XO 24 h after administration, whereas a slight or negligible increase in accumulation of PEG-XO was found in normal organs. The highest PEG-XO enzyme activity was detected in tumor compared with normal organs except blood; enzyme activity in tumor was 5.0, 3.9, and 9.4 times higher than that in liver, kidney, and spleen, respectively. Intratumor activity remained high even after 48 h. Administration of hypoxanthine, a substrate of XO, via i.p. route 12 h after the injection of PEG-XO resulted in significant suppression of tumor growth, with no tumor growth even after 52 days (Figure 8). No or very little side effect, if any at all, was observed after this treatment. These findings suggest the validity of PEG-XO as a novel anticancer agent.

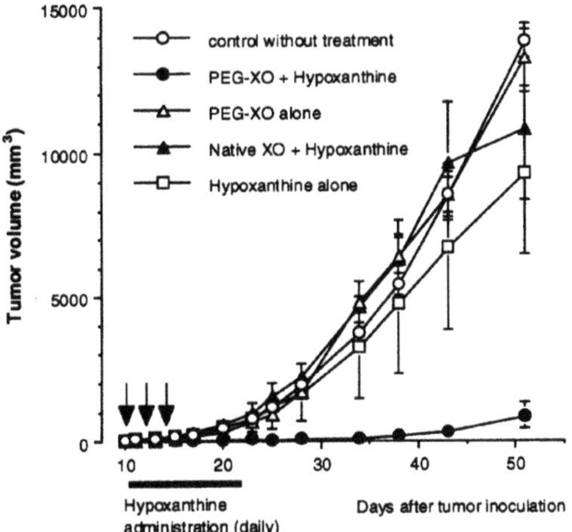

Figure 8. Antitumor activity of PEG-XO with or without hypoxanthine administration. *Arrowheads*, administration of native XO or PEG-XO (0.6 unit/mouse for the first and second administration and 0.2 unit/mouse for the third administration). Hypoxanthine was administered at 33 mg/kg body weight i.p. twice daily from days 11 to 21 after tumor inoculation, at 12 h or later after XO or PEG-XO injection. Data are means (n = 6-8); *bars*, SE. *, $P < 0.001$. #, The complete regression of tumor growth was observed in three of seven tumors in mice after treatment with PEG-XO plus hypoxanthine. See text for details. (From Ref. 58 with permission).

4.3 Poly(ethylene glycol) conjugated D-amino acid oxidase (PEG-DAO)

Along the line of PEG-XO, we have challenged an H_2O_2-generating enzyme, D-amino acid oxidase (DAO), by PEG conjugation [59]. The natural substrate of DAO is D-amino acids, which do not usually exist in mammalian organisms to a significant level. It is thus reasonable that H_2O_2 generation can be regulated by exogenous administration of D-amino acids, thus avoiding the possible induction of severe systemic side effects because of systemic generation of H_2O_2. However, DAO is relatively small protein (Mw 39 kDa), and it may be excreted gradually as previously observed for other small proteins or polymer drugs smaller than 40 kDa [6, 26, 28, 32]. Pegylation of DAO resulted in a 63 kDa molecule. Accordingly, the pharmacokinetic parameters in mice after i.v. injection was improved, compared with the native DAO: its *in vivo* half-life and the area under the concentration vs time curve increased 2.6- and 2.9-fold, respectively. PEG conjugation dramatically improved intratumor accumulation of DAO as well as plasma level of DAO, i.e., 3.2-fold relative to native DAO and 7.4-fold to untreated control in tumor (sarcoma 180); the plasma level was 2.4-fold for native DAO and 9.1-fold for PEG-DAO. In contrast, PEG-DAO injection showed no effect on the enzyme activity in normal organs and tissues. Animal experiments showed that administration of PEG-DAO (plus its substrate D-proline) significantly suppressed tumor growth. Growth suppression continued to at least 27 days after tumor implantation. In contrast, no significant antitumor effect was observed in mice treated with native DAO plus D-proline. In addition, oxidative metabolites were significantly increased in solid tumor by administration of PEG-DAO followed by D-proline, as evidenced by thiobarbituric acid-reactive substance assay, whereas this treatment did not affect results from the metabolites in the liver and kidney [59]. These results indicate the antitumor potential of PEG-DAO, by selective generation of H_2O_2 in tumor site. PEG-DAO, thus warrants further investigation for its clinical application.

4.4 Poly(ethylene glycol) conjugated zinc protoporphyrin IX (PEG-ZnPP)

Recently, we developed a PEG conjugate of zinc protoporphyrin IX (ZnPP), which is a strong inhibitor of heme oxygenase (HO) [60]. HO is an important antioxidative enzyme because of its production of bilirubin via biliverdin – a potent antioxidant. We recently found that tumor cells utilize HO to protect themselves from oxidative stress by producing the antioxidant bilirubin [61]. This result suggested antitumor potential of ZnPP by inhibiting HO activity, hence cancer cells become vulnerable to ROS induced by, such as anticancer drugs or leukocytes of the host. This concept was validated by using the intraarterial administration of ZnPP [61, 62]. However, ZnPP is sparsely soluble in water, but may be dissolved in non-physiological solution, alkaline at high pH, though it limits its practicality. PEG conjugation made ZnPP a water-soluble compound; more importantly, increased the molecular size to above 70 kDa in aqueous media. PEG-ZnPP injected i.v. significantly suppressed intratumor HO activity in murine solid tumor model, which suggested that tumor-targeted inhibition of HO is possible with the use of PEG-ZnPP [63]. In addition, from the preliminary studies, we found a tumor growth suppression by using one injection of PEG-ZnPP, to the extent about 50% (Fang *et al.*, unpublished data). Thus we anticipate its therapeutic use against tumor, especially in combination with ROS-generating systems and including traditional antitumor drugs. Further studies on this compound, i.e., pharmacokinetics, in vivo antitumor effect, are undergoing.

5. SUMMARY

Both enhanced vascular permeability and angiogenesis of tumor sustain rapid growth of tumor involving many vascular mediators and high vascular density. On the contrary, however, they can be utilized for macromolecular drug delivery to tumor. Impaired reticuloendothelial/lymphatic clearance of macromolecules from the tumor, or lack of such clearance, is another unique characteristic of tumor tissue, which results intratumor retention of macromolecular drugs thus delivered (Figure 1). Consequently, enhanced permeability and retention (EPR) effect is the basis for the selective targeting of macromolecular drugs to tumor, and the EPR concept is now utilized for selective delivery of many macromolecular anticancer agents in aqueous formation for i.v. or i.a. as well as oily formation for i.a. dosing, which is not possible for low-molecular-weight drugs because of rapid washout by capillary vascular blood flow. This EPR concept has been validated in clinical settings with hepatoma and other solid tumors [3, 8, 48-53]. In our laboratories, several promising macromolecular anticancer drugs after SMANCS, such as PEG-XO, PEG-DAO, PEG-ZnPP, were developed, warranting further investigation for clinical application.

More efficient drug delivery to tumor, especially of macromolecular drugs, may be possible by enhancing the EPR effect with the use of various vascular permeability mediators or potentiators. Suppression of the EPR effect by the use of appropriate inhibitors or antidotes, such as the bradykinin antagonist HOE 140 and protease inhibitors or NOS inhibitors, may also be possible. Thus, one may be able to suppress or retard tumor growth and tumor metastasis. Also, by suppressing vascular permeability with antidotes such as the bradykinin antagonist HOE 140, pleural fluid in lung cancer and ascitic fluid in abdominal carcinomatosis may be controlled and the clinical course of cancer patients may be improved.

In summary, tumor vasculature can be an excellent target for delivery of macromolecular anticancer drugs; the most beneficial class of drugs in view of tumor-selective targeting based on the EPR effect in solid tumor as well as compliance of patients and ultimate therapeutic efficacy [3, 4, 8, 50-54, 61].

ACKNOWLEDGEMENTS

We would like to thank our colleagues and friends for their collaboration in conducting the experiments described here, including Drs. Y. Matsumura,

J. Wu, and T. Akaike, R. Duncan, and T. Konno to name a few. Work was supported by the Japanese Ministry of Education, Science and Culture as Grant-in-Aid for Science Research in Cancer and General Section. A large part of this article is published in references 63, 64 by H. Maeda: Journal of Controlled Release 2001.

REFERENCES

1. Senger, D. R., Galli, S. J., Dvorak, A. M., Perruzzi, C. A., Harvey, V. S., and Dvorak, H. F., 1983, Tumor cells secrete a vascular permeability factor that promotes accumulation of ascites fluid. *Science* **219:** 983-985.
2. Asano, M., Yukita, A., Matsumoto, T., Kondo, S., and Suzuki, H., 1995, Inhibition of tumor growth and metastasis by an immunoneutralizing monoclonal antibody to human vascular endothelial growth factor/vascular permeability factor. *Cancer Res.* **55:** 5296-5301.
3. Maeda, H., and Matsumura, Y., 1989, Tumoritropic and lymphotropic principles of macromolecular drugs. *Crit. Rev. Ther. Drug Carrier Sys.* **6:** 193-210.
4. Maeda, H., 1991, SMANCS and polymer–conjugated macromolecular drugs: advantages in cancer chemotherapy. *Adv. Drug Deliv. Rev.* **6:** 181-202.
5. Maeda, H., 1994, Polymer conjugated macromolecular drugs for tumor-specific targeting. In *Polymer Site Specific Pharmacotherapy* (A. J. Domb, eds.) John Wiley & Sons Ltd., New York, USA, pp. 95-116.
6. Maeda, H., Seymour, L., and Miyamoto, Y., 1992, Conjugation of anticancer agents and polymers: advantages of macromolecular therapeutics in vivo. *Bioconjugate Chem.* **3:** 351-362.
7. Courtice, F. C., 1963, The origin of lipoprotein. In *Lymph and Lymphatic System* (H. S. Meyersen, Chairman) Charles C. Thomas, Springfield, IL, USA, pp. 89-126.
8. Muggia, F. M., 1999, Doxorubicin–polymer conjugates: further demonstration of the concept of enhanced permeability and retention. *Clin. Cancer Res.* **5:** 7-8.
9. Folkman, J., 1971, Tumor angiogenesis: therapeutic implications. *N. Engl. J. Med.* **285:** 1182-1186.
10. Folkman, J., and Shing, Y., 1992, Angiogenesis, *J. Biol. Chem.* **267:** 10931-10934.
11. Maeda, H., Matsumura, Y., and Kato, H., 1988, Purification and identification of [hydroxyprolyl ^{3}] bradykinin in ascitic fluid from a patient with gastric cancer. *J. Biol. Chem.* **263:** 16051-16054.
12. Matsumura, Y., Kimura, M., Yamamoto, T., and Maeda, H., 1988, Involvement of the kinin-generating cascade in enhanced vascular permeability in tumor tissue. *Jpn. J. Cancer Res.* **79:** 1327-1334.
13. Matsumura, Y., Maruo, K., Kimura, M., Yamamoto, T., Konno, T., and Maeda, H., 1991, Kinin-generating cascade in advanced cancer patients and in vitro study. *Jpn. J. Cancer Res.* **82:** 732-741.
14. Wu, J., Akaike, T., and Maeda, H., 1998, Modulation of enhanced vascular permeability in tumors by bradykinin antagonist, a cyclooxygenase inhibitor, and a nitric oxide scavenger. *Cancer Res.* **58:** 159-165.
15. Maeda, H., Noguchi, Y., Sato, K., and Akaike, T., 1994, Enhanced vascular permeability in solid tumor is mediated by nitric oxide and inhibited by both nitric oxide scavenger and nitric oxide synthase inhibitor. *Jpn. J. Cancer Res.* **85:** 331-334.
16. Doi, K., Akaike, T., Horie, M., Noguchi, Y., Fujii, S., Beppu, T., Ogawa, M., and Maeda, H., 1996, Excessive production of nitric oxide in rat solid tumor and its implication in rapid tumor growth. *Cancer* **77:** 1598-1604.

17. Ferratra, N., and Henzel, W. J., 1989, Pituitary follicular cells secrete a novel heparin-binding growth factor specific for vascular endothelial cells. *Biochem. Biophys. Res. Commun.* **161:** 851-858.
18. Rosenthal, R. A., Megyesi, J. F., Henzel, W. J., Ferrara, N., and Folkman, J., 1990, Conditioned medium from mouse sarcoma 180 cells contains vascular endothelial growth factor. *Growth Factors* **4:** 53-59.
19. Leung, D. W., Cachianes, G., Kuang. W-J., Goeddel, D. V., and Ferrara, N., 1989, Vascular endothelial growth factor is a secreted angiogenic mitogen. *Science* **246:** 1306-1309.
20. Keck, P. J., Hauser, S. D., Krivi, G., Sanzo, K., Warren, T., Feder, J., and Connolly, D. T., 1989, Vascular permeability factor, an endothelial cell mitogen related to PDGF. *Science* **246:** 1309-1312.
21. Reichman, H. R., Farrell, C. L., and Del Maestro, F. R., 1986, Effect of steroids and nonsteroid anti-inflammatory agents on vascular permeability in a rat glioma model. *J. Neurosurg.* **65:** 233-237.
22. Wu, J., Akaike, T., Hayashida, K., Okamoto, T., Okuyama, A., and Maeda, H., 2001, Enhanced vascular permeability in solid tumor involving peroxynitrite and matrix metalloproteinases. *Jpn. J. Cancer Res.* **92:** 439-451.
23. Suzuki, M., Takahashi, T., and Sato, T., 1987, Medial regression and its functional significance in tumor–supplying host arteries. *Cancer* **59:** 444-450.
24. Skinner, S. A., Tutton, P. J. M., and O'brien, E., 1991, Microvascular architecture of experimental colon tumors in the rats. *Cancer Res.* **50:** 2411-2417.
25. Kuruppu, D., Christophi, C., Maeda, H., and O'Brien, P. E., 2002, Changes in the microvascular architecture of colorectal liver metastases following the administration of SMANCS/lipiodol. *J. Surg. Res.* **103:** 47-54.
26. Matsumura, Y., and Maeda, H., 1986, A new concept for macromolecular therapeutics in cancer chemotherapy: mechanism of tumoritropic accumulation of proteins and the antitumor agent SMANCS. *Cancer Res.* **46:** 6387-6392.
27. Iwai, K., Maeda, H., and Konno, T., 1984, Use of oily contrast medium for selective drug targeting to tumor: enhanced therapeutic effect and X-ray image. *Cancer Res.* **44:** 2115-2121.
28. Noguchi, Y., Wu, J., Duncan, R., Strohalm, J., Ulbrich, K., Akaike, T., and Maeda, H., 1998, Early phase tumor accumulation of macromolecules: A great difference in clearance rate between tumor and normal tissues. *Jpn. J. Cancer Res.* **89:** 307-314.
29. Iwai, K., Maeda, H., Konno, T., Matsumura, Y., Yamashita, R., Yamasaki, K., Hirayama, S., and Miyauchi, Y., 1987, Tumor targeting by arterial administration of lipids: rabbit model with VX2 carcinoma in the liver. *Anticancer Res.* **7:** 321-328.
30. Maeda, H., Matsumoto, T., Konno, T., Iwai, K., and Ueda, M., 1984, Tailor-making of protein drugs by polymer conjugation for tumor targeting: a brief review on Smancs. *J. Prot. Chem.* **3:** 181-193.
31. Maeda, H., Matsumura, Y., Oda, T., and Sasamoto, K., 1986, Cancer selective macromolecular therapeutics: tailoring of antitumor protein drugs. In *Protein Tailoring for Food and Medical Uses* (R. E. FEENEY and J. R. WHITAKER, eds.) Marcel Dekker Inc., New York, USA, pp. 353-382.
32. Sawa, T., Sahoo, S. K., and Maeda H., 2002, Water-soluble polymer therapeutics with special emphasis on cancer chemotherapy. In *Polymers in Medicine and Biotechnology* (Ashady, eds.), Am. Chem. Soc., Washington D. C., Monograph, in press.
33. Suzuki, M., Hori, K., Abe, Z., Saito, S., and Sato, H., 1981, A new approach to cancer chemotherapy: selective enhancement of tumor blood flow with angiotensin II. *J. Natl. Cancer Inst.* **67:** 663-669.
34. Li, C. J., Miyamoto, Y., Kojima, Y., and Maeda, H., 1993, Augmentation of tumor delivery of macromolecular drugs with reduced bone marrow delivery by elevating blood pressure. *Br. J. Cancer* **67:** 975-980.

35. Maeda, H., and Yamamoto, T., 1996, Pathogenic mechanisms induced by microbial proteases in microbial infections. *Biol. Chem. Hoppe-Seyler.* **377:** 217-226.
36. Nakano, S., Mastukado, K., and Black, K. L., 1996, Increased brain tumor microvessel permeability after intracarotid bradkinin infusion is mediated by nitric oxide. *Cancer Res.* **56:** 4027-4031.
37. Hu, D. E., and Fan, T. P., 1993, [Leu^8]des-Arg^9-bradykinin inhibits the angiogenic effect of bradykinin and interleukin-1 in rats. *Br. J. Pharmacol.* **109:** 14-17.
38. Maeda, H., Wu, J., Okamoto, T., Maruo, K., and Akaike, T., 1999, Kallikrein-kinin in infection and cancer. *Immunopharmacology.* **43:** 115-128.
39. Hori, K., Saito, S., Takahashi, H., Sato, H., Maeda, H., and Sato, Y., 2000, Tumor-selective blood flow decrease induced by an angiotensin converting enzyme inhibitor, temocapril hydrochloride. *Jpn. J. Cancer Res.* **91:** 261-269.
40. Strausser, H. R., and Humes, J. L., 1975, Prostaglandin synthesis inhibition: effect on bone changes and sarcoma tumor induction in BALB/c mice. *Int. J. Cancer* **15:** 724-730.
41. Trevisani, A., Ferretti, E., Capuzzo, A., and Tomasi, V., 1980, Elevated levels of prostaglandin E_2 in Yoshida hepatoma and the inhibition of tumor growth by non-steroidal anti-inflammatory drugs. *Br. J. Cancer* **41:** 341-347.
42. Greengberg, E. R., Baron, J. A., Freeman, D. H., Mandel, J. S. Jr, and Haile, R., 1993, Reduced risk of large-bowel adenomas among aspirin users. *J. Natl. Cancer Inst.* **85:** 912-916.
43. Meyer, R. E., Shan, S., Deangelo, J., Dodge, R. K., Bonaventura, J., Ong. E. T., and Dewhirst, M. W., 1995, Nitric oxide synthase inhibition irreversibly decreases perfusion in the R3230Ac rat mammary adenocarcinoma. *Br. J. Cancer* **71:** 1169-1174.
44. Tozer, G. M., Prise, V. E., and Chaplin, D. J., 1997, Inhibition of nitric oxide synthase induces a selective reduction in tumor blood flow that is reversible with L-arginine, *Cancer Res.* **57:** 948-955.
45. Gallo, O., Masini, E., Morbidelli, L., Franchi, A., Fini-Storchi, I., Vergari, W. A., and Ziche, M., 1998, Role of nitric oxide in angiogenesis and tumor progression in head and neck cancer. *J. Natl. Cancer Inst.* **90:** 587-596.
46. Garcia-Cardena, G., and Folkman, J., 1998, Is there a role for nitric oxide in tumor angiogenesis. (Editorial) *J. Natl Cancer Inst.* **90:** 560-561.
47. Jackson, J. R., Seed, M. P., Kirchen, C. H., Willoughby, D. A., and Winkler, J. D., 1997, The codependence of angiogenesis and chronic inflammation. *FASEB J.* **11:** 457-465.
48. Maeda, H., Takishita, J., and Kanamaru, R., 1979, A lipophilic derivative of neocarzinostatin. A polymer conjugation of an antitumor protein antibiotic. *Int. J. Pept. Protein Res.* **14:** 81-87.
49. Maeda, H., Ueda, M., Morinaga, T., and Matsumoto, T., 1985, Conjugation of poly(styrene-co-maleic acid) derivatives to antitumor protein neocarzinostatin: pronounced improvements in pharmacological properties. *J. Med. Chem.* **28:** 455-461.
50. Konno, T., Maeda, H., Iwai K., Maki, S., Tashiro, S., Uchida, M., and Miyauchi, Y., 1984, Selective targeting of anti-cancer drug and simultaneous image enhancement in solid tumors by arterially administered lipid contrast medium. *Cancer* **54:** 2367-2374.
51. Konno, T., Maeda, H., Iwai, K., Tashiro, S., Maki, S., Marinaga, T., Mochinaga, M., Hiraoka, T., and Yokoyama, I., 1983, Effect of arterial administration of high-molecular-weight anticancer agent SMANCS with lipid lymphographic agent on hepatoma: a preliminary report. *Eur. J. Cancer Clin. Oncol.* **19:** 1053-1065.
52. Maki, S., Konno, T., and Maeda, H., 1985, Image enhancement in computerized tomography for sensitive diagnosis of liver cancer and semiquantitation of tumor selective drug targeting with oily contrast medium. *Cancer* **56:** 751-757.

53. Tsuchikya, K., Uchida, T., Kobayashi, M., Maeda, H., Konno, T., and Yamanaka, H., 2000, Tumor-targeted chemotherapy with SMANCS in Lipiodol for renal cell carcinoma: longer survival with larger size tumors. *Urology* **55:** 495-500.
54. Maeda, H., and Miyamoto, Y., 1994, SMANCS approach – Oily formulation of protein drugs for arterial injection and oral administration. In *Drug Absorption Enhancement: Concepts, Possibilities, Limitations, and Trends* (A. G. DE BOER, ed.) Harwood Academic Publishers, Chur, Switzerland, pp. 221-247.
55. Konno, T., and Maeda, H., 1987, Targeting chemotherapy of hepatocellular carcinoma: arterial administration of SMANCS/Lipiodol. In *Neoplasms of the Liver* (K. OKUDA, K.G. ISHAK, eds.), Springer-Verlag, Tokyo, Berlin, New York, pp. 343-352.
56. Konno, T., 1992, Targeting chemotherapy for hepatoma: arterial administration of anticancer drugs dissolved in Lipiodol. *Eur. J. Cancer* **28:** 403-409.
57. Maeda, H., and Konno, T., 1997, Metamorphosis of neocarzinostatin to SMANCS: chemistry, biology, pharmacology and clinical effect of the first prototype anticancer polymer therapeutic. In *Neocarzinostatin: The Past, Present, and Future of an Anticancer Drug* (H. MAEDA, K. EDO and N. ISHIDA, eds.) Springer-Verlag, Tokyo, Berlin, New York, pp. 227-267.
58. Sawa, T., Wu, J., Akaike, T. and Maeda H., 2000, Tumor-targeting chemotherapy by a xanthine oxidase-polymer conjugate that generates oxygen-free radicals in tumor tissue. *Cancer Res.* **60:** 666-671.
59. Fang, J., Sawa, T., Akaike, T., and Maeda, H., 2002, Tumor-Targeted Delivery of PEG-Conjugated D-Amino Acid Oxidase for Antitumor Therapy via Enzymatic Generation of Hydrogen Peroxide. *Cancer Res.* 62: 3138-3143.
60. Sahoo, S. K., Sawa, T., Fang, J., Tanaka, S., Miyamoto, Y., Akaike, T., and Maeda H., 2002, Pegylated zinc protoporphyrin: a water-soluble heme oxygenase inhibitor with tumor-targeting capacity. *Bioconjug. Chem.* **13:** 1031-1038.
61. Doi, K., Akaike, T., Fujii, S., Tanaka, S., Ikebe, S., Beppu, N., Shibahara, T., Ogawa, S., and Maeda, H., 1999, Induction of haem oxygenase-1 by nitric oxide and ischaemia in experimental solid tumours and implications for tumour growth. *Br. J. Cancer* **80:** 1945-1954.
62. Tanaka, S., Akaike, T., Fang, J., Beppu, T., Ogawa, M., Tamura, F., Miyamoto, Y., and Maeda, H., 2002, Antiapoptotic effect of haem oxygenase-1 induced by nitric oxide in experimental solid tumour. *Br. J. Cancer* (in press).
63. Maeda, H., Sawa, T., and Konno, T., 2001, Mechanism of tumor-targeted delivery of macromolecular drugs, including the EPR effect in solid tumor and clinical overview of the prototype polymeric drug SMANCS. *J. Controlled Release* **74:** 47-61.
64. Maeda, H., 2002, Enhanced permeability and Retention (EPR) Effect: Basis for Drug Targeting to Tumor. In Biomedical Aspects of Drug Targeting (V. Muzykantov and V. Torchilin, eds.), Kluwer Academic Publishers, Dordrecht.

PEG-Adenosine Deaminase and PEG-Asparaginase

FRANK F. DAVIS
Biotechnology Consultant, 1407 Rifle Range Road, El Cerrito, CA 94530, USA

In two 1977 papers, Abuchowski *et al.*[1,2] showed that the covalent attachment of polyethylene glycol (PEG) to exogenous proteins produced conjugates with greatly reduced immunogenicities and extended circulating lives in rabbits and mice. PEG was chosen for these studies because of its properties: hydrophilicity (three water molecules are bound per oxyethyl unit[3]), linearity, lack of charge, and availability in a spectrum of molecular weights. The availability of monomethoxy PEGs facilitated the activation and coupling processes as it eliminated the possibility of crosslinking.

Since this pioneering work, so many proteins, peptides, small bioactive molecules, Liposomes, surfaces, etc. have been modified by PEGs of various sizes, types, and linkages that the term "pegnology" is sometimes used to describe work in this field. Here, two PEG-enzymes will be discussed. The first, PEG-adenosine deaminase (PEG-ADA) is designated as an "orphan drug" by the Food and Drug Administration.

1. PEG-ADENOSINE DEAMINASE

1.1 Introduction

Thirty years ago Giblett and coworkers[4] reported a deficiency of adenosine deaminase (ADA) in two patients with greatly impaired cellular immunity. This condition of severe combined immunogenicity (SCID) is a rare autosomal recessively inherited disorder which results in low levels of

Polymer Drugs in the Clinical Stage, Edited by Maeda et al.
Kluwer Academic/Plenum Publishers, New York, 2003

immunoglobulins, B and T lymphocytes, and killer cells. Later studies have shown that ADA deficiency affects mainly rapidly growing and dividing lymphoid cells. Intracellular accumulation of adenosine (ADO), and deoxyadenosine (dADO) results in part in their phosphorylation to ATP and dATP. Of the various negative effects produced by accumulation of purine metabolites, the most damaging may be the programmed cell death of immature lymphocytes (apoptosis) caused by dATP accumulation[5]. The result is a major decrease in lymphoid cells and, if the mutated ADA is completely inactive, loss of immune function.

1.2 Synthesis and Properties of PEG-Adenosine Deaminase

ADA, a protein of 41,000 daltons from bovine intestine, is used; PEG is monomethoxy PEG of 5,000 daltons. In an early study of PEG-ADA by Davis *et al.*[6], the conjugate was prepared using PEG activated by reaction with cyanuric chloride. PEG-ADA was attached to 60% of the amino groups, with retention of 28% of the original activity. In mice, PEG-ADA had a half-life of 28 hours on initial i.v.injection, and 30 hours after 13 weekly i.v.injections. ADA, on the other hand, was cleared very rapidly, with a calculated half-life of only 30 minutes on first injection and after 13 injections less than 30 minutes. These results encouraged Enzon, Inc. to initiate a clinical trial of PEG-ADA. The synthesis of PEG-ADA again featured the use of bovine intestinal ADA and monomethoxy PEG of 5,000 daltons. However, to increase the activity of the conjugate, succinimidyl succinate-PEG was used[7] (PEG-enzymes prepared using cyanuric chloride-PEG often exhibit greatly decreased activities). Although the company has not released exact figures, attachment of PEG to half or more of the lysine amino groups of the enzyme generally yields a product with good activity and circulating life, and very little immunogenicity or antigenicity. The half-life of PEG-ADA in humans is 3-6 days[8].

1.3 Clinical Results

The number of patients undergoing PEG-ADA treatment is less than 100 at any time; thus, it is truly an orphan drug. In an early clinical trial Hershfield *et al.*[8] found that treatment with **Adagen**[tm] (Enzon's trade name for PEG-ADA) of two children afflicted with SCID due to ADA deficiency resulted in almost complete reversal of biochemical consequences. It should be noted that continuous diffusion of ADO and dADO across cell membranes into plasma and their resultant deamination results eventually in the reduction of, especially, dATP in lymphoid cells, with a major decrease in their apoptotic death, and eventual restoration of immune function. Later studies have confirmed the efficacy of PEG-ADA in treating SCID due to ADA deficiency.

1.4 Final Comments

The restoration of immune function may take several weeks or months, and treatment must be continuous during this time. If treatment is discontinued either during or after restoration of immune function, buildup of dATP, apoptotic death of lymphoid cells, and loss of immune function will occur. This means that patients must receive one or two weekly i.m. injections of PED-ADA to maintain blood levels sufficient to prevent loss of immune function.

For various reasons, treatment of ADA deficiency by gene therapy has attracted groups involved in this activity. Progress over several years has been gradual, but a recent paper[9] looks promising. The abstract does not indicate whether the two patients who received gene therapy were completely ADA-deficient, or whether their mutated ADA had a few percent of activity, which would allow them survive, possibly not in the best of health, without PEG-ADA treatment. This is of some importance as no PEG-ADA had been administered either before or after stem/progenitor cell gene therapy. The absence of circulating PEG-ADA provided a selective pressure for increase of the transduced cells. Results look good, as the first patient, who was enrolled in the study at 7 months of age has, 11 months after treatment, recovered ADA activity in lymphoid cells and is at home, with normal growth and development, as is the second patient, 4 months after gene transfer. With children born with no ADA activity however, the situation may be different. They require PEG-ADA treatment shortly after birth, and even then some die before their immune systems become active. If given gene therapy it would seem that they would require continuing PEG-ADA treatment until their transduced cells are sufficient in number to provide immune protection. If nothing else, this might require a longer time, as selective pressure for growth of transduced cells would be more or less eliminated.

For a more detailed discussion of SCID the reader is referred to excellent reviews by Hershfield[10] and Hirschhorn[11].

ACKNOWLEDGEMENT

Supported in part by a Small Business Innovative Research grant from the United States Food and Drug Administration to Enzon, Inc.

2. PEG-ASPARAGINASE

2.1 Introduction

In 1961 Broome[12] reported that the antilymphoma activity in guinea pig serum observed earlier by Kidd[13] was due to L-asparaginase, which converts L-asparagine to L-aspartic acid and ammonia. Broome also noted that asparagine, a nonessential amino acid for most cells, was essential for the growth of several tumors. This led to a search for asparaginases with antilymphoma activity, especially from a source that could be grown for the production of large amounts of the enzyme. Campbell *et al.*[14] purified two asparaginases from *Escherichia coli (E.coli)* and showed that one of them (EC2) exhibited antitumor activity comparable to guinea pig asparaginase. *E. coli* asparaginase EC2 then was produced in large quantities for preclinical and clinical studies, with eventual approval by the FDA as an anticancer agent for treatment of acute lymphoblastic leukemia (ALL) and other lymphoid malignancies. An asparaginase from *Erwinia chrysanthemi* also is available for patients who become allergic to the *E. coli* enzyme. A comprehensive clinical review of the asparaginases has been published by Kurtzberg[15].

This discussion will focus on PEG-asparaginase (Oncaspar™) the Enzon, Inc. trade name for the product), which was developed to provide an asparaginase with extended circulating life and reduced immunogenicity. Such a product should require fewer injections and have fewer allergic responses.

2.2 Synthesis of PEG-Asparaginase

E.coli asparaginase, a 140,000 dalton monomer, is composed of four subunits, each with an active site. PEG-asparaginase (Oncaspar) is prepared by reacting *E. coli* EC2 asparaginase with succinimidyl succinate-PEG, essentially as described by Abuchowski *et al.*[16]. PEG is attached to 64% of the 88 amino groups, or 14 PEG groups per subunit. The conjugate retains 51% of the original activity. A later paper by Ho *et al.*[17] on the clinical pharmacology of PEG-asparaginase contains footnote data that can be used to calculate 15 PEGs per subunit.

The properties of Oncaspar are summarized in the review by Kurtzberg[15]: Oncaspar and asparaginase have similar K_m values, and ratios of glutaminase/asparaginase activities (0.03). The low glutaminase activity is desirable, as excessive hydrolysis of glutamine to glutamic acid and ammonia can lead to neurological problems

2.3 Preclinical studies

PEG conjugates of asparaginases from *E. coli* and *Vibrio succinogenes* were evaluated for immunogenicity and circulating life in mice and rabbits[18]. Immunogenicities of the PEG-asparaginases were a small fraction of the native asparaginases. In mice, the circulating half-life of *E. coli* asparaginase was 5 hours, and *E. coli* PEG-asparaginase was 3.75 days; *Vibrio* asparaginase half-life was too short to be measured, while that of *Vibro* PEG-asparaginase was 4.0 days. Ho *et al.*[7] reported a half-life in rabbits of 20 hours for *E. coli* asparaginase, and 144 hours for PEG-asparaginase. MacEwen and coworkers [19] evaluated the effectiveness of PEG-asparaginase alone or with combination chemotherapy against canine malignant melanoma, and reported antotumor activity.

2.4 Clinical Studies

The clinical pharmacology of PEG-asparaginase was evaluated in 31 patients.[17] The half-life of asparaginase was approximately 20 hours, and for PEG-asparaginase, 357 hours. Anaphylaxis, a problem with asparaginase, was not eliminated, although the three reactions that occurred were with the first of four preparations of PEG-asparaginase that were used in the study; two of the patients had shown prior hypersensitivity to asparaginase. The greatly increased half-life of PEG-asparaginase means that fewer injections are necessary to maintain a level of activity in the blood sufficient to reduce asparagine to extremely low or undetectable levels. Summaries of clinical trials follow.

In a combination chemotherapeutic protocol including asparaginases for treatment of patients with relapsed ALL, Abshire *et al.*[20] found that PEG-asparaginase produced a higher reinduction rate than asparaginase.

In a Phase II clinical trial[22] patients with relapsed ALL were given Oncaspar as monotherapy for a period of two weeks prior to combination chemotherapy, which also included Oncaspar. During monotherapy, 22% of patients achieved complete or partial remission, and combination chemotherapy for a period of 35 days produced 78% complete or partial remission. Anaphylaxis did not occur.

Muss and others[23] conducted a Phase II trial of Oncaspar in the treatment of non-Hodgkin's lymphoma (NHL), and found modest activity in a heterogeneous group of patients.

Children with ALL or NHL were treated with Oncaspar under German protocols[24]. Seventy children were given 1,000 U/m^2 in contrast to 10,000 U/m^2 of asparaginase. Toxicity of Oncaspar was low, and no allergic reaction was seen.

Children with relapsed ALL were treated with low-dose Oncaspar [25]. These children had been treated with E. coli or Erwinia asparaginases in earlier protocols, and several of the 35 patients had experienced allergic reactions. Pharmacokinetics of Oncaspar was not influenced by prior hypersensitivity of these patients. However, some "silent" inactivation without clinical manifestations, which produced rapid lowering of Oncaspar blood levels, did occur. In a large-scale Consortium Protocol26 involving 377 patients, E. coli asparaginase were randomized. Patients experiencing a mild allergic event to one was switched to the other. Erwinia asparaginase was substituted if a patient became allergic to the other two. Oncaspar was associated with a lower incidence of mild allergic reactions.

Fu *et al.*[27] report that the addition of Oncaspar to the combination of cytosine arabinoside and 6-thioguanine results in a 15.6-fold synergism over the effectiveness of the two drugs alone in tissue culture studies with human leukemiacell lines. A pilot Phase I trial is in progress.

Patients with advanced solid tumors were studied in a Phase I and pharmacodynamic evaluation of PEG-asparaginase (Oncaspar). In vitro evaluations of tumor samples incubated with PEG-asparaginase indicated that malignant melanoma and multiple myeloma might be good targets for PEG-asparaginase therapy. Patients were given escalating i.m. injections of PEG-asparaginase (250-2,000U/m^2). No partial or complete tumor responses were found[16].

2.5 Conclusions

Because of its extended blood circulating life, fewer injections of smaller amounts of Oncaspar than unmodified asparaginases are required to maintain blood asparagine levels at low, therapeutically effective levels. While immune responses do occur with Oncaspar they are fewer than with unmodified asparaginases. Oncaspar might be even more effective if given in the first level of treatment.

REFERENCES

1. Abuchowski, A., van Es, T., Palczuk, N.C., and Davis,F.F., 1977, Alteration of immunological properties of bovine serum albumin by covalent attachment of polyethylene glycol. *J. Biol. Chem.* 252: 3578-3581.
2. Abuchowski, A., McCoy, J.R., Palczuk, N.C., and Davis, F.F., 1977, Effect of covalent attachment of polyethylene glycol on immunogenicity and circulating life of bovine liver catalase. *J. Biol. Chem. 252*: 3582-3586.
3. Liu, K-J., and Parsons, J.L., 1969, Solution effects on the preferred conformation of poly(ethylene) glycols. *Macromol. 2*: 529-533.

4. Giblett, E.R., Anderson, J.E., Cohen, F., Pollara,B., and Meuwissen, H.J., 1972, Adenosine deaminase deficiency in two patients with severely impaired cellular immunity. *Lancet 2*: 1067-1069.
5. Benveniste, P., and Cohen, A., 1995, p53 expression is required for thymocyte apoptosis induced by adenosine deaminase deficiency. *Proc. Natl. Acad .Sci. USA 92:* 8373-9377.
6. Davis,S., Abuchowski, A., Park, Y.A., and Davis,F.F., 1981, Alteration of the circulating life and antigenic properties of bovine adenosine deaminase in mice by attachment of polyethylene glycol. *Clin. Exp. Immunol. 46*: 649-652.
7. Abuchowski, A., Kazo, G.M. Verhoest, Jr., C.R., van Es, T., Kafkewitz, D., Nucci, M.L., Viau, A.T. and Davis, F.F., 1984, Cancer therapy with chemically modified enzymes. 1. Antitumor properties of polyethylene glycol-asparaginase conjugates. *Cancer Biochem. Biophys. 7*: 175-186.
8. Hershfield, M., Buckley, R.H., Greenberg, M.L., Melton, A.L., Schiff, R., Hatem, C., Kurtzberg, J., Markert, M.L., Kobayashi, R.H., Kobayashi, A.L., Abuchowski, A.,1987, Treatment of adenosine deaminase deficiency with polyethylene glycol-modified adenosine deaminase. *New Eng. J. Med.. 310*: 589-586.
9. Aiuti, A. Slavin, S. Aker, M. Ficara, S., *et al.*, 2001, Correction of ADA-SCID defect without PEG-ADA therapy by stem/progenitor cell gene therapy combined with non-myeloablative conditioning. *Blood 98*: 780a.
10. Hershfield, M., 1997, Biochemistry and immunology of poly(ethylene glycol)-modified adenosine deaminase (PEG-ADA). In *Poly(ethyleneglycol) Chemistry and Biological Applications*(J. M. Harris and S. Zalipsky, eds.), ACS symposium series, 145-154.
11. Hirschhorn, R., 1993, Overview of biochemical abnormalities and molecular genetics of adenosine deaminase deficiency. *Pediat. Res. 33: Suppl.,* S35-41.
12. Broome J.D. 1961, Evidence that the L-asparaginase activity of guinea pig serum is responsible for its antilymphoma effects. Nature, 191: 1114-1115.
13. Kidd, J.G. 1953 Regression of transplanted lymphomas induced in vivo by means of normal guinea pig serum. I. Course of transplanted cancers of various kinds in mice and rats given guinea pig serum, horse serum, or rabbit serum. *J. Exp. Med.* 98: 565-582.
14. Campbell, H.A., Mashburn, L.T., Boyse, E.A., and Old, L.J., 1967, Two L-asparaginases from *Escherichia coli* B. Their separation, purification, and antitumor activity. *Biochem.* 6: 721-729.
15. Kurtzberg, J., 2,000, Asparaginase. In *Holland-Frei Cancer Medicine e.* 5(R. C. Bast, Jr., et al., eds.) B.C. Decker, Inc., Hamilton, Ontario, Canada, pp. 699-705.
16. Abuchowski, A., Kazo, G., Verhoest, Jr., C.R., van Es, T., Kafkewitz. D., Nucci, M.L., Viau, A.T., and Davis, F.F. 1984, Cancer therapy with chemically modified enzymes.I. Antitumor properties of polyethylene glycol-asparaginase conjugates. *Cancer Biochem. Biophys.* 7: 175-186.
17. Ho, D.H., Brown, N.S., Yen, A., Holmes, R., Keating, M., Abuchowski, A., Newman, R.A., and Krakoff, I.H., 1986, Clinical pharmacology of polyethylene glycol-L-asparaginase. *Drug Metab. Dispos.* 14: 349-352.
18. Ho, D.S.W., Wang, C., Lin, J.R., Brown, N., Newman, R.A., Krakoff, I.H., 1988, Polyethylene glycol-L-asparaginase and L-asparaginase studies in rabbits. *Drug Metab. Dispos.* 16: 27-29.
19. MacEwen, E.G., Rosenthal, R., Matus, R., Viau, A.T., Abuchowski, A., A preliminary study on the evaluation of asparaginase. *Cancer 59:* 2011-2015.
20. Abshire, T.C., *et al.,* Weekly polyethylene glycol conjugated (PEG) L-asparaginase ASP) produces superior induction remission rates in childhood relapsed acute lymphoblastic leukemia (rALL): a pediatric oncology group (POG) study 9310. *Proc. AM. Soc. Clin. Oncol.* 14: 344.

21. Ettinger,L.J., Kurtzberg, J., Voute, P.A., Jurgens, H., Halpern, S.L., 1995, an open-label, multicenter study of polyethylene glycol-L-asparaginase for the treatment of acute lymphoblastic leukemia. *Cancer* 75: 1176-1181.
22. Muss, H.B., Spell, N., Scudiery, D., Capizzi, R.L, Cooper, M.R., Cruz, J., Jackson, D.V., Richards, F., Spurr, C.L., White, R., Zekan, P.J., Franklin, A.J., 1990. A phase II trial of PEG-L-asparaginase in the treatment of non-Hodkin's lymphoma. *Invest.New Drugs* 8: 125-130.
23. Muller, H-J., Loning, L., Horn, A., Schwabe, D., Gunkel, M., Schrappe, M., Schutz, V.V., Henze, G., Palma., J.C., Ritter, J., Pinhiero, J.P.V., Winkelhorst., M., Boos, J., 2,000, Pegylated asparaginase (Oncaspar) in children with ALL: drug monitoring in reinduction according to the ALL/NHL-BFM 95 protocols. *Br. J. Haematol.* 110: 379-384.
24. Pinheiro, J.P.V., Muller,H.J., Schwabe, D., Gunkel, M., Palma, J.C., Henze, G., Shutz, V.V., Winkelhorst, M., Wurthwein, G., Boos, J., 2,001, Drug monitoring of low-dose PEG-asparaginase (Oncaspar) in children with relapsed acute lymphoblastic leukemia. *Br. J. Haematol.* 113: 115-119.
25. Silverman, L.B., et al., 2,001, Improved outcome for children with acute lymphoblastic leukemia: results of Dana-Farber consortium protocol 91-01. *Blood* 97: 1211-1218.
26. Fu, C.H., *Martin*-Aragon,S. Weinberg, K.I., *et al.*, 2,001, Reversal of cytosine arabinoside (ARA-C) resistance by the synergistic combination of 6-thioguanine plus ara-C plus PEG-asparaginase (TGAP) in human leukemia lines lacking or expressing p53 protein. *Cancer Chemother. Pharmacol.* 48: 123-133.
27. Taylor, C.W., Dorr, R.T., Fanta, P., *et al.*, 2001, A phase I and pharmacodynamic evaluation of polyethylene glycol-conjugated L-asparaginase in patients with advanced solid tumors. *Cancer Chemother.Pharmacol.* 47: 83-88.

Peginterferon alfa-2a (40KD): A Potent Long-Acting Form of Interferon alfa-2a for the Treatment of Hepatitis C

MARLENE W. MODI, MATTHEW W. LAMB, and MARI SHIOMI*
*Department of Clinical Pharmacology, Hoffmann-La Roche, Inc., Nutley NJ, USA; *Clinical Pharmacology Group, Nippon Roche K.K.,Tokyo Japan*

1. INTRODUCTION

Hepatitis C viral infection is a major cause of liver disease worldwide. The real burden of this disease is not in the initial or acute, mild phase of the infection, but rather in the sequelae that are associated with chronic hepatitis C infection[1]. Up to 90% of acute cases progress to persistent infection[1,2], and between 60% to 80% of those who are persistently infected will develop chronic infection. Within 5 years of infection, one-third of patients develop chronic active hepatitis, with one-third of these patients eventually progressing to cirrhosis[3,4]. Many patients develop cirrhosis, hepatic failure, and/or hepatocellular carcinoma after 10 or more years of indolent, asymptomatic infection[5]. Although the incidence of newly acquired hepatitis C infection is decreasing, tens of thousands of seriously ill patients who were infected decades ago are likely to experience complications of this infection in the future, which might include a hepatitis-related death[5]. The need for new therapies and the better use of current treatment options are clearly recognised.

Polymer Drugs in the Clinical Stage, Edited by Maeda et al.
Kluwer Academic/Plenum Publishers, New York, 2003

1.1 Interferon alfa-2a and its Limitations as a Therapeutic Agent

A cornerstone of the treatment regimen for chronic hepatitis C infection is an alpha interferon (IFN). IFNs are endogenous glycoproteins produced by a variety of cells, usually in response to a viral infection. The mechanism by which IFN acts against the hepatitis C virus is not completely understood. Possible actions include a direct antiviral effect and to a lesser extent, immune system modulation[6,7]. Immune system modulation by IFN may be important in that decreases in liver inflammation and fibrosis are considered to be long-term goals in the disease's management.

Clearly, an immediate goal in the treatment of chronic hepatitis C infection is the eradication of the virus from the serum. A sustained virological response is defined as the inability to detect hepatitis C virus in the serum 6 months after treatment has been completed. The antiviral effect of IFN in patients with chronic hepatitis C infection is well established[8]. The standard therapeutic schedule of IFN consists of 3 MIU administered subcutaneously three times a week for up to 48 weeks. IFN therapy alone produces a sustained virological response in less than 20% of patients[9].

IFN's pharmacokinetic characteristics limit its therapeutic efficacy. IFN is rapidly absorbed from the subcutaneous injection site, and peak serum concentrations occur 3 to 8 hours after dosing. IFN is rapidly cleared by renal filtration, reabsorption and catabolism in the kidney[10, 11]. The rapid absorption and avid renal clearance of IFN produce the large fluctuations in IFN serum concentrations that are seen after each dose (Figure 1). IFN's therapeutic efficacy is limited by its relatively brief residence time in a patient's circulation. Indeed, the amount of IFN left in the body after 24 hours is so insignificant that the three times weekly regimen is unlikely to maintain serum levels that are required for adequate antiviral or immunomodulatory activity.

A rapid and dose-dependent decline in serum HCV RNA titre is seen within the first 24 hours of subcutaneous administration of the first IFN dose[12, 13]. Viral titres continue to decline 36 to 48 hours after the first IFN dose, but at a more variable and slower rate. At 48 hours after the first IFN dose, the HCV RNA viral titre is elevated again. The viral titre appears to rebound during periods of time when IFN serum concentrations are declining[13]. The rates of both the first and second phase of viral decline are much faster in patients infected with hepatitis C virus genotype 2, and may explain why a greater proportion of patients with genotype non-1 hepatitis C viral infection experience a sustained virological response compared to those infected with genotype 1 virus[12]. Patients with the genotype 1 virus are considered harder-to-treat.

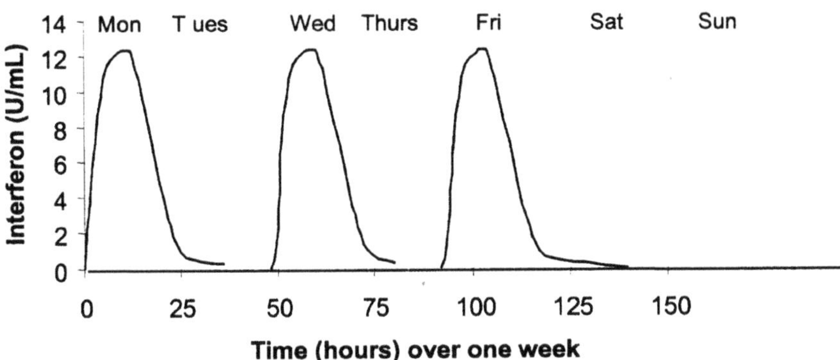

Figure 1. Conceptual View of IFN Serum Concentration Profile During the First Week

Conceptually, patients treated with IFN 3 MIU three times weekly experience a subtherapeutic antiviral response throughout much of the time that they are being treated. In addition, Zhi and colleagues[14] showed that the intensity of flu-like symptoms was greatest between 8 to 12 hours after a single dose of IFN. IFN peak exposure is reached around 8 hours and concentrations decline sharply after 8 hours. These data suggest that the intensity of flu-like symptoms are related to the steep fluctuations in IFN concentrations that are seen during the first 24 hours after dosing.

1.2 History of Pegylating Interferon alfa-2a

The efficacy of exogenously administered proteins is often limited by the relatively short time that the protein is present in the circulation[15]. Polyethylene glycol (PEG)-conjugated proteins have better physical and thermal stability as the protein portion of the conjugate is protected by PEG moiety against rapid enzymatic degradation. The systemic clearance, or removal of the PEG-protein conjugate from the circulation, is reduced compared to the unmodified protein as the protein portion is protected from metabolism and the size of the PEG-protein conjugate often limits renal filtration of the molecule. Greater efficacy may be seen compared to the unmodified protein as the PEG-protein conjugate circulates for a longer period of time at more constant levels throughout a dosing interval. The

PEG-protein conjugate may have safety advantages compared to the unmodified protein as there is less fluctuation in the peak to trough concentrations of the new molecule, and the volume of distribution of the new and larger molecule may be more restricted to the circulation[2].

The aim of pegylating IFN has been to optimize the pharmacological activity of the protein such that efficacy is enhanced, adverse effects minimized, and patient compliance and quality of life are improved. In the early 1990's, Hoffmann-La Roche attempted to benefit from the advantages that pegylation could afford by developing a linear 5 kDa pegylated form of IFN alfa-2a. In 1994, the clinical development of this linear 5 kDa pegylated IFN alfa-2a was discontinued because with once weekly dosing, the efficacy of this linear 5 kDa pegylated IFN alfa-2a was not equivalent to IFNalfa-2a given three times a week in a comparative Phase II clinical trial in patients with chronic hepatitis C infection. Roche scientists with collaboration from Shearwater Corporation (Huntsville, Alabama) went back to the drawing board to develop an optimized pegylated alpha interferon.

2. PEGYLATION: BIOCHEMISTRY AND EFFECTS ON THE PHARMACOLOGY OF INTERFERON

2.1 Optimizing the Pegylation of Interferon alfa-2a

An optimal pegylated IFN for use in the treatment of hepatitis C infection would be absorbed in a sustained fashion, would be distributed predominantly to the liver and remain in the circulation and interstitial fluids, and would have a reduced clearance from the body compared to IFN. The pegylation of IFN would result in a less active molecule in vitro than that of the native endogenous protein, IFN, however; the in vivo pharmacological activity related to efficacy would be better than that of IFN because sustained therapeutic concentrations would be maintained throughout a one week dosing interval (Figure 2). Conceptually then, the size, branching and pegylation process needs to be optimized for each protein such that therapeutically active concentrations are maintained for the appropriate period of time.

The biochemical and pharmacological properties of a protein conjugate depend on the physiochemical properties of the PEG moiety, and the pegylation process (i.e., PEG molecular weight, linear or branched PEG structure, chemical method of attachment, number and location of PEG moieties attached to the protein). A PEG molecular mass of 40 to 60 KD (kilodaltons) substantially reduces the renal and cellular clearance of small protein molecules[16, 17]. Smaller pegylated proteins are filtered readily by the

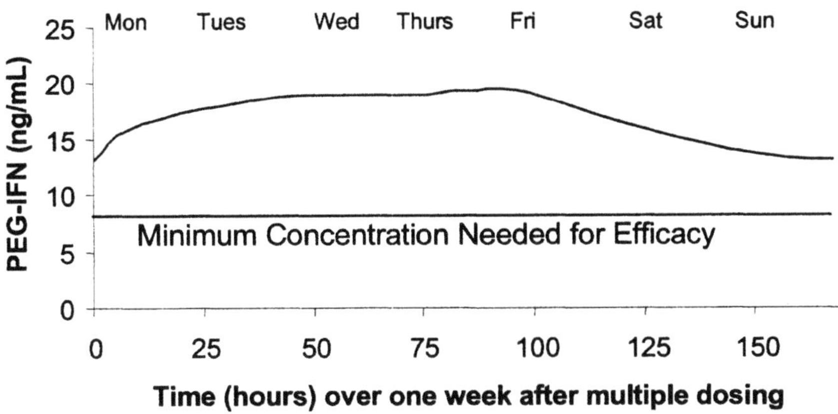

Figure 2. Conceptual Serum Concentration Profile for an Optimized Pegylated Interferon

kidney. Branched chain pegylated proteins are more stable against enzymatic proteolysis than linear moieties. PEG chains attached at a single site on the protein may be less likely to influence in vitro specific activity as attachment at a single site is less likely to obscure the active binding site on the protein. The size and the structure of the PEG moiety may also result in a more sustained absorption that is mediated via the lymphatics and a more restricted distribution within the body where the PEG-protein conjugate is limited to the circulation and interstitial fluids.

The paradigm that was used to optimize the pegylation of IFN required a multidimensional approach (Figure 3). Each parameter was optimized based on the constraints of pegylation and the cost of goods. Based on clinical pharmacology work with the 5 kDa pegylated interferon, it was understood that sustained concentrations above a given effective concentration were needed for stimulation of endogenous effector proteins and maintaining these effective concentrations would lead to the best efficacy profile[18]. Proof-of-concept studies could be performed in healthy subjects[19] by measuring the pegylated IFN-stimulation of effector proteins. Certain physico-chemical properties associated with PEG size and structure and the stability of the bond between the PEG moiety and IFN could lead to a molecule that exhibited sustained concentrations but no measureable in vitro activity. Thus, a balance between the in vitro potency and the in vivo properties of a pegylated IFN needed to be achieved. Preclinical work

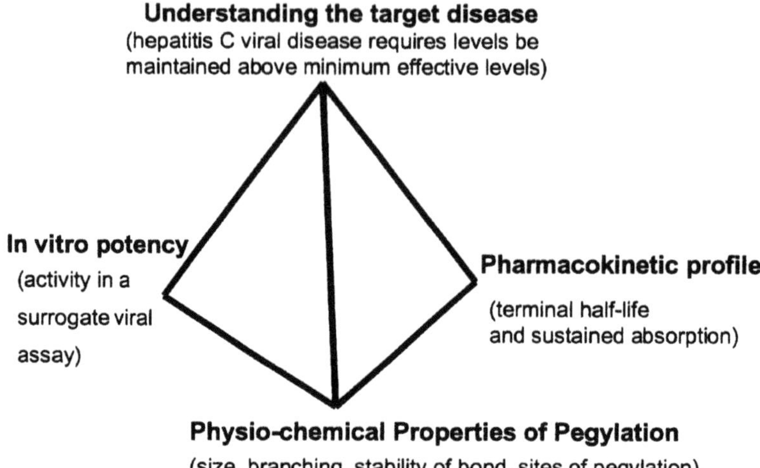

Figure 3. Multidimensional Approach used to Optimize Pegylation of Interferon alfa-2a

ensured that the selected pegylated IFN retained the antiviral, immunomodulatory and antiproliferative properties that are associated with IFN alfa-2a[20].

Pharmacokinetic studies in rats using conjugates of IFN alfa-2a with PEG moieties of varying molecular weights and different structures (branched and linear), including three linear (5, 20 and 40 KD) and two branched (20 and 40 KD) PEG moieties showed that the absorption of the pegylated IFNwas more sustained, the distribution more restricted and the clearance reduced as the size of the PEG moiety increased[21].

2.2 Chemistry of Peginterferon alfa-2a (40KD)

Peginterferon alfa-2a (40KD) contains a 40KD branched PEG chain, each with an average molecular weight of 20KD. The two monomethoxy chains are joined via hydrolytically stable urethane bonds to a lysine linker molecule, one at the lysine α-amino group and another at the lysine ε-amino group[20]. Linking the two 20KD chains via lysine is achieved in a one-step procedure by reacting lysine with monomethoxy PEG succinimidyl carbonate, and the resulting monomethoxy PEG-disubstituted lysine can then be purified by ion exchange chromatography[22]. The branched PEG structure is attached at a single site to IFN alfa-2a via a lysine linker molecule. The carboxyl group of the lysine linker is activated to an N-hydroxy succinimidyl ester than can then form stable amide bonds with amino groups located on lysine residues in the protein. The reaction conditions can be manipulated to favor generation of the monosubstituted conjugate, which can then be purified using ion exchange chromatography. Purified peginterferon alfa-2a (40 KD) contains 95-99% monopegylated conjugates[20].

3. CLINICAL PHARMACOLOGY OF PEGINTERFERON ALFA-2A (40KD)

The pharmacokinetic profile of peginterferon alfa-2a (40KD) in rats was predictive of the pharmacokinetic characteristics of the drug in humans. In a clinical study[23] in which serum concentrations of the drug were monitored, peginterferon alfa-2a (40KD) given as a single dose in healthy male subjects was absorbed in a sustained fashion and had a reduced clearance compared to IFN alfa-2a. These findings led researchers to conclude that continuous drug exposure would be seen throughout the week-long dosing period in patients. In patients with hepatitis C treated once weekly over 48 weeks, steady-state concentrations were reached after 5 to 8 weeks of treatment, the peak-to-trough ratio of peginterferon alfa-2a was around 1.5 to 2.0 and thus a constant drug concentration was present throughout the once-weekly dosing interval[24].

In a proof-of-concept study in healthy subjects[19], IFN-induced stimulation of serum 2',5'-oligoadenylate synthetase (OAS) activity, a widely used marker for IFN antiviral activity and endogenous effector protein, increased after a single 3 MIU dose of IFN alfa-2a, reached a peak at 24 hours and then declined rapidly. In contrast, higher OAS activity was induced within 48 hours after a dose of peginterferon alfa-2a (40KD) than seen with IFN and these higher OAS activities were maintained for a one-week period. Thus, the sustained peginterferon alfa-2a (40 KD) concentrations translated into a sustained antiviral effect.

4. PEGINTERFERON ALFA-2A (40KD) IN CLINICAL TRIALS

Once-weekly administration of peginterferon alfa-2a (40KD) has superior efficacy to three times weekly dosing of 3 MIU IFN alfa-2a[25] with a sustained virological response in more than 35% of patients. Sustained virological response was significantly greater in patients who received peginterferon alfa-2a (40KD) versus IFN alfa-2a, with a similar side-effect profile. Histological improvements were seen in patients who achieved sustained virological responses and were often seen among patients who did not achieve a sustained virological response. The efficacy and an acceptable safety profile were also seen in the difficult-to-treat patient with hepatitis C (patients with cirrhosis and hepatitis C genotype 1 virus)[25, 26].

Phase III efficacy and safety results confirmed that the optimization of pegylation of IFN and the optimization of the pharmacokinetics and pharmacodynamics of a pegylated interferon led to superior efficacy and a better benefit:risk ratio than that seen with IFN. Newer therapeutic regimens will include a pegylated interferon in combination with ribavirin or another antiviral agent so that greater than 50% of patients achieve a sustained virological response. Much progress in the treatment of hepatitis C has been made in the last 5 years and pegylated interferons play a significant role in this progress.

ACKNOWLEDGEMENTS

This work was sponsored by Hoffmann-La Roche, Inc.

REFERENCES

1. Sharara, A.I., Hunt, C.M., et al., 1996, Hepatitis C. *Ann Intern Med* **125**:658-68.
2. Koziel, M.J., 1996, Immunology of viral hepatitis. *Am J Med* **100**:98-109.
3. Kiyasu, P.K. and Caldwell, S.H., 1993, Diagnosis and treatment of the major hepatotropic viruses. *Am J Med Sci* **306**: 248-61.
4. Iwarson, S., Norkraus, G. et al., 1995, Hepatitis C: natural history of a unique infection. *Clin Infect Dis* **20**: 1361-70.
5. Alter, M., 1997, Epidemiology of hepatitis C. *Hepatology* **26**: (3 Suppl 1): 625-655.
6. Davis, G.L., 2000, Current therapy for chronic hepatitis C. *Gastroenterol* **118** (Suppl 1): S104-S114.
7. Lawrence, S.P., 2000, Advances in the treatment of hepatitis C. In *Advances in Internal Medicine.* Mosby, St. Louis.
8. Hoofnagle, J.H. and di Bisceglie, A.M., 1997, The treatment of chronic viral hepatitis. *N Engl J Med* **336**: 347-56.
9. McHutchinson, J.G., Gordon, S.C., et. al., 1998, Interferon alfa-2b or in combination with ribavirin as initial treatment for chronic hepatitis C. *N Engl J Med* **339**: 1485-92.
10. Wills, R.J., 1990, Clinical pharmacokinetics of interferons. *Clin Pharmacokinet* **19**: 390-399.
11. Bocci, V., Pacini, A. et. al., 1981, Renal filtration, absorption and catabolism of human alpha interferon. *J Interferon Res* **1**: 347-52.
12. Zeuzem, S., Herrmann, E. et. al., 2001, Viral kinetics with chronic hepatitis C patients treated with standard or peginterferon alfa-2a. *Gastroenterol* **120**: 1438-1447.
13. Lam, N.P. Neumann, A.U. et. al., 1997, Dose-dependent acute clearance of hepatitis C genotype 1 virus with interferon alfa. *Hepatology* **26**: 226-31.

14. Zhi, J., Teller, S.B. et al., 1995, Influence of human serum albumin content in formulations on the bioequivalency of interferon alfa-2b given by subcutaneous injection in healthy male volunteers. *J Clin Pharmacol* **35**: 281-4.
15. Harris, J.M., Martin, N.E., et. al., 2001, Pegylation: a novel process for modifying pharmacokinetics. *Clin Pharmacokinet* **40**: 539-51.
16. Yamaoka, T., Tabata, Y., et. al., 1994, Distribution and tissue uptake of poly(ethylene glycol) with different molecular weights after intravenous administration to mice. *J Pharm Sci* **83**: 601-6.
17. Fung, W.-J., Porter, J.E., et. al., 1997, Strategies for the preparation and characterization of polyethylene glycol vinyl sulfone. *Polymers Preprint:* 565-66.
18. Nieforth, K.A., Nadeau, R., et. al., 1996, Use of an indirect pharmacodynamic stimulation model of MX protein induction to compare in vivo activity of interferon alfa-2a and a polyethylene glycol-modified derivative in healthy subjects. *Clin Pharmacol Ther* **59**: 636-46.
19. Xu, Z.-X., Patel, I., et al., 1998, Single-dose safety, tolerability and pharmacokinetics of PEG-FIN alfa-2a and may explain its enhanced efficacy in chronic hepatitis C (CHC). *Hepatology* **28** (Suppl): 702.
20. Bailon, P., Palleroni, A., et al., 2001, Rational design of a potent, long-lasting form of interferon: a 40 kDa branched polyethylene glycol-conjugated interferon alpha-2a for the treatment of hepatitis C. *Bioconjugate Chem* **12**: 195-202.
21. Bailon, P., Spence, C., et al., 1999, Pharmacokinetic properties of five polyethylene glycol conjugates of interferon alfa-2a. *Antiviral Therapy* **4** (Suppl 4): 27.
22. Harris, N.J., Veronese, F.M., et al., 1999, Multiarmed, monofunctional, polymer for coupling to molecules and surfaces. *US Patent & Trademark Office*, USA.
23. Algranati, N.E., Sy, S., et. al., 1999, A branched methoxy 40 kDa, polyethylene glycol (PEG) moiety optimizes the pharmacokinetics of PEG-IFN alfa-2a and may explain its enhanced efficacy in chronic hepatitis C (CHC). *Hepatology* **40**: 190.
24. Modi, M.W., Fried, M.W., et. al., 2000, The pharmacokinetic behavior of pegylated (40 kDa) interferon alfa-2a (PEGASYS) in chronic hepatitis patients after multiple dosing. *Hepatology* **32** (4 Pt 2 of 2): 394A.
25. Zeuzem, S., Feinman, S.V., et al., 2000, Peginterferon alfa-2a in patients with chronic hepatitis C. *N Engl J Med* **343**: 1666-72.
26. Heathcote, E.J., Shiffman, M.J., et. al., 2000, Peginterferon alfa-2a in patieints with chronic hepatitis C and cirrhosis. *N Engl J Med* **345**: 1673-80.

PEG-Methioninase

ROBERT M. HOFFMAN
AntiCancer, Inc., 7917 Ostrow Street, San Diego, CA 92111, USA, E-mail: all@anticancer.com

1. INTRODUCTION

1.1 Background

Conjugation of protein therapeutics with polyethylene glycol (PEG) has been shown to confer important therapeutic benefits—most importantly, increased serum half-life and reduced antigenicity[1]. PEG-proteins enhance solubility, decrease antigenicity, decrease proteolysis, and reduce rates of kidney clearance as well as enhance selective tumor targeting. All of these effects are dependent on the molecular weight of the PEG conjugates[1]. To couple PEG to a protein, it is first necessary to activate the polymer by converting the hydroxyl terminus to a functional group capable of reacting typically with lysine and N-terminal amino groups[1]. The heterogeneity in lysine substitution and in PEG molecular weights is a concern for PEG-protein pharmaceuticals[1].

Each ethylene oxide unit associates with two to three water molecules, which results in the molecule behaving as if it were five to ten times as large as a protein of comparable molecular weight[1]. The clearance rate of PEGylated proteins is inversely proportional to molecular weight[1]. Below a molecular weight of about 20 000, the molecule is cleared in the urine. Higher-molecular-weight PEGs are cleared more slowly in the urine and the feces[2].

The type of PEG reagent is critical to the properties of the linked protein[1]. "First-generation" PEG chemistries were generally restricted to low-molecular-weight methoxy-PEGs because of diol contamination and resulting difunctional linkers[1]. Weak linkages and side reactions were additional problems[1]. "Second-generation" PEGylation reagents avoid weak linkages, side reactions, and diol contaminants, and, as a result, high-molecular-weight PEGs could be used[1].

1.2 PEG Proteins As Human Therapeutics

The FDA has approved the PEGylated forms of the protein therapeutics adenosine deaminase, asparaginase, α-interferon (IFN) and a growth hormone antagonist[3]. Linear PEGs with molecular weights of 12 000, including succinimidyl succinate (SS-PEG) and succinimidyl carbonate (SC-PEG) have been used on the first approved PEG-protein products. They possess the disadvantages of weak linkages between PEG and protein, side reactions, low-molecular-weight and diol contamination (HO-PEG-OH)[1]. The SS-PEG linkage used for asparaginase is susceptible to hydrolysis after the polymer has been attached to the protein[1]. An advantage of SC-PEG relative to SS–PEG is that SC–PEG does not contain a degradable ester linkage that can lead to hydrolytic removal of the PEG from the PEG-protein conjugate[1]. The linkage formed between SC–PEG and a protein lysine is a urethane linkage, stable to hydrolysis. However, SC–PEG couples at low pH to histidine moieties in a hydrolytically unstable linkage[4]. SC chemistry is restricted to low-M_w PEGs because of diol contamination[1]. High-molecular-weight, second-generation PEG reagents were used to generate PEG-α-IFN for treatment of hepatitis C.[1] Patients with refractory or recurrent acute lymphoblastic leukemia (ALL) are treated with a combination of PEG-asparaginase and methotrexate, vincristine, and prednisone[13]. A genetic defect of the enzyme adenosine deaminase (ADA) deficiency inhibits the development of the immune system, making patients vulnerable to almost any type of infection. PEG-ADA treatments strengthen the immune system considerably[14].

2. PEG-METHIONINASE

Elevated minimum methionine dependence of most and possibly all types of tumor cells relative to normal cells has been demonstrated[16-27]. The L-methionine α-deamino-γ-mercaptomethane lyase (methioninase, METase) gene from *Pseudomonas putida* has been previously cloned in *Escherichia coli*[27-29]. Recombinant METase (rMETase) is a homotetrameric pyridoxal 5'-phosphate enzyme of 172 kDa molecular mass.

The biochemical reaction catalyzed by L-methioninase is shown below:

$$
\begin{array}{ccccccccc}
 & COO^- & & & & COO^- & & & \\
 & | & & & & | & & & \\
H_3N^+ - & CH & & & & C{=}O & & & \\
 & | & & & & | & & & \\
 & CH_2 & & & & CH_2 & & & \\
 & | & + & H_2O & = & | & + & SH & + \quad NH_4^+ \\
 & CH_2 & & & & CH_3 & & | & \\
 & | & & & & & & CH_3 & \\
 & S & & & & & & & \\
 & | & & & & & & & \\
 & CH_3 & & & & & & & \\
\end{array}
$$

L-methionine α-ketobutyrate methanethiol ammonia

A scale-up rMETase production protocol has been established with high yield (60%), high purity (98%), high stability, and low endotoxin for preclinical and clinical studies targeting the methionine dependence of human cancer[27].

Studies of the antitumor efficacy of rMETase *in vitro* and *in vivo* on human tumors xenografted in nude mice demonstrated that all types of human tumors tested were sensitive to rMETase[27]. No toxicity was detected *in vivo* at the effective doses[27].

However, as with many other bacterial polypeptides and proteins, rMETase may be immunogenic in higher animals, which may limit the utility of rMETase especially with regard to multiple dosing. Anti-METase antibodies may accelerate methioninase clearance and consequently reduce its therapeutic effectiveness and may also reduce the enzyme potency by binding at the active site.

In order to prevent immunological reactions which might be produced by multiple dosing of rMETase and to prolong the serum half-life of rMETase, the N-hydroxysuccinimidyl ester of methoxypolyethylene glycol propionic acid (M-SPA-PEG 5000) has been coupled to rMETase. Molar ratios of M-SPA-PEG-5000 (PEG) to rMETase from 10 to 40 were used for PEGylation of rMETase. PEGylation reactions were run at 20°C for 30 to 60 min in reaction buffer (20 mM sodium phosphate buffer, pH 8.3). The PEGylated molecules (PEG-rMETase) were purified from unreacted PEG with Amicon

30 K Centriprep concentrators or by Sephacryl S-300 HR gel-filtration chromatography. Unreacted rMETase was removed by DEAE Sepharose FF anion-exchange chromatography. The resulting PEG-rMETase subunit, from a PEG/rMETase ratio of 30/1 in the synthetic reaction, had a molecular mass of approximately 53 kDa determined by matrix-assisted laser desorption/ionization (MALDI) mass spectrometry, indicating the conjugation of two PEG molecules per subunit of rMETase and eight per tetramer. PEG-rMETase molecules obtained from reacting ratios of PEG /rMETase of 30/1 had enzyme activities of 70% of unmodified rMETase. PEGylation of rMETase increased the serum half-life of the enzyme in rats to approximately 160 min compared to 80 min for unmodified rMETase. PEG-rMETase could deplete serum methionine levels to less than 0.1 μM for approximately 8 h compared to 2 h for rMETase in rats. PEG-rMETase injected intravenously in mice demonstrated a tumor/blood retention ratio of approximately 1/6 compared to 1/10 of unmodified enzyme, indicating that PEG-rMETase distributes to the tumor at least as effectively as rMETase[30].

2.1 Methods for PEGylation of rMETase with M-SPA-PEG-500030

2.1.1 PEGylation reaction

PEG reagents were dissolved in 20 mM sodium phosphate buffer (pH 8.3) at concentrations between 2 mM and 20 mM. The molar ratios of PEG to rMETase were varied from 10:1 to 60:1. For each condition, 0.3-0.5g rMETase (15 mg/ml) was used. PEGylation reactions were carried out in reaction buffer (20 mM sodium phosphate buffer, pH 8.3), at 20°C for 30 to 60 minutes. The reactions were stopped with one-tenth volume of stop buffer (1 M sodium phosphate buffer, pH 6.5) at 0°C[31]. PEG-rMETase was then concentrated by a Centriprep-30 (Amicon Inc. Beverly, MA).

2.1.2 Purification of PEG-rMETases

2.1.2.1 Sephacryl S-300. Unreacted PEG was removed with a size-exclusion chromatography Sephacryl S-300 HR column (HiPrep 26/60, Pharmacia), with a diameter of 26 nm and length of 60 cm[32]. 10 ml of PEGylation products (15 mg/ml) were loaded on the column which was equilibrated and eluted with 0.15 M sodium chloride in 10 mM sodium phosphate (pH 7.4) at a flow rate of 1 ml/min. The fractions containing PEG-rMETase and rMETase were eluted at approximately 150~250 ml and identified by activity assay.

2.1.2.2 DEAE Sepharose FF. PEGylated rMETase was separated from un-PEGylated rMETase by anion-exchange chromatography using a DEAE Sepharose FF column (XK 16 / 15, Pharmacia) with a diameter of 16 mm and length of 15 cm[27,33]. The column was equilibrated with equilibration buffer [50 mM NaCl in 10 mM Na phosphate (pH 7.4)] and eluted with a 0-60% linear gradient of 300 mM NaCl in 10 mM Na phosphate (pH 7.4) at a 3 ml/min flow rate. The fractions containing PEG-rMETase were eluted with approximately 50~80 ml equilibration buffer and were identified by activity assay and electrophoresis on SDS-PAGE[30].

2.1.2.3 Sterilization and stability of PEG-rMETase. The PEG-rMETases were sterilized by filtration with a 0.2 micron membrane filter. PEG-rMETase was stored at -80°C for 6 months without loss of activity[30].

2.1.3 Properties of M-SPA-PEG-5000-rMETase

The PEG-rMETase had a much larger molecular mass than rMETase which is 172 KdA on native-PAGE. The sub-units of PEG-rMETase were also larger than the sub-units of rMETase which have a molecular mass of 43 kDa on SDS-PAGE[30]. The migration rates of PEG-rMETase molecules were much slower than rMETase due to the conjugation of PEG molecules and subsequent hydration. SDS-PAGE demonstrated that the sub-units of rMETase were all linked with PEG at polymer/METase (P/M) ratios greater than 30. There were a slight band at 43 kDa on SDS-PAGE of PEG-rMETase synthesized at P/M ratios of 10-30, which might be due to PEG molecules released from some subunits during denaturation with SDS and heating to 94°C [30].

The enzyme activity of PEG-rMETase depended on the P/M ratio. The PEG-rMETase synthesized at P/M ratios of 20 to 30 had activities of approximately 60-70 % of that of rMETase. At higher P/M ratios of 60 to 120, the resulting PEG-rMETase had activities of approximately 20-40% of rMETase[30].

MALDI mass spectrometry results confirmed that rMETase is composed of four identical subunits of MW 43 kDa. MALDI results for PEG-rMETase indicated that PEG-rMETase contained mainly four broad peaks, corresponding to molecular weights 52,661±5,000 and 106,631±8,000 for the monomer and dimer, respectively. These molecular weights of are consistent with each subunit linked to two M-SPA-PEG 5,000 molecules[30].

The t½ in serum of PEG-rMETase after iv injection in rats was approximately 160 minutes compared to approximately 80 minutes of rMETase. The results demonstrated that the serum half-life of PEG-rMETase increased to approximately twice that of rMETase when given by iv injection[30].

The depletion of methionine in rat serum by iv injection of 180 units PEG-rMETase reached maximum depletion from 50 μM to 0.1 μM within 5 min after the start of the injection. Methionine depletion to approximately 0.1 μM was maintained for at least 8 hours after a single iv injection of PEG rMETase which was much more effective than rMETase, which could deplete methionine after one injection but could only maintain depletion at 0.1 μM for two hours[30].

After iv administration to nude mice, the tissue distribution of PEG-rMETase was found to be in the following decreasing order: blood, kidney, liver, spleen, heart, lung, tumor, intestine and muscle. Significant PEG-rMETase levels accumulated in the tumor. One hour after iv injection of 60 units of PEG-rMETase, levels were approximately 0.026 units/mg protein in human colon tumor HCT 15 growing subcutaneously in nude mice compared to 0.017 units/mg protein for rMETase. These results demonstrated that PEG-rMETase could accumulate in the tumor at least as well as rMETase[30].

2.2 New PEG-rMETases

rMETase was recently coupled to activated polyethylene methoxypolyethylene glycol succinimidyl glutarate-5000 (MEGC-PEG-5000). MEGC-PEG/rMETase, synthesized at a ratio of PEG/rMETase of 30/1, maintained activity at 40%. Plasma half-life in mice increased 20-fold and methionine depletion time increased 5-fold. To deplete plasma methionine for 24 hours, the effective protein dose of MEGC-PEG-rMETase was reduced to approximately 10% that of naked rMETase. The antigenicity in mice of MEGC-PEG-rMETase and rMETase was measured by ELISA. After administration of MEGC-PEG-rMETase, Ig M specific for rMETase was reduced by 90%, and total Ig E was reduced 50% compared to mice injected with rMETase[34].

Two comb-shaped co-polymers of PEG and maleic anhydride, having molecular weights of 15 kDa (AKM1510) and 100 kDa (APM2090), and two four-branched pentaerythritol monosuccinimidyl glutarate PEGs, having molecular weights of 10 kDa (PTE-10TGSQ) and 20 kDa (PTE-20TGSQ), were also conjugated to rMETase. The plasma half-life of rMETase modified with AKM1510, APM2090, PTE-10TGSQ, and PTE-20TGSQ was prolonged from 2h to 28h, 40h, 56h, and 56h, respectively. Following 100 U intravenous injection of the four types of PEGylated rMETase, plasma methionine concentration dropped from a baseline of 20-50 μM to undetectable levels for 20 h and remained at less than 5 μM up to 48h, which is 5-and 8-fold longer than native rMETase, respectively. Furthermore, the four types of PEGylated rMETase exhibited reduced reactivity toward polyclonal antibody raised against native rMETase. Enzyme activity of rMETase modified with AKM1510, APM2090, PTE-10TGSQ, and PTE-20TGSQ was maintained at 48%, 50%, 30%, and 31% of native rMETase, respectively. These results indicate that comb-shaped and branched activated PEGs greatly improve the pharmacokinetic and immunological properties of rMETase. The comb-shaped AKM1510 and APM2090 maintained rMETase enzyme activity most effectively[35]. Comb-shaped and linear PEGylated rMETase are now being compared for anti-tumor efficacy. A summary of the properties of new PEG-rMETases is listed in Table 1.

Table 1. Summary of PEGylation of recombinant methioninase with various PEG derivatives

PEG-rMETase conjugates	Serum half-life (hrs)	Serum methionine depletion time (hrs)*	Activity percent of naked rMETase (%)
MEGC-50HS-rMETase	38	72	68
AKM-1510-rMETase	28	48	48
APM-2090-rMETase	40	48	50
PTE-10TGSQ-rMETase	56	72	29
PTE-20TGSQ-rMETase	56	72	31
MENP-50H-rMETase	48	48	16
MENP-20T-rMETase	48	48	25
SPA-rMETase	35	72	70
SSA-rMETase	40	72	63

PEG derivatives:

1. MEGC-50HS: PEG succinimidyl glutarate, MW 5 kd
2. AKM-1510: Comb-shaped copolymer of polyethylene glycol derivative and maleic auhydride, MW 15 kd.
3. APM-2090: Comb-shaped copolymer of polyethylene glycol derivative and maleic anhydride, MW 100 kd.
4. PTE-10TGSQ: Four-branched pentaerythritol polyethylene glycol ether monosuccinimidyl glutarate, MW 10 kd.
5. PTE-20TGSQ: Four-branched pentaerythritol polyethylene glycol ether monosuccinimidyl glutarate, MW 20 kd.
6. MENP-50H: PEG p-nitrophenyl carbonate, MW 5kd.
7. MENP-20T: PEG p-nitrophenyl carbonate, MW 20 kd
8. SPA: PEG succinimidyl propionate, MW 5 KD.
9. SSA: PEG succinimidyl succinamide, MW 5 kd.

3. PERSPECTIVES OF rMETase

A novel approach to the treatment of brain tumors with the combination of rMETase chemotherapeutic regimens that are currently used against such tumors has recently been carried out. The growth of Daoy, SWB77, and D-

54 xenografts implanted subcutaneously in athymic mice was arrested after the depletion of mouse plasma methionine (MET) with a combination of MET- and choline-free diet and rMETase. The treated tumor-bearing mice were rescued from the toxic effects of MET withdrawal with daily i.p. homocystine (HCYSS). This regimen suppressed plasma MET to levels below 5 μM for several days, with no treatment-related deaths. MET depletion for 10-12 days induced mitotic and cell cycle arrest, apoptotic death, and wide-spread necrosis in tumors but did not prevent tumor regrowth after cessation of the regimen. However, when a single dose of 35 mg/m^2 of *N,N'*-bis(2-chloroethyl)-*N*-nitrosourea (BCNU), which was otherwise ineffective as a single therapy in any of the tumors tested, was given at the end of the MET depletion regimen, a more than 80-day growth delay was observed for Daoy and D-54, whereas the growth of SWB77 was delayed by 20 days. MET-depleting regimens also trebled the efficacy of temozolomide (TMZ) against SWB77 when TMZ was given to animals as a single dose of 180 mg/m^2 at the end of a 10-day period of MET depletion[36].

MET depletion was shown to inhibit the growth in brain tumors implanted orthotopically in nude mice. MET depletion was induced by treatment with rMETase and dietary withdrawal of MET, homocysteine (HCYS) and choline. HCYSS was administered intraperitonealy daily to prevent toxicity. SWB77 and D-54 glioblastomas, implanted orthotopically in nude mice, showed marked regression, widespread necrosis, complete loss of mitotic activity and failure to infiltrate the brain parenchyma under MET depletion. MET depletion thus is effective against high-grade, more aggressive gliomas, growing orthotopically[37]. The PEG-rMETases described above will be evaluated on these orthotopic tumors which can be evaluated by whole-body imaging when transduced by green or red fluorescent proteins[38-40].

ACKNOWLEDGEMENT

This study was funded in part by the National Cancer Institute grant No. 1 R43 CA86166-01

REFERENCES

1. Kozlowski, A., Harris, J.M., 2001, Improvements in protein PEGylation: pegylated interferons for treatment of hepatitis C. *J. Control Release* 72:217-224.
2. Yamaoka, T., Tabata, Y., Ikada, Y., 1994, Distribution and tissue uptake of poly(ethyleneglycol) with different molecular weights after intravenous administration to mice. *J. Pharm. Sci.* 83:601-606.

3. Olson, K., Gehant, R., Mukku, V., et al., 1997, Preparation and characterization of poly(ethyleneglycol)ylated human growth hormone antagonist. In: *Poly(ethyleneglycol): Chemistry and Biological Applications* (J.M. Harris, S. Zalipsky, eds.), ACS Books, Washington, DC, pp. 170-181.
4. Park, C.W.G., Chuo, M. Interferon polymer conjugates. US Pat. 5,951,974, September 14, 1999.
5. Algranati, N.E., Sy, S., Modi, M., 1999, A branched methoxy 40 kDa polyethyeneglycol (PEG) moiety optimizes the pharmacokinetics (PK) of PEG-interferon α2a (PEG-IFN) and may explain its enhanced efficacy in chronic hepatitis C (CHC). *Hepatology* 40 (Suppl.): 190A.
6. Heathcote, E.J., Shiffman, M.L., Cooksley, W.G., Dusheiko, G.M., Lee, S.S., Balart, L., Reindollar, R., Reddy, R.K., Wright, T.L., Lin, A., Hoffman, J., De Pamphilis, J., 2000, Peginterferon alfa-2a in patients with chronic hepatitis C and cirrhosis. *N. Engl. J. Med.* 343:1673-1680.
7. Zeuzem, S., Feinman, S. V., Rasenack, J., Heathcote, E. J., Lai, M. Y., Gane, E., O'Grade, J., Reichen, J., Diago, M., Lin, A., Brunda, M. J., 2000, Peginterferon alfa-2a in patients with chronic hepatitis C. *N. Engl. J. Med.* 343:1666-1672.
8. Wang, Y.S., Youngster, S., Bausch, J., Zhang, R., McNemar, C., Wyss, D.F., 2000, Identification of the major positional isomer of pegylated interferon alpha-2b. *Biochemistry* 39:10634-10640.
9. Grace, M., Youngster, S., Gitlin, G., Sydor, W., Xie, L., Westreich, L., Jacobs, S., Brassard, D., Bausch, J., Bordens, R., 2001, Structural and biologic characterization of pegylated recombinant IFN-alpha2b. *J. Interferon Cytokine Res.* 21:1103-1015.
10. MacEwen EG, Rosenthal R, Matus R, Viau AT, Abuchowski A., 1987, A preliminary study on the evaluation of asparaginase. Polyethylene glycol conjugate against canine malignant lymphoma. *Cancer* 59:2011-2015.
11. Park YK, Abuchowski A, Davis S, Davis F., 1981, Pharmacology of Escherichia coli-L-asparaginase polyethylene glycol adduct. *Anticancer Res.* 1:373-376.
12. Ettinger LJ, Kurtzberg J, Voute PA, Jurgens H, Halpern SL., 1995, An open-label, multicenter study of polyethylene glycol-L-asparaginase for the treatment of acute lymphoblastic leukemia. *Cancer* 75:1176-1181.
13. Aguayo A, Cortes J, Thomas D, Pierce S, Keating M, Kantarjian H., 1999, Combination therapy with methotrexate, vincristine, polyethylene-glycol conjugated-asparaginase, and prednisone in the treatment of patients with refractory or recurrent acute lymphoblastic leukemia. *Cancer* 86:1203-1209.
14. Pool R., 1990, "Hairy enzymes" stay in the blood. *Science* 248:305.
15. Hershfield MS., 1995, PEG-ADA replacement therapy for adenosine deaminase deficiency: an update after 8.5 years. *Clin Immunol Immunopathol.* 76:S228-S232.
16. Hoffman, R.M. and Erbe, R.W., 1976, High *in vivo* rates of methionine biosynthesis in transformed human and malignant rat cells auxotrophic for methionine. *Proc. Natl. Acad. Sci., USA* 73:1523-1527.
17. Hoffman, R.M., 1984, Altered methionine metabolism, DNA methylation and oncogene expression in carcinogenesis: a review and synthesis. *Biochem. Biophys. Acta, Reviews on Cancer* 738:49-87.
18. Mecham, J.O., Rowitch, D., Wallace, C.D., Stern, P.H. and Hoffman, R.M., 1983, The metabolic defect of methionine dependence occurs frequently in human tumor cell lines. *Biochem. Biophys. Res. Commun.* 117:429-434.
19. Guo, H.Y., Herrera, H., Groce, A., and Hoffman, R.M., 1993, Expression of the biochemical defect of methionine dependence in fresh patient tumors in primary histoculture. *Cancer Res.* 53:2479-2483.
20. Kreis, W., and Goodenow, M., 1978, Methionine requirement and replacement by homocysteine in tissue cultures of selected rodent and human malignant and normal cells. *Cancer Res.* 38:2259-2262.

21. Guo, H., Lishko, V., Herrera, H., Groce, A., Kubota, T., and Hoffman, R.M., 1993, Therapeutic tumor-specific cell-cycle block induced by methionine starvation *in vivo*. *Cancer Res.* 53:5676-5679.
22. Goseki, N., Yamazaki, S., Shimojyu, K., Kando, F., Maruyama, M., Endo, M., Koike, M., and Takahashi, H., 1995, Synergistic effect of methionine-depleting total parenteral nutrition with 5-fluorouracil on human gastric cancer: A randomized, prospective clinical trial. *Jpn. J. Cancer Res.* 86:484-489.
23. Goseki, N., Yamazaki, S., Endo, M., Onodera, T., Kosaki, G., Hibino, Y., and Kuwahata, T., 1992, Antitumor effect of methionine-depleting total parenteral nutrition with doxorubicin administration on Yoshida sarcoma-bearing rats. *Cancer* 69:1865-1872.
24. Lishko, V.K., Lishko, O.V., and Hoffman, R.M., 1993, The preparation of endotoxin-free L-methionine-α-deamino-γ-mercaptomethane-lyase (L-methioninase) from *Pseudomonas putida. Protein Expression and Purification* 4:529-533.
25. Tan., Y., Xu, M., Guo, H., Sun, X., Kubota, T., and Hoffman, R.M., 1996, Anticancer efficacy of methioninase *in vivo*. *Anticancer Res* 16:3931-3936.
26. Tan, Y., Zavala Sr., J., Xu, M., Zavala Jr., J., and Hoffman, R.M., 1996, Serum methionine depletion without side effects by methioninase in metastatic breast cancer patients. *Anticancer Res* 16:3937-3942.
27. Tan, Y., Xu, M., Tan, X.Z., Tan, X., Wang., X., Saikawa, S., Nagahama, T., Sun, X., Lenz, M., and Hoffman, R.M., 1997, Overexpression and large-scale production of recombinant L-methionine-α-deamino-γ-mercaptomethane-lyase for novel anticancer therapy. *Protein Expression and Purification* 9:233-245.
28. Inoue, H., Inagaki, K., Sugimoto, M., Esaki, N., Soda, K., and Tanaka, H., 1995, Structural analysis of the L-methionine γ-lyase gene from *Pseudomonas putida. J. Biochem.* 117:1120-1125.
29. Hori, H., Takabayashi, K., Orvis, L., Carson, D.A., and Nobori, T., 1996, Gene cloning and characterization of *Pseudomonas putida* L-methionine-α-deamino-γ-mercaptomethane lyase. *Cancer Res.* 56:2116-2122.
30. Tan, Y., Sun, X., Xu, M., An, Z., Tan, X-Z., Tan, X-Y., Han, Q., Miljkovic, D.A., Yang, M., and Hoffman, R.M., 1998, Polyethylene glycol conjugation of recombinant methioninase for cancer therapy. *Protein Expression and Purification* 12:45-52.
31. Katre, N.V., Knauf, M.J., and Laird, W.J., 1987, Chemical modification of recombinant interleukin 2 by polyethylene glycol increases its potency in the murine Meth A sarcoma model. *Proc. Natl. Acad. Sci. USA* 84:1487-1491.
32. Bovara, R., Carrea, G., Gioacchini, A.M., Riva, S., and Secundo, F., 1997, Activity, stability and conformation of methoxypoly(ethylene glycol)-subtilisin at different concentrations of water in dioxane. *Biotechnol. Bioeng.* 54:50-57.
33. Brumeanu, T-D., Zaghouani, H., and Bona, C., 1995, Purification of antigenized immunoglobulins derivatized with monomethoxypolyethylene glycol. *J. Chromatogr. A*, 696:219-225.
34. Sun, X., Yang, Z., Li, S., Tan, Y., Zhang, N., An, Z., Yagi, S, Yoshioka, T., Suginaka, A., and Hoffman, R.M., 2002, Advantages of MEGC-PEG-5000 coupled recombinant methioninase for methionine depletion cancer therapy. *Proceedings of AACR 93rd Annual Meeting*, 43:1091.
35. Yang, Z., Li, S., Sun, X., Tan, Y., An, Z, Zhang, N., Yagi, S., Yoshioka, T., Suginaka, A., and Hoffman, R.M., 2002, Novel comb-shaped and branched conjugated polyethylene glycols improve pharmacokinetics, enzyme activity maintenance, and reduce immunoreactivity of coupled recombinant methioninase. *Proceedings of AACR 93rd Annual Meeting*, 43:273.
36. Kokkinakis, D.M., Hoffman, R.M., Frenkel, E.P., Wick, J.B., Han, Q., Xu, M., Tan, Y., Schold, S.C., 2001, Synergy between methionine stress and chemotherapy in the treatment of brain tumor xenografts in athymic mice. *Cancer Res* 61:4017-4023.

37. Kokkinakis, D.M., Wick, J.W., Zhou, Q.X., Tan, Y., Hoffman, R.M., and Frenkel, E., 2002, Response to methionine stress of orthotopic human brain tumors in nude mice. *Proceedings of AACR 93rd Annual Meeting,* 43:746.
38. Yang, M., Baranov, E., Jiang, P., Sun, F-X., Li, X-M., Li, L., Hasegawa, S., Bouvet, M., Al-Tuwaijri, M., Chishima, T., Shimada, H., Moossa, A.R., Penman, S., Hoffman, R.M., 2000, Whole-body optical imaging of green fluorescent protein-expressing tumors and metastases. *Proc. Natl. Acad. Sci. USA* 97:1206-1211.
39. Hoffman, R.M. , 2002, Green fluorescent protein imaging of tumor cells in mice. *Lab Animal* 31:34-41.
40. Yang, M., Baranov, E., Wang, J-W., Jiang, P., Wang, X., Sun, F-X., Bouvet, M., Moossa, A.R., Penman, S., and Hoffman, R.M., 2002, Direct external imaging of nascent cancer, tumor progression, angiogenesis, and metastasis on internal organs in the fluorescent orthotopic model. *Proc. Natl. Acad. Sci. USA* 99:3824-3829.

Poly-(L)-Glutamic Acid-Paclitaxel (CT-2103) [XYOTAX™], a Biodegradable Polymeric Drug Conjugate

Characterization, Preclinical Pharmacology, and Preliminary Clinical Data

JACK W. SINGER*, BRIAN BAKER, PETER DE VRIES, ANIL KUMAR, SCOTT SHAFFER, ED VAWTER, MARY BOLTON, AND PAMELA GARZONE
Cell Therapeutics, Inc., 201 Elliott Avenue West, Suite 400, Seattle, Washington, 98119, USA
**Corresponding author: e mail jsinger@ctiseattle.com*

1. INTRODUCTION

Cytotoxic therapies for cancer have relatively low therapeutic ratios and limited efficacy due to the non-selective nature of their molecular targets and the inability to selectively deliver anti-cancer agents to tumour tissue. To increase the selectivity of delivery of therapeutics to tumour tissues, both highly selective and non-selective methods of targeting tumour tissue have been explored. An example of successful delivery of a cytotoxic agent to tumours tissue through active targeting is the use of monoclonal antibodies to antigens with relatively restricted expression as stand-alone therapeutics or as carriers for pharmaceuticals to treat haematologic neoplasia. Unfortunately, this approach has proven less viable for the treatment of solid tumours due to limitations in specificity of targeting epitopes and the inability to deliver targeted therapeutics to tumour tissue distant from microvasculature.

An alternative strategy to enhance the therapeutic ratio of cancer therapeutics is to passively increase the distribution of drugs to tumour tissue

Polymer Drugs in the Clinical Stage, Edited by Maeda et al.
Kluwer Academic/Plenum Publishers, New York, 2003

by exploiting the increased permeability of tumour vasculature to macromolecules and the inability of the trapped molecules to return to the systemic circulation due to the lack of lymphatic vessels in tumour tissues[1-3]. These phenomena have been called the "enhanced permeability and retention" or the EPR effect[1,2]. As demonstrated in preclinical models and in a recent clinical study, conjugation of cytotoxic drugs such as doxorubicin to a macromolecular polymer through an enzymatically degradable linker resulted in a substantial enhancement of the percentage of a dose of the cytotoxic agent reaching tumour tissue[4,5]. The inactive drug conjugate then can enter tumour cells by pinocytosis and free drug is released by lysozomal enzymatic action[6]. These therapeutics promise improved efficacy without a concomitant increase in toxicity because exposure to the active compound is maximised in the tumour tissue but is systemically limited[7,8].

For a polymeric conjugate to have enhanced efficacy, several characteristics are critical:

1. The polymeric conjugate should be inactive.
2. The polymer should be biodegradable in order to be able to optimise its molecular weight. Molecular weights of 50 to 80kD are optimal for the EPR effect [1,7].
3. The conjugate should be stable in circulation and thus keep distribution of the active (free) cytotoxic drug and related toxic effects to normal tissues at a minimum[8].
4. The conjugate should be non-immunogenic[1].
5. The conjugate should release the active agent in tumour tissue in a predictable fashion[8].
6. The conjugate should be soluble in aqueous solutions and thus easy to deliver.

The present report describes the covalent conjugation of paclitaxel to γ-carboxylic acids of poly-L-glutamic (PG) acid (CT-2103). Paclitaxel is a particularly appropriate molecule for conjugation to a polymer carrier because it is broadly active as an anti-tumour agent, yet it is difficult to deliver because it is highly hydrophobic. The commercial preparations of paclitaxel use Cremophor and ethanol as solubilising agents. These have inherent toxicities and require slow infusions and premedications with corticosteroids and histamine receptor blockers.

PG has several unique properties when compared with other polymers in development.

1. PG is a protein and therefore subject to cleavage by proteolytic enzymes. The enzymatic degradation of CT-2103 has been demonstrated in cell free systems and in tumour tissues both *in vitro* and *in vivo*. The biodegradable nature of PG has allowed molecular weight optimisation to

levels above the renal clearance threshold. Non-biodegradable polymers accumulate in phagocytic cells if they are not renally excreted.

2. Unlike most other polymeric drug carriers in development, PG is a polyanion at physiological pH. This greatly enhances its ability to render hydrophobic molecules water-soluble and allows relatively high molar ratios of active drug to glutamate residues (approximately 1 in 11 for paclitaxel). The negative charge also may have important effects on biodistribution and the rate of cellular uptake.
3. PG is non-immunogenic, even when conjugated to paclitaxel, possibly because paclitaxel is directly linked to a polyanionic homopolymer, thus providing minimal antigenic epitopes other than those on native paclitaxel.
4. When coupled to paclitaxel by an ester-linkage formed between the 2' hydroxyl and a γ-carboxylate of glutamate, a stable conjugate is formed which is not subject to cleavage by plasma esterases, possibly due to steric hindrance[9]. Because the 2' hydroxyl is in the tubulin binding domain, until paclitaxel is released from polyglutamate, it is inactive. Therefore, systemic exposure to active paclitaxel only occurs following the release of free paclitaxel from the polymer in tissues and redistribution. Following administration of CT-2103, it accumulates and is broken down in tumour tissues and in reticuloendothelial organs such as the liver, spleen and to a lesser extent, in the lung. Presumably, the cells involved in degradation of the polymer in each of these tissues are the fixed macrophages.

Several publications have described the striking efficacy of PG-paclitaxel prepared at the MD Anderson Cancer Research Center. This material contained approximately 20% paclitaxel by weight and used PG of 20-35 kD by viscosity. Single doses of this preparation were curative in established Fisher rat mammary cancers[10] and murine Oca-1 ovarian cancers[10]. Enhanced efficacy over free paclitaxel at its maximally tolerated dose was repeatedly demonstrated in both syngeneic tumours and in human tumour xenografts[11]. The increase in therapeutic ratio was thought to result from enhanced biodistribution to tumour tissue through a presumed EPR mechanism[12]. Administration of the same dose of ^{3}H paclitaxel (20 mg/kg) to mice either in Cremaphor ethanol or linked to PG demonstrated at least a 7 fold enhancement in paclitaxel distribution of subcutaneous OCa-1 tumours with slow release of free paclitaxel over 7 days compared with rapid disappearance of paclitaxel given by the standard method from tumour tissues. Similar results were observed in experiments using CT-2103 (see below).

A series of optimisation studies were undertaken prior to clinical development of CT-2103. In these studies, the molar ratio of paclitaxel to glutamate and the MW of PG were varied. To assess the efficacy of these preparations, a rapid syngeneic screening model using Lewis lung cancer in immunocompetent C57BL/6 mice was utilized[13,14]. This is a relatively paclitaxel-insensitive model that has a modest but significant and reproducible tumour growth delay in response to CT-2103 but not to free paclitaxel. In a series of experiments it was determined that efficacy increased as the molar ratio of paclitaxel increased until solubility began to decrease when paclitaxel loading increased to over 40 percent by weight. The drug candidate that resulted from these studies is designated CT-2103. Its chemistry, preclinical pharmacology and results of a Phase I clinical study are described in subsequent sections.

2. CHARACTERIZATION AND SYNTHESIS OF CT-2103

2.1 Synthetic Route

CT-2103 is synthesized by converting Na-PG from its salt form to its protonated form followed by formation of an ester between the gamma carboxylate of the polymer and the 2' alcohol of paclitaxel. A minor modification of combining the 2 steps via in situ formation of the PG acid has been investigated with success. Carbodiimide coupling catalysed by DMAP was chosen as the appropriate reagent. Based on solubility, DMF was chosen as the reaction solvent.

2.2 Physical Properties and Characterization

2.2.1 Structural formula

A representative structure for CT-2103 is shown in Figure 1. CT-2103 is a random condensation product of α-poly-(L)-glutamic acid and paclitaxel. The structure shown is illustrative of a fragment of the molecule, but specific conjugation sites are not implied. On average, there are approximately 10.4 non-conjugated monomer (m) glutamic acid units per paclitaxel conjugate glutamic acid units (n).

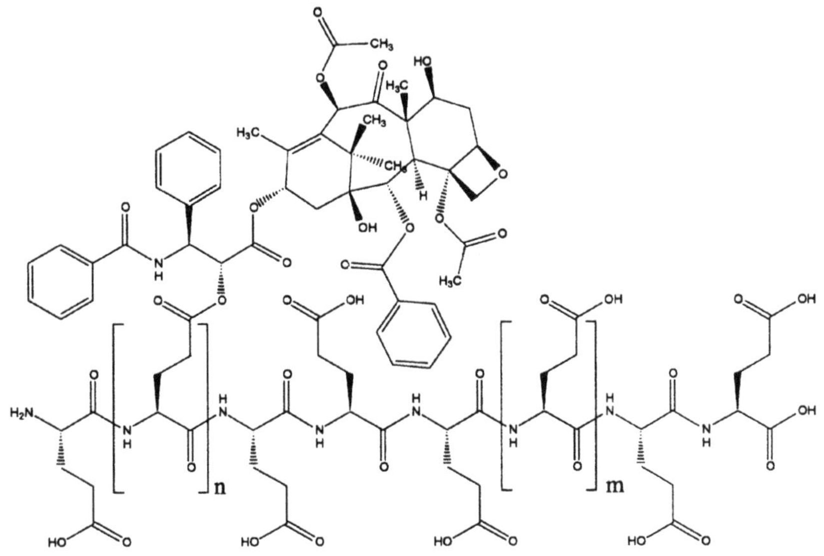

Figure 1. Representative CT-2103 Structure

2.2.2 Molecular formula

The molecular formula of CT-2103 is a distribution since the α-poly-(L)-glutamic acid degree of polymerization and the number of conjugation sites with paclitaxel are variable. A generalized molecular formula is shown.

N-Terminus	C-Terminus	Unconjugated Monomer Unit	Conjugated Monomer Unit	Conjugated Paclitaxel
$(C_5H_8NO_3)$ -	$(C_5H_8NO_4)$-	$(C_5H_7NO_3)_m$-	$(C_5H_6NO_2)_n$-	$(C_{47}H_{50}O_{14}N)_n$

N is the number of paclitaxel groups conjugated to the α-poly-(L)-glutamic acid backbone, and m + n is the number of glutamic acid monomer units other than the N-terminus and the C-terminus. The ratio of m to n varies from 8.3 to 13.2. Because paclitaxel is the active molecule in CT-2103, it avoids confusion to consider the conjugate in terms of conjugated paclitaxel, i.e. the actual amount of paclitaxel contained within a dose of CT-2103.

2.2.3 Physical form

White to off-white powder

2.2.4 Solubility

0.1M HCl	Practically Insoluble
0.1M NaOH	Soluble
0.1N Na_2HPO_4 (pH=6.5)	Soluble
Methanol	Slightly Soluble
Dimethylsulfoxide	Slightly Soluble
Dimethylformamide	Slightly Soluble
Acetonitrile	Practically Insoluble
Ether	Insoluble

2.2.5 Ionisation constant

pK_a of the gamma carboxylate of monoglutamate is approximately 4.5.

2.2.6 Molecular form and weight

Poly-L-glutamate is known to exist in random coil configuration in water at neutral pH. In acidic solutions where the carboxyl groups are not ionized, PG adopts an α-helical conformation. Paclitaxel conjugation also results in a right-hand α-helical conformation as measured in DMSO. The molecular weight of CT-2103 is approximately 80 kD as determined by gel permeation chromatography with multi-angle light scatter detection.

3. PRECLINICAL PHARMACOLOGY

3.1 Biodistribution of CT-2103 in C57BL/6 Mice Bearing Subcutaneous B16 Melanomas

To determine the biodistribution and pharmacokinetics of CT-2103 and to compare them with paclitaxel administered in Cremophor EL/ethanol, female mice (C57BL/6) with approximately 100 mm^3 subcutaneous B16 melanomas were allocated to two groups, 75 animals per group. One group received a PG-[^{3}H]TXL dose equivalent to 40 mg/kg conjugated paclitaxel and the second group received 40 mg/kg [^{3}H]TXL in Cremophor-ethanol. This dose was selected because it was below the MTD and had anti-tumour effects in this model. Five animals per time point per group were sacrificed at 0, 0.5, 1.0, 1.5, 2, 4, 8, 12, 24, 48, 72, 96, 120, or 144 hours post injection. Plasma, tumour, and various organs were harvested from each animal at each time point and analysed individually[15].

The total taxane (TTAX) concentration, a sum of the concentrations for CT-2103, TXL, and TXL-metabolites was determined from scintillation counting of the plasma or tissue sample homogenates. Extractable taxanes, including TXL and organically extractable TXL metabolites, were determined by scintillation counting of ethyl acetate extractions of the plasma, tumour, liver, and spleen samples. Plasma and tissue TXL concentrations were also determined by HPLC/radiometric analysis of the extracts. Metabolites were identified by HPLC followed by mass spectrometry on a Quattro II (Micromass, Manchester, UK) triple quadrupole mass spectrometer fitted with an electrospray orthogonal "Z" spray ion interface operating in the positive ion mode[15].

The total taxane (TTAX) plasma exposure (Cmax and AUC) was markedly higher for animals receiving PG-[^{3}H]TXL as compared to those receiving [^{3}H]TXL (Table 1, Figure 2). In all cases, the Cmax was observed immediately post-injection (time 0). In the PG-[^{3}H]TXL treated animals, the extractable taxanes (ETAX) and TXL levels were < 0.2% of the TTAX amount as measured by Cmax and < 0.5% as indicated by AUC, thus reflecting a negligible amount of TXL release from the polyglutamate backbone in the plasma compartment. As expected, following [^{3}H]TXL treatment, the Cmax and AUC values were similar between the TTAX, ETAX, and TXL determinations. The t1/2 for TTAX was 3-times greater following PG-[^{3}H]TXL treatment (5.0 hr) when compared with [^{3}H]TXL (1.7 hr). The values for TTAX volume of distribution (Vd) were 1.3 ml for PG-[3H]TXL, approximately the blood volume of a mouse, compared with 5.1 ml for [^{3}H]TXL suggesting extensive tissue distribution or protein binding[15].

Table 1. Plasma Pharmacokinetics

	C_{MAX} (μg/mL)	$AUC_{0\text{-}Last}$
CT-2103 (40 mg/kg TXL)		
Total Taxane	1218	4563
Free Taxane	2.3	19.9
Free TXL (HPLC)	2.1	20.1
Paclitaxel (40 mg/kg)		
Total Taxane	564	397
Free Taxane	679	329
Free TXL (HPLC)	579	330

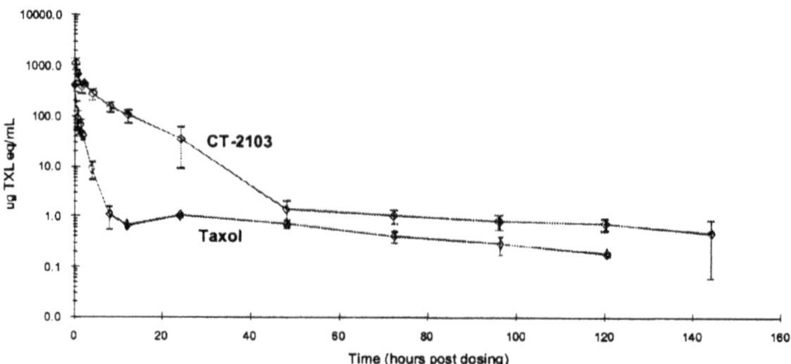

Figure 2. Plasma Concentration of ^{3}H Paclitaxel Following CT-2103 or Taxol

Table 2. Tumour Pharmacokinetics

	T_{MAX} (hour)	C_{MAX} (μg/gm)	$AUC_{0\text{-}Last}$ (μg*hr/gm)
CT-2103 (40 mg/kg TXL)			
Total Taxane	4	72	4545
Free Taxane	72	8.3	611
Free TXL (HPLC)	72	4.3	368
Paclitaxel (40 mg/kg)			
Total Taxane	1.5	27	384
Free Taxane	1.5	25	297
Free TXL (HPLC)	1.5	24	283

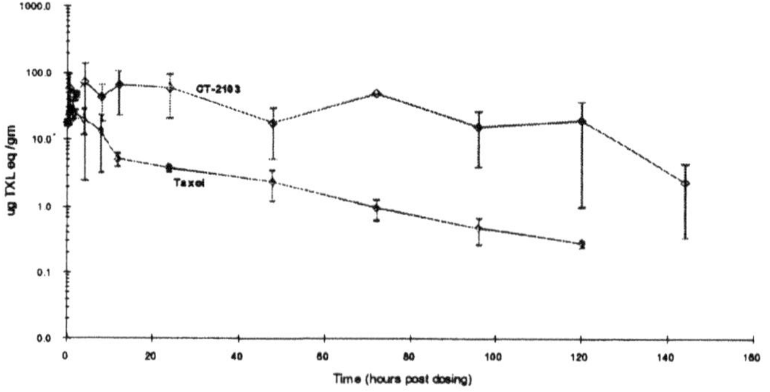

Figure 3. Tumour Concentration of ^{3}H Paclitaxel Following CT-2103 or Taxol

The exposure of B16 melanoma tumours to TTAX was greatly enhanced following PG-[^{3}H]TXL treatment when compared with [^{3}H]TXL, the former yielding 170% higher Cmax and 1,100% higher AUC (Table 2, Figure 3). The overall exposure as indicated by AUC to ETAX and TXL was higher, 97% and 32% respectively, following PG-[^{3}H]TXL administration. Mean residence times were 122%, 232%, and 288% higher, for TTAX, ETAX, and TXL, respectively, for the PG-[^{3}H]TXL group and correlated with the observed increases in AUC15. Although conjugated paclitaxel is inert, it can be assumed that slow breakdown of the remaining conjugate continued after the experiment was terminated at 144 hours. Paclitaxel-2′-γ-glutamic acid ester was identified as a metabolite in tumour, liver and spleen, but not plasma, in the PG-[^{3}H]TXL treated animals. This abundant metabolite is formed during proteolysis of the polyglutamate backbone, the apparent initial step in CT-2103 metabolism by both tumour and reticuloendothelial tissues.

These study results indicate that distribution of CT-2103 to tumour tissue and tumour exposure to TXL were enhanced compared with TXL administered alone, and provide at least a partial explanation for enhanced efficacy of CT-2103 compared to free paclitaxel[15].

3.2 *In Vitro* and *In Vivo* Metabolism of CT-2103

When incubated in the presence of human HT-29 colon cancer cells or murine RAW macrophages, CT-2103 is taken up by the cells and increased levels of free paclitaxel are found in the medium than in control cultures without cells. When the washed cellular fractions were tested for extractable Taxanes, increasing amounts of paclitaxel 2' monoglutamate and free paclitaxel were observed over several days (Figure 4). These observations suggest that the polymeric conjugate is taken up by the cells, and the PG backbone is cleaved by proteolysis and is followed by hydrolysis of the monoglutamate to yield free paclitaxel. To determine which proteolytic enzymes might be involved in this process, CT-2103 was exposed to a variety of proteases under cell free conditions. Of the enzymes tested, only cathepsin B was capable of degrading CT-2103 to paclitaxel-diglutamates[16]. The enzyme responsible for cleavage to the paclitaxel-monoglutamate was not identified. The 2' paclitaxel monoglutamate is unstable and breaks down spontaneously to paclitaxel and glutamic acid.

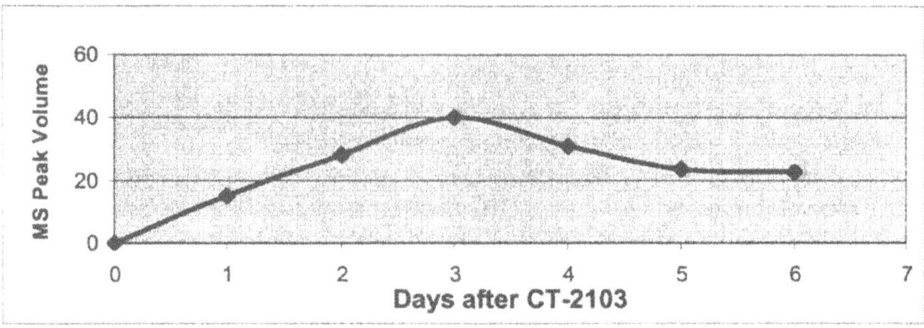

Figure 4. Accumulation of Paclitaxel Monoglutamate in HT-29 Cells *In Vitro*

To determine if paclitaxel monolglutamate was detectable as a metabolite in vivo, a series of tumours explants were extracted and assayed 24 hours after a single intravenous dose of CT-2103 (Figure 5A). As seen in Figure 5B, increasing amounts of the paclitaxel-monoglutamate were detected over several days in HT-29 colon cancers. Similar data were obtained from analysis of liver and spleen, suggesting that reticuloendothelial cells are also able to break down CT-2103 by a similar mechanism[17].

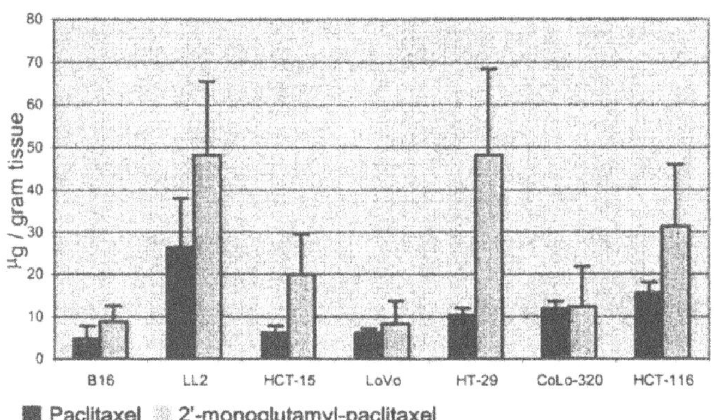

Figure 5A. Extractable Metabolites in Tumour Tissue from Mice with Various Tumours 24 Hours After a Single Dose of CT-2103

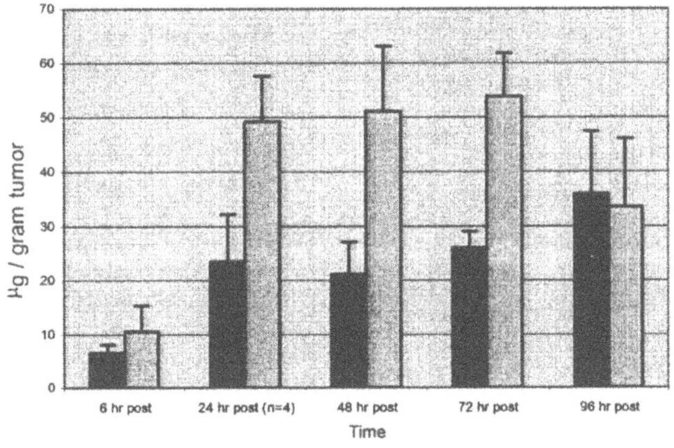

Figure 5B. Changes in CT-2103 Metabolites in HT-29 Tumours with Time After a Single Dose (5 Animals/Group)

Note: The heights of the bars do not represent absolute values since only a paclitaxel standard was used. Later studies with authentic standards determined that the relative values are about 50% of the 2'-monoglutamyl-paclitaxel bar heights.

Taken in sum, these data suggest that the CT-2103 is taken up by tumour tissues and cells within the reticuloendothelial system. Free paclitaxel is slowly released following cleavage of the PG backbone by cathepsin B. In circulation, CT-2103 does not release paclitaxel in appreciable quantities. An important parameter for a successful polymeric conjugate is a slow rate of release only outside of circulation. This spares normal organs high levels of exposure to free paclitaxel[15].

3.3 *In Vivo* Efficacy Evaluations

CT-2103 has been studied in a wide variety of syngeneic and xenogeneic tumour models (Tables 3A and 3B). In all cases it has enhanced efficacy when its maximum tolerated dose (MTD) was compared to that of free paclitaxel administered in Cremophor EL/ethanol. In the mouse strains that were evaluated, the single dose IV or IP MTD for CT-2103 was approximately twice that of paclitaxel administered in Cremophor EL/ethanol [80 mg/kg for paclitaxel in immunocompetent mice (syngeneic models) and 60-70 mg/kg in nu/nu mice respectively compared with 160-200 mg/kg in syngeneic mice and 120-150 mg/kg in nu/nu mice for CT-2103[11,18]. An example of the enhanced efficacy of CT-2103 in nude mice bearing the HT-29 human colon cancer is shown in Figure 6.

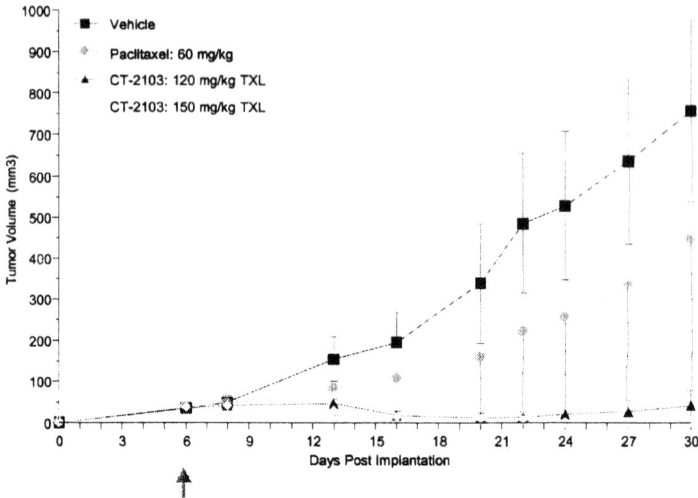

Figure 6. Effect of CT-2103 vs. Paclitaxel on the Growth of Human HT-29 Colon Carcinomas in *Nude* Mice

The MTD and tumour growth delay (TGD) in Lewis lung cancer (LL/2) [13] and B16 melanoma syngeneic tumours in female C57BL/6 mice[19] after a single IP injection were used to evaluate the biological consistency of CT-2103. In these studies the paclitaxel-equivalent MTD varied between 160 and 240 mg/kg, and the mean ± SD [range] for TGD to 500 mm^3 was 3.8 ± 1.8 [range 0.4 - 9.8] days for Lewis lung tumours and 6.2 ± 3.2 [range1.3 - 13.2] for B16 tumors[13,19]. The TGD to 500 mm^3 for paclitaxel in Cremophor-ethanol at its MTD of 80 mg/kg was 2.0 +/-0.9 [range 0.4-3.5] days (n=16) in mice bearing the LL/2 and 2.0 +/- 1.1 [range 0.7-4.3] days (n=10) in B-16 model ($p<0.01$ compared to CT-2103 for both models).

Studies in mice using the murine P388 leukemia sub-line selected for mdrl overexpression and the human colon cancer cell lines that express mdrl (Table 3B) suggest that intracellular paclitaxel derived from breakdown of CT-2103 is less subject to the multidrug resistance pump than is paclitaxel that enters the cell by diffusion of free paclitaxel[20]. As has been shown for other polymeric drug conjugates, this is probably due active uptake of the conjugate by tumour cells with breakdown of the PG backbone and release of free paclitaxel at sites distant from the plasma membrane where they cannot be exported by intrinsic plasma membrane pumps.

Studies in mice bearing the OCa-1 ovarian cancer demonstrated that CT-2103 is synergistic when co-administered with gemcitabine, doxorubicin, irinotecan, and carboplatin in a schedule independent manner (data not shown). Preliminary data indicate that it is also a substantially more potent radiosensitiser than paclitaxel in Cremophor EL/ethanol with an enhancement factor in a curative model of multidose radiation reported to be >8.0 compared to approximately 2 for paclitaxel reported in the same model by the same investigator [12,21-24]. Of great interest was the observation that unlike free paclitaxel, CT-2103 did not sensitise normal skin or gastrointestinal mucosa to radiation[25].

Table 3A. Effect of CT-2103 on Syngeneic Rodent Tumour Models

Cell line/	**CT-2103 Test**	**Paclitaxel-Equivalent MTD, mg/kg Route of Administration**		**Tumour growth delay (TGD) at MTD, days**	**Ratio of TGDs, days**
Derivation	**Material**	**Paclitaxel**	**CT-2103**	**CT-2103 Group**	**CT-2103 / paclitaxel**
Single Dose Studies					
OCA-1 murine ovarian [10]	PG MW 36,200; 20% paclitaxel w/w	80 IV	160 IV	Histological cure in 25 / 26 mice	10 day growth delay with paclitaxel at 80 mg/kg
13762F rat mammary [10]		20 IV	60 IV	Complete regression at 40 and 60 mg/kg	5 day growth delay with paclitaxel at 20 mg/kg
Mca-4 murine mammary		60 IV	120 IV	39.6	39.6 / 4.5
Mca-35 murine mammary		80 IV	160 IV	16	16 / 7
Hca1 murine hepatoma		80 IV	160 IV	4 (estimated)	4 / 1
Fsa-II murine fibrosarcoma		80 IV	160 IV	2 (estimated)	2 / 1
LL/2 murine Lewis lung carcinoma[A)]	PG MW 33,000; 37% paclitaxel w/w	80 IP	160 to 240 IP	3.7 at 160 mg/kg	3.7 / 1.2
B16 Melanoma [B)]		80 IP	160 to 200 IP	5.2 at 160 mg/kg	5.2 / 0.9
P388/dox [C)] Murine doxorubicin-resistant lymphoid leukemia		80 IP	160 IP	5.7	5.7 / -0.1

Table 3B. Effect of CT2103 on Human Tumour Xenografts

Cell line/ Derivation	**Paclitaxel - Equivalent MTD, mg/kg Route of Administration**		**TGD at MTD, days; Other Results**	**Ratio of TGDs, days CT-2103/ paclitaxel**
	Paclitaxel	**CT-2103**		
NCI-H460 non small lung cancer	60 IP	120 IP	13.3	13.3 / 1.4
PC3: Prostate adenocarcinoma	60 IP	150 IP	Experiment terminated 4 weeks after drug administration). 80% (8/10) of the mice in the CT-2103 and 10% (1/10) of the mice in the paclitaxel group no longer had detectable tumours.	
DU-145: Metastatic prostate carcinoma	60 IP	120 IP	>6.6 Exp. terminated 74 days post drug administration. 25% (2/8) mice had tumours <500 mm^3	Paclitaxel was too toxic at this dose in this model
LS174t: mdr-1$^-$ colon adenocarcinoma	75 IP	169 IP	>39 Exp. terminated 45 days post drug administration: 100% (10/10) mice had tumours <500 mm^3	>39 / 12.3
HT-29: mdr-1$^-$ colon adenocarcinoma	Not done	135 IP	>58.8 12 weeks post dosing 80% (8/10) of the mice no longer had detectable tumours	Not applicable
HCT-116: mdr-1$^-$ colon adenocarcinoma	80 IP	150 IP	>96.4 16 weeks post dosing 60% (6/10) of the mice in the CT-2103 group and 10% (1/10) in the paclitaxel group no longer had detectable tumours.	>96.4 / 28.1
CaCO-2: mdr-1$^+$ colon adenocarcinoma	60 IP	120 IP	3.8	3.8 / 0.1
LoVo: mdr-1$^+$ colon adenocarcinoma	60 IP	120 IP	37.4	37.4 / 11.6
HCT-15: mdr-1$^+$ colon adenocarcinoma	60 IP	120 IP	5.4	5.4 / -0.4
Colo 320DM: mdr-1$^+$ colon adenocarcinoma	60 IP	135 IP	>14.6 Exp. terminated 67 days post drug administration: 14% (1/7) mice had tumours <500 mm^3	>14.6 / 1.8
CT-2103 test material in all experiments described in Table 3B: PG MW 38,000; 37% paclitaxel w/w				

3.4 Preclinical Toxicology

Following single doses or 5-day repeat dosing in rodents, CT-2103 induced effects that were consistent with those previously reported for paclitaxel[26-29], including dose-related effects on clinical condition, haematology, clinical chemistry, tissues with normally active cell mitosis, and neural tissues. Single IV dose MTD in mice and rats was >280 mg/M^2. Local tolerance tests of CT-2103 in rabbits showed minimal to mild concentration-dependent irritation with intravenous, peri-venous, or subcutaneous dosing, and a slightly more severe reaction with intra-arterial dosing. Sensitisation studies in guinea pigs and rabbits revealed no evidence of sensitisation or specific antibody formation against CT-2103[19].

3.5 Preliminary Clinical Data

CT-2103 is currently under evaluation as a single agent in Phase II clinical trials in patients with relapsed ovarian cancer, primary non-small-cell lung cancer in the aged and in patients with a poor performance status, and in patients with relapsed colon cancer. It is also under evaluation in ovarian and lung cancer in combination with platinates[19].

A Phase I clinical study, performed in the U.K. under the auspices of the Cancer Research Campaign, completed enrolment in August 2001[30,31]. The primary objectives of this study were to determine pharmacokinetics, tolerance, and maximum tolerated dose of CT-2103 when administered every 21 days, and to propose a suitable dose for further evaluation in Phase II studies. A secondary objective was to observe for potential antitumour effects in taxane-naïve patients[19].

Eighteen adult patients with advanced solid tumours who had failed conventional therapy and who had not been treated with taxanes were enrolled. A rapid dose escalation plan was used, with one patient treated at each dose level until a drug-related grade 2 toxicity was observed in cycle 1; thereafter, 3 to 6 patients were to be treated at each dose level[19].

CT-2103 was administered as a 30-minute intravenous infusion once every 21 days starting at a dose of 11 mg/m^2 paclitaxel-equivalent. The dose was doubled in each successive patient through doses of 22, 44, 89, and 176 mg/m^2. The dose was then increased by 50% to 266 mg/m^2, and 6 patients were enrolled at that dose. Two patients had dose-limiting toxicities at that dose. One patient with an unusual, abrupt onset sensorimotor neuropathy that was consistent with a paraneoplastic syndrome, and an uncomplicated neutropenia[32]. A cohort of six patients was treated at the next lower dose of 233 mg/m^2. Two patients experienced uncomplicated grade 4 neutropenia lasting more than 5 days. Thus the MTD for heavily pre-treated patients lies between 175 and 233 mg/m^2. Higher doses are likely to be tolerated in less heavily treated patients or if uncomplicated neutropenia is considered an acceptable side effect[19].

In contrast to the near complete alopecia observed with the marketed preparation of paclitaxel, only minimal alopecia was noted at all doses, even after multiple cycles of therapy. Neuropathy was infrequent with occasional patients with non-specific tingling in fingers and toes, which resolved quickly and did not recur. In subsequent trials, clinically significant neuropathy appears to be quite rare. Eight of the eighteen patients received 3 or more cycles of therapy indicating that they had at least stable disease. There was one partial remission lasting 7 months in a patient with a mesothelioma. The pharmacokinetic analyses done as part of this study showed a prolonged half-life (greater than 80 hrs), and increased exposure to both CT-2103 and to free paclitaxel as the dose increased[19].

Phase I studies in conjunction with cisplatin at 75 mg/m2 and carboplatin AUC 5-6 are currently in progress. Preliminary reports from a Phase I-II study in patients with advanced ovarian cancer demonstrate single agent responses[19].

4. CONCLUSIONS

These data describing the preclinical and early clinical development of CT-2103 demonstrate the feasibility of using polyglutamic acid homopolymers to create macromolecular cytotoxic drug conjugates. PG has the characteristics of an ideal polymeric drug carrier including biodegradability, the ability to solubilise hydrophobic agents even at high loading, stability in circulation, and apparent lack of immunogenicity. Preliminary clinical data indicate that CT-2103 is well tolerated by short infusion and has what appears to be reduced toxicity to neural tissue and hair follicles compared with paclitaxel delivered in the standard formulation. In preclinical studies, the MTD was approximately twice that of standard paclitaxel and the antitumour efficacy in was improved. Preliminary clinical data from Phase II studies indicate that the MTD will be higher than that of paclitaxel and that CT-2103 has activity, even in patients who have failed prior taxane therapy. The potentially enhanced efficacy and apparently reduced toxicity of CT-2103 can be predominantly ascribed to its improved distribution to tumour tissue through the EPR effect and the reduced exposure of normal tissues. Taken together, these data suggest that PG is an excellent polymeric backbone for the delivery of oncologic therapeutics and is likely to improve the therapeutic indices of a number of other agents. A second PG conjugate designated CT-2106, a PG camptothecin with an interposed glycine linker, will enter clinical trials shortly.

REFERENCES

1. Maeda, H. 2001. The enhanced permeability and retention (EPR) effect in tumour vasculature: the key role of tumour-selective macromolecular drug targeting. *Adv.Enzyme Regul.* 41:189-207.
2. Maeda, H., J. Wu, T. Sawa, Y. Matsumura, and K. Hori. 2000. Tumour vascular permeability and the EPR effect in macromolecular therapeutics: a review. *J.Control Release* 65:271-284.
3. Matsumura, Y. and H. Maeda. 1986. A new concept for macromolecular therapeutics in cancer chemotherapy: mechanism of tumoritropic accumulation of proteins and the antitumor agent smancs. *Cancer Res* 46:6387-6392.
4. Pimm, M. V., A. C. Perkins, J. Strohalm, K. Ulbrich, and R. Duncan. 1996. Gamma scintigraphy of the biodistribution of 123I-labelled n-(2-hydroxypropyl)methacrylamide copolymer-doxorubicin conjugates in mice with transplanted melanoma and mammary carcinoma. *J Drug Targeting* 3:375-383.
5. Vasey, P. A., S. B. Kaye, R. Morrison, C. Twelves, P. Wilson, R. Duncan, A. H. Thomson, L. S. Murray, T. E. Hilditch, T. Murray, S. Burtles, D. Fraier, E. Frigerio, and J. Cassidy. 1999. Phase I clinical and pharmacokinetic study of PK1 [N-(2-hydroxypropyl)methacrylamide copolymer doxorubicin]: first member of a new class of chemotherapeutic agents-drug-polymer conjugates. Cancer Research Campaign Phase I/II Committee. *Clin Cancer Res* 5:83-94.
6. McCormick-Thomson, L. A. and R. Duncan. 1989. Poly(amino acid) copolymers as a potential soluble drug delivery system. 1. pinocytic uptake and lysosomal degradation measured in vitro. *J Bioactive and Compatible Polymers* 4:242-251.
7. Duncan, R. 1992. Drug-polymer conjugates: potential for improved chemotherapy. *Anticancer Drugs* 3:175-210.
8. Duncan, R. and F. Spreafico. 1994. Polymer conjugates. Pharmacokinetic considerations for design and development. *Clin.Pharmacokinet.* 27:290-306.
9. Gueritte-Voegelein, F., D. Guenard, F. Lavelle, M. T. Le Goff, L. Mangatal, and P. Potier. 1991. Relationships between the structure of taxol analogues and their antimitotic activity. *J.Med.Chem.* 34:992-998.
10. Li, C., D. F. Yu, R. A. Newman, F. Cabral, L. C. Stephens, N. Hunter, L. Milas, and S. Wallace. 1998. Complete regression of well-established tumours using a novel water-soluble poly(L-glutamic acid)-paclitaxel conjugate. *Cancer Res* 58:2404-2409.
11. Li, C., Price, J. E., Milas, L., Hunter, N. R., Ke, S., Yu, D. F., Chusilp, C., and Wallace, S. Antitumor activity of Poly(L-glutamic acid)-Paclitaxel on syngeneic and xenografted tumours. Proc Am Assoc Cancer Res 40, 1909. 1999.
12. Li, C., R. A. Newman, Q. P. Wu, S. Ke, W. Chen, T. Hutto, Z. Kan, M. D. Brannan, C. Charnsangavej, and S. Wallace. 2000. Biodistribution of paclitaxel and poly(L-glutamic acid)-paclitaxel conjugate in mice with ovarian OCa-1 tumour. *Cancer Chemother.Pharmacol.* 46:416-422.
13. de Vries, P., Kumar, A., Heasley, E., and Singer, J. W. Optimisation of the anti-tumour activity of water-soluble poly L-glutamic acid (PG)-paclitaxel (TXL) conjugates. AACR - NCI - EORTC 92, 451. 11-17-1999. Washington DC.

14. Singer, J. W., de Vries, P., Kumar, A., Baker, B., Lynn, S., Li, C., and Wallace, S. Poly-L-Glutamic Acid Paclitaxel Conjugate (PG-TXL): A water-soluble biodegradable conjugate with decreased toxicity and enhanced efficacy. 4th International Symposium on Polymer Therapeutics . 2000.
15. Baker, B., Bellamy, G., Nudelman, E., Shaffer, S., de Vries, P., Heasley, E., Stone, I., Reigh, C., Burke, S., Kumar, A., Klein, P., Brannan, M., and Singer, J. W. Biodistribution of poly-L-glutamic acid-paclitaxel (CT-2103), and paclitaxel in C57BL/6 mice bearing subcutaneous B16 melanomas. Cancer Research . 2001.
16. Shaffer, S. A., Baker Lee, C., Nudelman, E., Kumar, A., Coon, M., Stone, I., de Vries, P., and Singer, J. Metabolism of poly-L-glutamic acid (PG) paclitaxel (CT-2103); proteolysis by lysosomal cathepsin B and identification of intermediate metabolites. Proc Amer Assoc Cancer Res . 2002.
17. Shaffer, S., Baker Lee, C., de Vries, P., Bellamy, G., Heasley, E., Stone, I., Kumar, A., Bhatt, R., Nudelman, E., Reigh, C., Baker, B., and Singer, J. *In vivo* identification of monoglutamyl paclitaxel metabolite from poly-L-glutamic acid-paclitaxel (CT-2103) in tumour bearing mice. Proceedings of the 49th ASMS Conference on Mass Spectrometry and Allied Topics , A010970. 2001.
18. Li, C., J. E. Price, L. Milas, N. R. Hunter, S. Ke, D. F. Yu, C. Chusilp, and S. Wallace. 1999. Antitumor activity of Poly(L-glutamic acid)-Paclitaxel on syngeneic and xenografted tumours. *Clin Cancer Res* 5:891-897.
19. CTI. Investigator Brochure CT-2103. 2001.
20. de Vries, P., Kumar, A., Heasley, E., Stone, I., and Singer, J. CT-2103: A water soluble poly-L-glutamic acid (PG)- Paclitaxel (TXL) conjugate has enhanced efficacy on MDR-1^+ human colon carcinoma cell line xenografts compared to free TXL. Proc Am Assoc Cancer Res 42, 462. 2001.
21. Li, C., S. Ke, Q. Wu, W. Tansey, N. Hunter, L. M. Buchmiller, L. Milas, C. Charnsangavej, and S. Wallace. 2000. Potentiation of ovarian OCa-1 tumour radioresponse by poly (L-glutamic acid)-paclitaxel conjugate. *Int.J Radiat.Oncol.Biol.Phys.* 48:1119-1126.
22. Li, C., S. Ke, Q. Wu, W. Tansey, N. Hunter, L. Buchmiller, L. Milas, C. Charnsangavej, and S. Wallace. 2000. Tumour irradiation enhances the specific-specific distribution of poly(L-glutamic acid)-conjugated paclitaxel and its antitumor efficacy. *Clin Cancer Res* 6:2829-2834.
23. Ke, S., Oldham, E., Milas, L., Hunter, N. R., Tansey, W., Charnsangavej, C., Wallace, S., and Li, C. Schedule-independent radiosensitization of a murine ovarian OCa-1 tumour by PG-TXL. Proc Am Assoc Cancer Res 40, 4223. 1999.
24. Li, C., Ke, S., Oldham, E., Milas, L., Hunter, N. R., Tansey, W., Charnsagavej, C., and Wallace, S. Enhancement of tumour radioresponse of a murine ovarian carcinoma by poly(L-glutamic acid)-paclitaxel conjugate. Ninth International Symposium on Recent Advances in Drug Delivery Systems. 1999.
25. Mason, K. A., Hunter, N., Wallace, S., and Milas, L. Poly (L-glutamic Acid)-paclitaxel dramatically enhances the anti-tumour efficacy of radiotherapy. AACR - NCI - EORTC , 397. 2001. Miami Beach, Florida.
26. Cavaletti, G., E. Cavalletti, P. Montaguti, N. Oggioni, O. De Negri, and G. Tredici. 1997. Effect on the peripheral nervous system of the short-term intravenous administration of paclitaxel in the rat. *Neurotoxicology* 18:137-145.
27. Cavaletti, G., G. Tredici, M. Braga, and S. Tazzari. 1995. Experimental peripheral neuropathy induced in adult rats by repeated intraperitoneal administration of taxol. *Exp.Neurol.* 133:64-72.

28. Kadota, T., H. Chikazawa, H. Kondoh, K. Ishikawa, S. Kawano, K. Kuroyanagi, N. Hattori, K. Sakakura, S. Koizumi, E. Hiraiwa, and . 1994. [Toxicity studies of paclitaxel. (II)--One-month intermittent intravenous toxicity in rats]. *J.Toxicol.Sci.* 19 Suppl 1:11-34.
29. Kadota, T., H. Chikazawa, H. Kondoh, K. Ishikawa, S. Kawano, K. Kuroyanagi, N. Hattori, K. Sakakura, S. Koizumi, E. Hiraiwa, and . 1994. [Toxicity studies of paclitaxel. (I)--Single dose intravenous toxicity in rats]. *J.Toxicol.Sci.* 19 Suppl 1:1-9.
30. Todd, R., Sludden, J., Boddy, A. V., Griffin, M. J., Robson, L., Cassidy, J., Bissett, D., Main, M., Brannan, M. D., Elliott, S., Fishwick, K., Verrill, M., and Calvert, H. Phase I and pharmacological study of CT-2103, a poly (L-glutamic Acid)-paclitaxel conjugate. Journal of Clinical Oncology , #439. 2001.
31. Bolton, M. G., Cassidy, J., and Calvert, H. Phase I studies of PG-Paclitaxel (CT-2103) as a single agent and in combination with cisplatin. 5th International Symposium on Polymer Therapeutics . 2002.
32. Sludden, J., Boddy, A. V., Griffin, M. J., Robson, L., Todd, R., Cassidy, J., Bissett, D., Main, M., Brannan, M. D., Elliott, S., Verrill, M., and Calvert, H. Phase I and pharmacological study of CT-2103, a poly(L-glutamic acid)-paclitaxel conjugate. Proc Amer Assoc Cancer Res 42, 535. 2002.

HPMA Copolymer Delivery of Chemotherapy and Photodynamic Therapy in Ovarian Cancer

C. MATTHEW PETERSON, JANE-GUO SHIAH, YONGEN SUN, PAVLA KOPEČKOVÁ, TAMARA MINKO, RICHARD C. STRAIGHT, and JINDRICH KOPEČEK
Departments of Obstetrics and Gynecology, Pharmaceutics and Pharmaceutical Chemistry, Utah Center for Photo-Medicine, University of Utah and the Veteran's Administration Medical Center Salt Lake City, Utah, USA

1. INTRODUCTION

Ovarian cancer is diagnosed in approximately one in 55-70 women in the United States. [1] It is the fourth leading cause of death in women and is the most lethal neoplasm of the female genital tract. [1] Current prevalence rates indicate more than 23,000 cases will be diagnosed, and over 14,000 women will die from ovarian cancer this year. Currently, primary and metastatic tumor nodules are treated by aggressive cytoreductive surgery, however, micronodular disease and floating tumor colonies within the peritoneal cavity are inadequately treated by surgery, and result in recurrent disease in the majority of treated women. [2-4]

The majority of ovarian cancers (>70%) are diagnosed when intraperitoneal metastases (Stage III) are present. The presence of intra-abdominal metastases at the time of diagnosis results in persistent or recurrent tumor in 25-60%, despite maximal initial debulking and multiple courses of adjuvant chemotherapy. [5-6] Cytoreductive surgery with adjuvant chemotherapeutic treatments (combination therapy: cisplatin or carboplatin and Taxol; or, doxorubicin and hexamethylmelamine) provide only marginal 5 year survivals (Clinical Stage IIIa: 30-40%; IIIb: 20%; IIIc-IV: 5%, respectively) and are associated with significant anticancer drug related morbidity and mortality. [6-8] Recent analyses document only a minimal improvement in overall mortality rates from 1979 to 1995. [1]

An NIH panel on ovarian cancer advised that "innovative approaches to the treatment of advanced primary as well as recurrent ovarian cancer must be identified and studied". [2] Williams reached similar conclusions, namely that "there are two striking needs in the therapy of ovarian carcinoma: new more effective drugs and development of best current therapy using drugs presently available". [9]

2. N-(2-HYDROXYPROPYL)METHACRYLAMIDE (HPMA) COPOLYMERS FOR THE DELIVERY OF ANTICANCER AGENTS

The use of polymeric drug delivery systems is rapidly becoming an established approach for improvement of cancer chemotherapy. The covalent binding of low molecular weight drugs to water-soluble polymer carriers offers a potential mechanism to enhance the specificity of drug action. The major distinction between low molecular weight anticancer drugs and their macromolecular conjugates is the mechanism of cell entry. While low molecular weight drugs may penetrate into all cell types by diffusion, their attachment to macromolecules such as N-(2-hydroxypropyl)methacrylamide (HPMA) copolymer, limits cellular uptake of the polymer-drug conjugates to the endocytic route. Internalized macromolecules are then transferred via endosomes into the lysosomal compartment of the cell. [10] The rate of (fluid-phase) pinocytosis is low. Consequently, in normal tissue the polymer-drug conjugate is largely confined to the bloodstream. [11] However, the abnormal tissue vasculature found in tumors allows the uptake of large molecules to proceed more efficiently than in normal tissues. Furthermore, the poor lymphatic drainage of tumors allows higher concentrations of macromolecular therapeutics to accumulate. [12-14] Maeda coined the phrase "enhanced permeability and retention (EPR) effect" to describe this phenomenon. [12] The alternative mechanism of cellular entry afforded by HPMA copolymer delivery provides a number of documented benefits and advantages over standard methods of cancer therapy. (Figure 1)

These favorable advantages include: control of biodistribution and accumulation via molecular weight limitations; biodegradability of side chains; minimal immunogenicity; subcellular localization of anticancer drug release; targeting capabilities; enhanced permeability and retention; increased apoptosis, lipid peroxidation, and DNA damage; significantly reduced nonspecific toxicity; and applicability to a wide range of anticancer agents. [10,14-17]

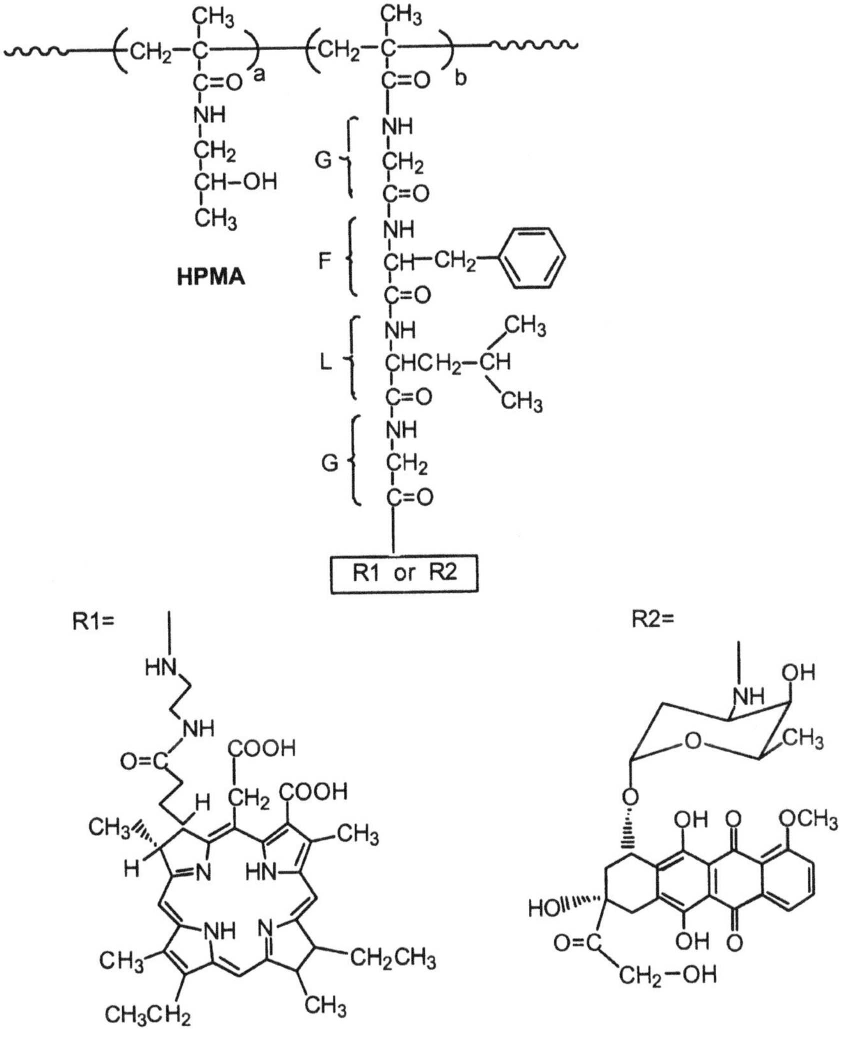

Figure 1. Structure of N-(2-hydroxypropyl)methacrylamide (HPMA) copolymers: R1 = mesochlorin e 6; R2 = doxorubicin.

2.1 Biocompatibility and Control of Biodistribution of Poly [N-(2-hydroxypropyl)methacrylamide]

In multiple experiments, biocompatibility and the absence of toxicity was noted with the use of HPMA copolymer alone. (17) The macromolecular HPMA copolymer is capable of facilitating the delivery of multiple agents (drugs and/or targeting moieties), which are then incorporated intracellularly through pinocytotic pathways. [9] Present methods of anticancer drug delivery to ovarian cancer cells are routinely limited to simple passive diffusion. Pinocytosis, in contrast to passive diffusion, facilitates specific targeting through the subcellular localization (lysosomal) of anticancer drug release. Furthermore, the unique design features of the HPMA copolymer allow the addition of targeting moieties capable of cell specific localization. [10,14,15]

2.2 Biodegradability of Tetrapeptide Attachment/ Release Sites Resulting in Subcellular Delivery

The sequence of the oligopeptide drug attachment/release site, or spacer, is a critical factor contributing to the success of HPMA copolymer drug delivery. This peptide spacer, glycine-phenylalanine-leucine-glycine (G-F-L-G), has been designed to allow the HPMA copolymer-drug conjugate to maintain stability in the circulation [16], yet, retain susceptibility to enzymatically catalyzed degradation in the lysosomal compartment of the cell. [18,19] Recently, a key advantage provided by the subcellular delivery of anticancer drugs was demonstrated when HPMA copolymer bound doxorubicin delivery to the lysosome was shown to overcome the energy driven P-glycoprotein efflux pump found in multi-drug resistant ovarian carcinoma cell lines. [20] The control of anticancer drug release at the subcellular level also results in a substantial reduction in nonspecific toxicity of the polymer-bound drugs compared to the free drugs. [18,19] Examples of selective targeting utilizing N-acylated galactosamine (GalN) or monoclonal OV-TL16 antibodies with doxorubicin in human hepatocarcinoma HepG2 and ovarian carcinoma OVCAR-3 cell lines, respectively, demonstrate cell specific enhancement of HPMA copolymer-drug conjugate recognition, internalization, localization to lysosomes, release and subsequent diffusion via the cytoplasm to the cell nuclei. [20] Multiple selective targeting moieties for ovarian carcinoma are being investigated including monoclonal antibodies and folic acid. [21,22]

2.3 Enhanced Permeability and Retention (EPR) of HPMA Copolymer-Anticancer Agents

Compounding interest in the efficacy of HPMA copolymer delivery is the fact that regardless of the presence or absence of a selective targeting moiety, HPMA copolymer-drug conjugates accumulate preferentially in solid tumors, through the enhanced permeability and retention (EPR) effect conceptualized by Maeda. [13,14,23] The EPR effect is attributed to:1) high vascular density in the tumor secondary to abnormal vascular architecture and angiogenesis; 2) increased permeability of tumor vessels due to a number of vasoactive compounds including: VEGF, bFGF, bradykinin, nitric oxide, peroxynitrite, prostaglandins, cytokines, and uPA; and 3) poor and/or defective lymphatic drainage inherent in solid tumors. The higher molecular weights (approximately 30,000 Daltons) of HPMA copolymer bound drugs are uniquely suited to capitalize on EPR effects in ovarian cancer through the enhancement of subcellular localization in these solid tumors. Additional design features of HPMA copolymers which make them ideal vehicles for the delivery of anticancer drugs include: the ability to control the molecular weight of the copolymer to remain under the renal threshold, thus avoiding long term accumulation in the body; controllable pH sensitivity and degradability, and biodegradability of oligopeptide drug attachment/release sites. [10, 24] Finally, the HPMA copolymer has minmal immunogenicity and is biocompatible. [25] Thus, the HPMA copolymer-anticancer drug delivery system has great potential to enhance the biodistribution, subcellular release, metabolism, cell specificity, and therapeutic safety of many suitable anticancer drugs.

2.4 HPMA copolymer-Anticancer Agents Currently in Human Trials

Presently there are seven polymer-drug conjugates which have entered Phase I/II clinical trials as anti-cancer agents in the U.K (five of which are HPMA copolymer-drug conjugates). These include N-(2-hydroxy-propyl)methacrylamide (HPMA) copolymer doxorubicin (PK1, FCE 28068), HPMA copolymer-paclitaxel (PNU 166945), HPMA copolymer-camptothecin, PEG-camptothecin, poly(glutamic acid)-paclitaxel, HPMA copolymer-platinate (AP 5280), and HPMA copolymer-doxorubicin conjugates bearing galactosamine (PK2). The rapid proliferation of HPMA copolymer anti-cancer agents is evidence of the promising potential of HPMA copolymer carried agents.

3. DOXORUBICIN FOR TREATMENT OF OVARIAN CANCER-BENEFITS OF HPMA COPOLYMER CONJUGATION

Doxorubicin (adriamycin), a well studied anticancer agent, has shown efficacy in the treatment of human ovarian epithelial carcinoma. [26] Doxorubicin acts by reversibly stabilizing covalent adducts between topoisomerase II and DNA and additionally generates free radicals. These activities result in DNA breaks, cellular membrane damage and cell death. [27, 28]

Doxorubicin possesses two specific dose-limiting toxicities: cardiotoxicity and bone marrow supression. [29, 30] It has been suggested that the dose-limiting cardiotoxicity of doxorubicin is mediated by oxygen radical formation which damages mitochondrial membranes and decreases superoxide dismutase activity, resulting in the further generation of reactive oxygen species and additional cellular damage. [31] HPMA copolymer delivery of doxorubicin reduces these risks, and demonstrates efficacy, reduced toxicity and immunogencity and great promise in human trials.

3.1 Efficacy-*In Vitro* and *In Vivo* models

The efficacy and reduced nonspecific toxicity of HPMA copolymer bound doxorubicin for the treatment of ovarian cancer has been demonstrated in numerous preclinical in vitro and in vivo investigations. In the OVCAR-3 cell line, doxorubicin bound to the HPMA copolymer demonstrated a ten-fold increase in the drug concentration required compared to free doxorubicin in order to obtain equivalency in cell growth inhibition in vitro. [32] The reduced specific toxicity of HPMA copolymer doxorubicin was consistent with the slower pinocytotic uptake mechanism required by higher molecular weight drugs and predicted a reduced non-specific toxicity which has been subsequently documented in vivo. [33] A greater reduction in thymidine incorporation over mitochondrial respiration in free and HPMA copolymer bound doxorubicin was consistent with a primary activity on cellular DNA in these in vitro studies. [32] HPMA copolymer bound doxorubicin also demonstrated a 15-fold longer intravascular half-life and 100-fold lower peak initial cardiac level compared to free drug, resulting in a notable 15-fold reduction in nonspecfic toxicities during in vivo studies. [14] In mouse models of ovarian carcinoma, HPMA copolymer-doxorubicin conjugate at 2.2 mg/kg of free doxorubicin equivalent caused no toxic deaths and an 8% maximal weight loss which was regained completely within three weeks. [33] This dosage of HPMA copolymer bound doxorubicin (2.2 mg/kg of free doxorubicin equivalent) provided tumor response equivalency to a dose of 1 mg/kg of free doxorubicin in this nude mouse model. Free doxorubicin administered at doses over 1.5 mg/kg was uniformly fatal in the nude mouse model. To summarize, HPMA copolymer-doxorubicin demonstrates efficacy and reduced nonspecific toxicity in experimental models of ovarian carcinoma and other tumor models. [33, 34] The efficacy and safety of HPMA copolymer bound doxorubicin in the nude mouse model is demonstrated in Figure 2.

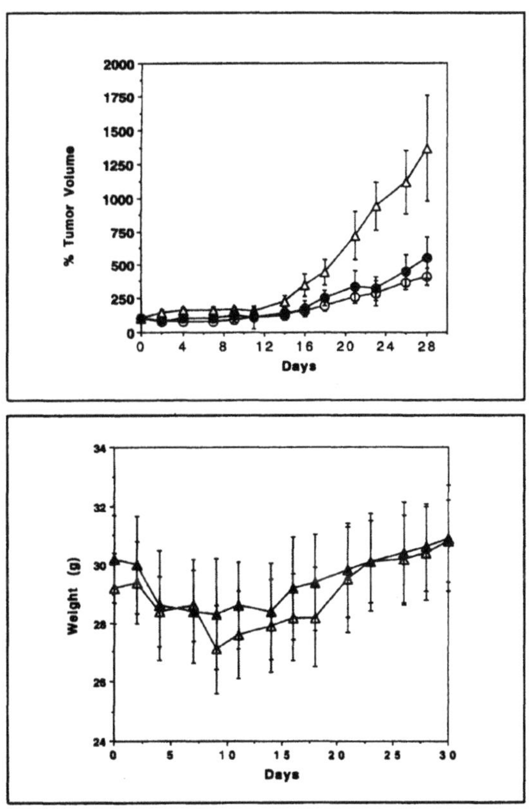

Figure 2. Figure 2. Panel A. Inhibition of OVCAR-3 tumors heterotransplanted in nude mice by doxorubicin (1mg/kg; O) and HPMA copolymer-doxorubicin or P-A (30 mg/kg, 2.2mg/kg doxorubicin equivalent; ●) compared with controls (△). Tumor volumes from day 10 forward were significantly less than controls (all P<0.045). There was no significant difference between P-A (30 mg/kg, 2.2 mg/kg doxorubicin equivalent) and doxorubicin (1 mg/kg). Although tumor growth was inhibited, there were no cures. *Bars*, SE. Panel B. Weight changes in mice receiving free doxorubicin (1 mg/kg; △) and P-A (30 mg/kg; 2.2 mg/kg doxorubicin equivalent; ▲). Weight losses were less than 8% for both drugs. There were no statistically significant differences between the drug forms. *Bars*, SE. [33]

Presently, HPMA copolymer bound doxorubicin is undergoing very promising Phase I and II clinical trials in the U.K. for the treatment of solid tumors. [35] Quantitative signature gene expression studies between free and HPMA copolymer bound drugs are underway to document the enhancement derived from HPMA copolymer subcellular localization, and to reveal specific modes of action on a molecular level which may be further amplified or augmented by design features of the HPMA copolymer. One such example of the specific advantages of HPMA copolymer bound doxorubicin is that free doxorubicin up-regulates genes encoding the ATP driven efflux pumps (MDR1, MRP) while HPMA copolymer bound doxorubicin overcomes these existing pumps and downregulates the MRP gene. Furthermore, free doxorubicin activates the expression of genes responsible for detoxification and DNA repair which are suppressed or activated to a lesser degree by HPMA copolymer bound doxorubicin (glutathione-GST-pi, UDP transferase-BUDP, Topoisomerase II- alpha and beta, thymidine kinase isoform 1- TK-1, heat shock protein 70-HSP-70). Finally, both free and HPMA copolymer bound doxorubicin induce the p53 gene central death signal as well as the c-fos and c-jun pathways activating cell death. To complete cell death, bcl-2, the inhibitor of apoptosis, is also down-regulated by HPMA copolymer bound doxorubicin. [36] Figure 3 details the findings described above.

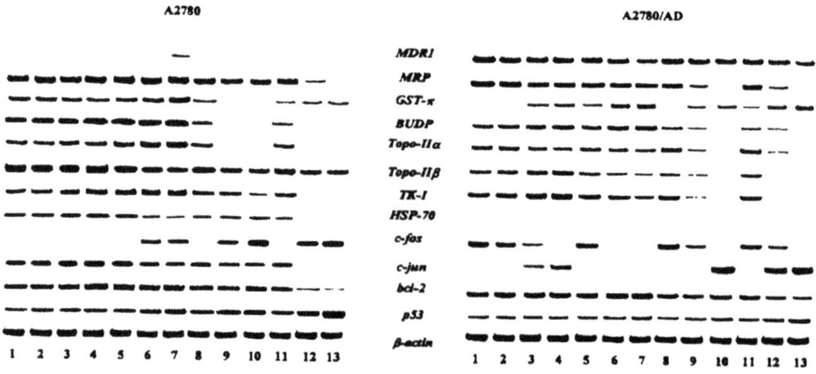

Figure 3. Typical images of gel electrophoresis of RT-PCR products form A2780 sensitive (left panel) and A2780/AD doxorubicin (DOX) resistant (right panel) human ovarian carcinoma cells. Identical numbers of cells, amounts of RT products and volumes of PCR products were used for each analysis. Primers and PCR regimens used for individual genes are listed in the reference [36]. RT-PCR products from cells indicated below were loaded and electrophoresed in 0.6-4.0% MetaPhor agarose gell: Lane 1, control cells; Lane 2, cells after 24 hr incubation with an 1X IC_{50} dose of free DOX; Lane 3, cells after 48 hr incubation with a 1X IC_{50} dose of free DOX; Lane 4, cells after a 72 hr incubation with a 1 X IC_{50} of free DOX; Lane 5, cells after a 24 hr incubation with 10 X IC_{50} dose of free DOX; Lane 6, cells after a

48 hr incubation with a 10 X IC_{50} dose free DOX; Lane 7, cells after a 72 hr incubation with a 10 X IC_{50} free DOX; Lane 8, cells after a 24 hr incubation with a 1 X IC_{50} dose of P(GFLG)-DOX; Lane 9, cells after a 48 hr incubation with a 1 X IC_{50} dose of P(GFLG)-DOX; Lane 10, cells after a 72 hr incubation with a 1 X IC_{50} dose of P(GFLG)-DOX;Lane 11, cells after a 24 hr incubation with a 10 X IC_{50} dose of P(GFLG)-ADR; Lane 12, cells after a 48 hr incubation with a 10 X IC_{50} dose of P(GFLG)-DOX; Lane 13, cells after a 72 hr incubation with a 10 X IC_{50} dose of P(GFLG)-DOX. P(GFLG) = HPMA copolymer with GFLG spacer/attachments sites. [36]

3.2 Toxicity/Immunogenicity in Animal Models

Conjugation of anti-cancer agents to hydrophilic polymers provides the ability to solubilize minimally water soluble drugs, enhance efficacy through improved drug delivery and reduced toxicity, and avoid immunogenicity associated with free drug administration. The HPMA copolymer main chain has a molecular weight well below the renal threshold of 40-50 kDa, thus allowing rapid renal clearance and the avoidance of toxicity. [37] Immunogenicity studies previously conducted show HPMA copolymers to be very weak thymus-independent immunogens. The intensity of the immune response is dependent on many factors including the molecular weight of the conjugate, the composition of the oligopeptidic side chains, and the genetic background of the immunized animals. [38-40]

Multiple studies demonstrate minimal IgM antibody response, the absence of activation of complement, and a minimal antibody response (one to three dilutions of sera) to HPMA copolymer-doxorubicin conjugates, which was not due to a diminution of responsiveness secondary to toxicity of the HPMA copolymer bound doxorubicin. [39,41, 42]

3.3 Results of Human Clinical Trials

In Phase I trials in the UK, HPMA copolymer doxorubicin (PK1) given once every three weeks, had significantly reduced toxicity when compared to free doxorubicin. The maximum tolerated dose, toxicity profile, and pharmacokinetics of PK1 as an i.v. infusion every 3 weeks to patients with refractory or resistant cancers was determined. In the most recent report, 100 cycles were administered (range, 20-320 mg/m^2 [free drug equivalent]) to 36 patients (20 males and 16 females) with a mean age of 58.3 years (age range, 34-72 years). The maximum tolerated dose was 320 mg/m^2, and the dose-limiting toxicities were febrile neutropenia and mucositis. This maximum tolerated dose was a 4-5 fold increase over the usual clinical doses (60-80 mg/m^2). No congestive cardiac failure was seen despite individual cumulative doses up to 1680 mg/m^2. Other anthracycline-like toxicities were attenuated. Pharmacokinetically, PK1 had a distribution t(1/2) of 1.8 h and an elimination t(1/2) averaging 93 h. ^{131}I-labeled PK1 imaging demonstrate PK1 is taken up by solid tumors. Responses (two partial and two minor responses) were seen in four patients with non-small cell lung cancer, colorectal cancer, and anthracycline-resistant breast cancer. PK1 demonstrated antitumor activity in refractory cancers, no polymer-related toxicity, and proof of principle that polymer-drug conjugation decreased known doxorubicin dose-limiting toxicities. The recommended Phase II dose justified by these studies was 280 mg/m^2 every 3 weeks. [43,44] PK-1 is currently undergoing Phase II evaluations for the treatment of breast, colon, and non-small cell lung cancer. [43,44]

HPMA copolymer-doxorubicin may have additional unique advantages in the treatment of ovarian cancer. It is now recognized that particularly aggressive solid tumors, such as ovarian cancer, have high levels of cysteine proteases which cleave the oligopeptide spacer Gly-Phe-Leu-Gly to release the drug. Thus, inherent properties of this and other solid tumors are particularly suited to HPMA copolymer doxorubicin delivery. [46]

4. PHOTODYNAMIC THERAPY FOR OVARIAN CANCER- BENEFITS OF HPMA COPOLYMER CONJUGATION OF MCE6

Photodynamic therapy (PDT) of superficially spreading ovarian cancer holds promise as a less toxic treatment through the controlled administration of light. Combining the activities of HPMA copolymer bound doxorubicin and mesochlorin e_6 photodynamic therapy provides cooperativity, synergy, and additivity in vitro, and results in tumor suppression in animal models which could not be achieved individually and accomplished this with significantly reduced nonspecific toxicity.

4.1 Efficacy of HPMA Copolymer Bound Mce6

We have previously demonstrated the efficacy of photodynamic therapy utilizing the hematoporphyrin derivative, Photofrin II on the human ovarian carcinoma cell line, OVCAR-3, xenografted in nude mice. [47] Microcirculatory damage caused by arteriolar constriction and venous thrombosis are the notable histopathologic markers of cellular damage attributed to photodynamic therapy. [48,49] Cell membrane and mitochondrial damage are the primary cellular mechanisms of cytotoxicity resulting from singlet oxygen formation. [50] In our Photofrin II study, the nonselective uptake of the photoactivatable hematoporphyrin derivative through simple diffusion resulted tumor ablation, but was also associated with significant toxicity and morbidity.

Mesochlorin e_6 monoethylene diamine (Mce_6) is a photoactivatable chemical which exhibits pharmacologic and photophysical properties better suited to PDT. [51] In vitro studies using HPMA copolymer delivery of Mce_6 documented, as with doxorubicin, a reduced specific toxicity compared to free drug. [32] The need for higher HPMA copolymer bound Mce_6 concentrations compared to free [Mce_6] to achieve equivalent inhibition of cell growth after light administration is consistent with the different mechanisms of cellular entry of the two forms of Mce_6, respectively: passive or simple diffusion for low molecular weight drugs in contrast to endocytosis for the higher molecular weight HPMA copolymer-drug conjugates. Increasing concentrations of HPMA copolymer-Mce_6 with light (up to 100X free [Mce_6] with light) demonstrated increased cytotoxicity in all assays consistent with a toxicity which was not restricted by cleavage from the HPMA copolymer tetrapeptide spacer for activity. Thus, photosensitizing agents in combination with known cytotoxic agents may be carried via the HPMA copolymer vehicle to reduce nonspecific toxicities and improve the therapeutic safety margins of both agents. HPMA copolymer delivery therefore allows: photosensitizer action which is independent of release from the HPMA copolymer carrier; a longer intravascular half life; higher accumulation in tumors; and a degree of targetability through the controlled administration of light. Figure 4 demonstrates the in vivo activities of free and HPMA copolymer delivered Mce_6. In nude mice xenografted with OVCAR-3 a significant reduction of HPMA copolymer bound Mce_6 toxicity compared to free Mce_6 was noted.

To summarize, HPMA copolymer-drug conjugates significantly broaden the therapeutic window, in vivo, of diverse anticancer agents possessing different cytotoxic pathways. The HPMA carrier system also allows one to design single agent and multiple drug combinations which maximize efficacy through capitalizing upon cellular processing requirements, control of light administration for targeting, and specific toxicities unique to each anticancer agent. Wider therapeutic indices for photosensitizers and many other potential drug combinations are expected to enhance response and cure rates without a parallel increase in nonspecific toxicity.

No human clinical and pharmacokinetics trials have been performed with this photosensitizer pending the results of the preclinical investigations proposed.

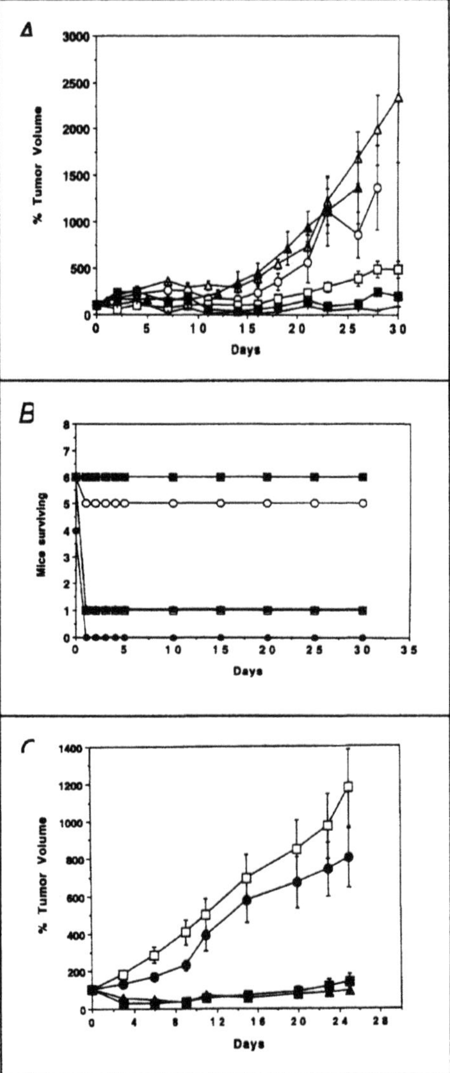

Figure 4. Panel A. Percentage of tumor volume in nude mice treated with Mce_6 and light (650 nm, 220 J/cm^2): 1.25 mg/kg (- O-), 2.5 mg/kg (- □-), 5 mg/kg (- +-), and 10mg/kg (- ■-) i.v., 2.5 mg/kg with no light (- ▲-) and controls (- △-). The lack of a significant response to 1.25 mg/kg Mce_6 and light (- O-) by human ovarian epithelial carcinoma is demonstrated. With Mce_6 and light at 2.5 mg/kg (-□-), the human OVCAR-3 tumor was destroyed (all P< 0.01 compared with controls). This dose caused mortality (shock syndrome) to one of six mice (17%). Eighty percent of tumors responded to therapy, with regression of tumor volume. Continued growth in nonresponding tumors became evident by day 21, but mean tumor volumes remained significantly less than control tumors (all P< 0.01). Mce_6 with light at 5 mg/kg(- +-) and 10 mg/kg (- ■-) caused mortality in five of six (83%) mice. A shock syndrome developed within 24 h after irradiation. Autopsy specimens revealed Mce_6

aggregation in the liver and lungs without evidence of acute toxicity or hemorrhagic necrosis. The surviving mice (5 and 10 mg/kg) had complete ablation of treated tumors. *Bars*, SE. *Panel B.* Mortality plot for Mce_6 administered at 1.25 mg/kg (- ■-), 2.5 mg/kg (- O-) ,5 mg/kg(-□-), and 10 mg/kg (- ▲-) i.v. and 2.5 mg/kg (- ●-) given i.p. followed by light (650 nm, 220 J/cm^2). Mortality (shock syndrome) was noted in doses of ≥2.5 mg/kg. *Panel C.* Inhibition of OVCAR-3 tumors heterotransplanted in nude mice treated with P-C and light (650 nm, 220 J/cm^2) at 12.5 mg/kg (1.5 mg/kg Mce_6 equivalent; (- ●-); 25 mg/kg (2.9 mg/kg Mce_6 equivalent, (- ■-); and 75 mg/kg (8.7 mg/kg Mce_6 equivalent, (- ▲-). Tumor volumes for 12.5 mg/kg P-C (1.5 mg/kg Mce_6 equivalent) were not significantly different compared with controls (-□-). Tumor volumes for 25 mg/kg (2.9 mg/kg Mce_6 equivalent) and 75 mg/kg (8.7 mg/kg Mce_6 equivalent) P-C were significantly less than controls ($P < 0.003$) but not significantly different from each other. Tumor recurrence became evident after day 20 for P-C at 25 mg/kg (2.9 mg/kg Mce_6 equivalent) and 75mg/kg (8.7 mg/kg Mce_6 equivalent). Two toxic deaths were noted with P-C at 25 mg/kg (2.9 mg/kg Mce_6 equivalent), but none was noted at 75 mg/kg (8.7 mg/kg Mce_6 equivalent). *Bars*, SE. [33]

4.2 Solution and Photoproperties of HPMA Copolymer Bound Mce_6

A recent study proposes a macromolecular conformation for HPMA copolymer bound Mce_6. Dynamic light scattering measurements indicate that intermolecular aggregation of Mce_6 within copolymers is not significant. Both absorption and fluorescence spectra confirm the existence of intramolecularly associated Mce_6. Fluorescence quenching measurements also indicate the presence of hydophobic Mce_6 domains which are identical with cores of unimeric micelles consisting of random copolymers. Fluorescence lifetime measurements also indicate the formation of Mce_6 aggregation. These findings support the notion that: 1) the covalent bonding of Mce_6 to HPMA copolymers significantly facilitates the formation of intramolecular micelle aggregates in aqueous solutions above that of free Mce_6; 2) there is a progressive dissociated into monomeric Mce_6 species when the volume percentage of ethanol is increased; and, 3) the more hydrophobic G-F-L-G side chains of the HPMA copolymer assist in the aggregation of Mce_6 within the copolymer conjugate. [52]

5. COMBINATION DOXORUBICIN AND PDT FOR OVARIAN CANCER-BENEFITS OF HPMACOPOLYMER CONJUGATION

The efficacy of combining doxorubicin with a photosensitizer in the treatment of a human carcinoma (mesothelioma cell line H-MESO-1) was first reported by Brophy and Keller. [53] In vitro studies with the combination of free doxorubicin and Mce_6 using both dose and effect addition isobolographic analysis demonstrated independent activity, cooperativity, synergy and additivity in their combined toxicity against OVCAR- 3 (Figure 5). [54]

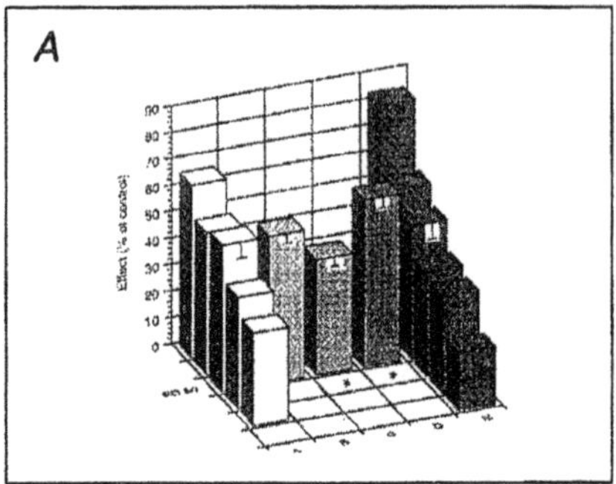

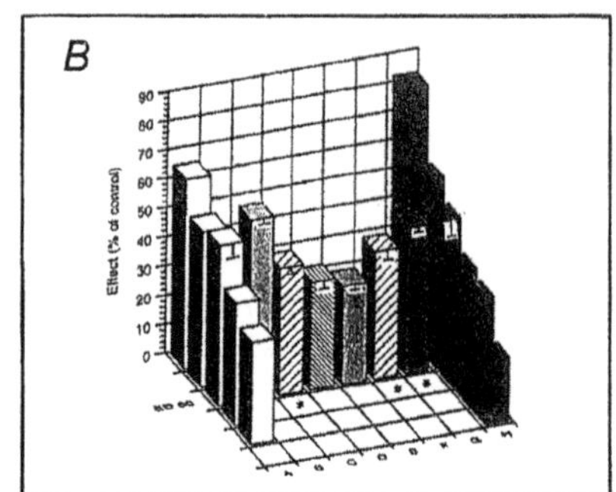

Figure 5. Panel A. The dose-addition isobole analysis for the MTT 72-hour assay and interactions. Columns A and E are the dose-response values for Mce_6/light and doxorubicin, respectively. Columns B, C, and D represent the 75% median effective concentration (ED_{50}) doxorubicin with 25% ED_{50} Mce_6/light which was additive (P = 0.62); 50% ED_{50} doxorubicin with 50% ED_{50} Mce_6/light, which was synergistic (*P = 0.027); and 25% ED_{50} doxorubicin with 75% ED_{50} Mce_6/light (*P = 0.035), which was antagonistic. Panel B. The effect-addition isobole analysis for the MTT 72-hour assay and interactions. Columns A and H are the dose-response values for Mce_6 and doxorubicin, respectively. Columns B-G represent various combinations as follows: B = 25% median effective concentration (ED_{50}) Mce_6/light with 50% ED_{50} doxorubicin, additive; C and F = 50% doxorubicin with 50% ED_{50} Mce_6/light, synergistic (* $P < 0.03$); D = 50% ED_{50} doxorubicin with 75% ED_{50} Mce_6/light, additive; E = 75% doxorubicin with 50 ED_{50} Mce_6/light, additive; and G = 25% ED_{50} adriamycin with 50% ED_{50} Mce_6/light, synergistic (*$P < 0.03$). [54]

For example, the ED_{50} of free doxorubicin combined with the ED_{50} of free Mce_6 resulted in a significant synergistic inhibition (27.5 %+ 1.57 of controls) of cell growth compared to approximately 40% inhibition for a twofold concentration of either free drug alone.

In vitro studies using HPMA copolymer-bound doxorubicin and Mce_6, in combination, have demonstrated a 10-fold increase in each drug concentration to be equally or more effective than free drug in the models used. These in vitro findings suggest the potential attenuation of combined nonspecific toxicities through HPMA copolymer conjugation. [54] This has been subsequently established in vivo. [33] Using a mouse model of ovarian cancer, HPMA copolymer delivery of doxorubicin or Mce_6 resulted in a 2-30 fold increase in the free drug equivalent dose delivered without increasing the nonspecific toxicity of either drug. [33] The combination of HPMA copolymer bound doxorubicin and Mce_6 resulted in significantly reduced nonspecific toxicity and a notable improvement in tumor cures which could not be obtained by either agent alone. (Figure 6)

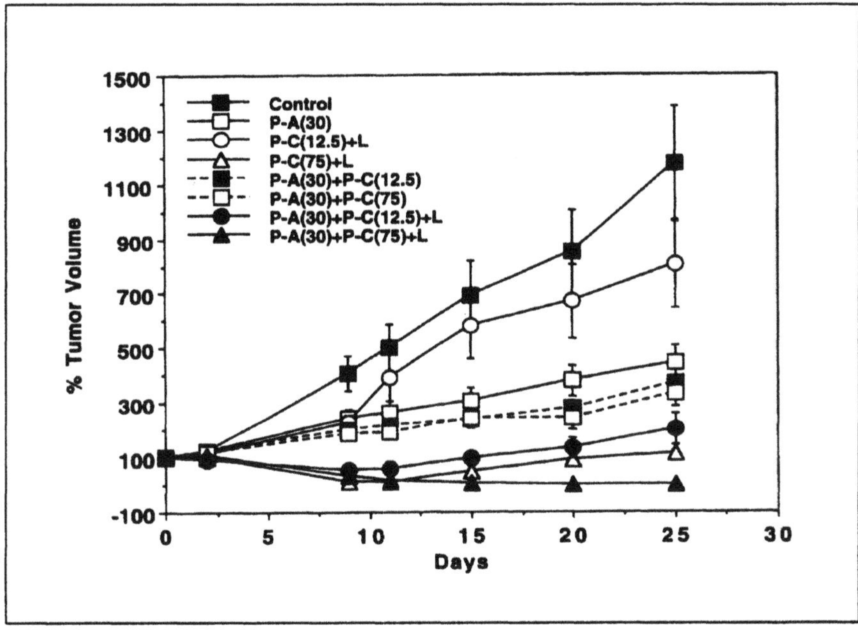

Figure 6. Combination chemotherapy and PDT of OVCAR-3 tumors heterotransplanted in nude mice treated with HPMA copolymer-bound anticancer drugs: control (-■-); P-C (12.5 mg/kg, 1.5 mg/kg Mce_6 equivalent) with light (-O-); P-A (30 mg/kg, 2.2 mg/kg Doxorubicin equivalent) (-□-); P-A (30 mg/kg, 2.2 mg/kg Doxorubicin equivalent) plus P-C (12.5 mg/kg, 1.5 mg/kg Mce_6 equivalent) without light (-■-); P-A (30 mg/kg, 2.2 mg/kg Doxorubicin equivalent) plus P-C (75 mg/kg, 8.7 mg/kg Mce_6 equivalent) without light (-□-); P-A (30 mg/kg, 2.2 mg/kg Doxorubicin equivalent) plus P-C (12.5 mg/kg, 1.5 mg/kg Mce_6 equivalent) with light (-●-); P-C (75 mg/kg, 8.7 mg/kg Mce_6 equivalent) with light (-△-); and P-A (30 mg/kg, 2.2 mg/kg Doxorubicin equivalent) plus P-C (75 mg/kg, 8.7 mg/kg Mce_6 equivalent) with light (-▲-). Bars. SE. P = HPMA copolymer bound. [33]

6. PRECLINICAL BIODISTRIBUTION STUDIES OF COMBINATION FREE AND HPMA COPOLYMER BOUND DRUGS

Biodistribution studies of copolymer-bound doxorubicin and Mce_6 in nude mice bearing human ovarian carcinoma, OVCAR-3 xenografts, have been performed using high pressure liquid chromatography and spectrophotometry, respectively.[9] The circulation lifetimes of both HPMA copolymer conjugate drugs were three times longer than the respective free drugs. Tumor concentrations peaked at 18 hours post-injection with intravenous administration. Preferential accumulation of HPMA copolymer drugs in tumor tissues is attributed to the enhanced permeability and retention effect in solid tumors. [9]

In vivo studies in nude mice bearing OVCAR-3 tumors have also provided additional insight into potential optimization of treatment regimens using HPMA copolymer doxorubicin and Mce_6. The least to most effective regimens were: (1) Multiple doses of HPMA copolymer doxorubicin, (2) single HPMA copolymer Mce_6/irradiation plus multiple HPMA copolymer doxorubicin treatments, (3) multiple HPMA copolymer Mce_6/irradiation, (4) multiple HPMA copolymer Mce_6/irradiation plus multiple HPMA copolymer doxorubicin. [55] Figure 7

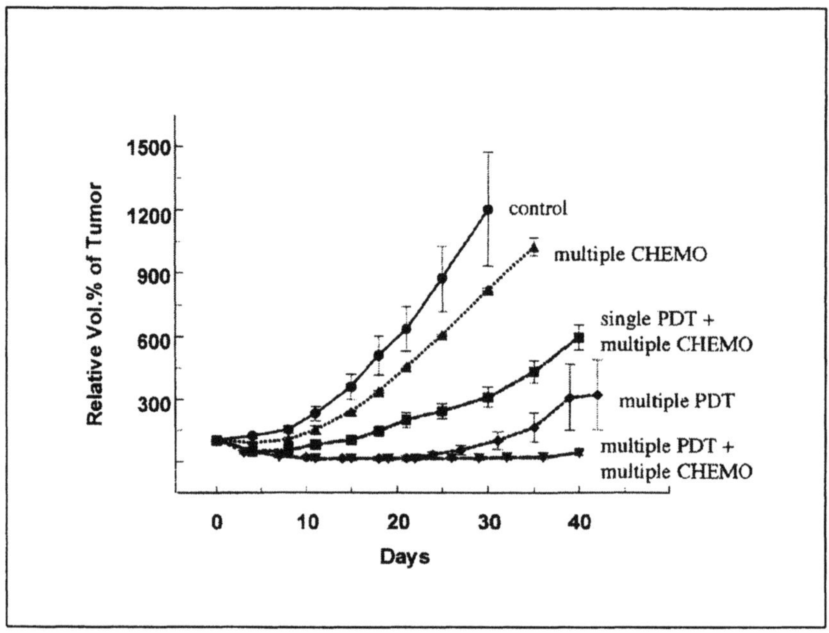

Figure 7. Growth inhibition of human ovarian OVCAR-3 carcinoma heterotransplanted in nude mice by multiple combination therapies of P-DOX (CHEMO = 2.2 mg/kg Doxorubicin equivalent) and/or PDT with P-Mce 6. The solutions were given to mice on days 0, 5, and 10. In PDT, the tumor was irradiated with laser light (110 J/cm^2, 650 nm) at 12 and 18 h, respectively, after i.v. administration of drug solution: control O; multiple CHEMO on days 0, 5, and 10; single PDTMC on day 0 plus multiple CHEMO on days 0, 5, and 10; multiple PDTMC on days 0, 5, and 10; and multiple PDTMC on days 0, 5, and 10 plus multiple CHEMO on days 0, 5, and 10. The control group received saline buffer. n = 12 tumors in each group. *Bars*, SD.

7. SUMMARY

Our studies document a unique and unexpected advantage of the combination of HPMA copolymer bound doxorubicin with mesochlorin e_6 /photodynamic therapy in the treatment of ovarian cancer. Each drug's activity is individually enhanced when compared with free (low molecular weight) drugs, furthermore, in combination these HPMA copolymer bound agents act synergistically to create an unexpected biological effect. Figure 8 depicts the known activities of each agent which may play synergistic roles.

HPMA copolymer-doxorubicin has been widely evaluated in preclinical and clinical studies. It demonstrates marked advantages over free doxorubicin: control of biodistribution and accumulation via molecular weight restrictions [10,16,35,37,45], biodegradability [16-19,24,25,39,42], minimal immunogenicity [17-19, 25,38-44], subcellular localization [15-20], anticancer activity [33-36,43-46,54,55,57], enhanced permeability and retention [9,14,57,58], increased apoptosis [36], lipid peroxidation [57], DNA damage [57], and reduced nonspecific toxicity [14,33-35,43-46]. Recent clinical trials in the UK provide "proof of principle" of the "enhanced permeability and retention effect" for solid tumors and the unique advantages of this novel drug delivery system for the treatment of ovarian cancer. [35,43-46]

With regards to photodynamic therapy using the photosensitizer mesochlorin e_6, the preclinical evaluations thus far document: control of biodistribution and accumulation via molecular weight restrictions [10,11,16,33], biodegradability [14,43], subcellular localization [15-19], anticancer activity [33,55,56], enhanced permeability and retention [55], and reduced nonspecific toxicity [33].

Ongoing microarray studies document unique cellular pathways and new pharmaceutical properties which are initiated by the HPMA copolymer delivery delivery of these agents, and predict an exciting future for this novel drug delivery system.

Figure 8. (see next page) Proposed mechanisms of the unexpected biological activity and reduced nonspecific toxicity associated with the combination of HPMA copolymer doxorubicin and mesochlorin e_6 in the treatment of ovarian cancer.

HPMA copolymer delivery of doxorubicin and mesochlorin e_6 requires internalization within membrane limited organelles (lysosomes) via pinocytosis. Because the rate of pinocytosis is slow the polymer drug conjugates are effectively confined to the blood stream. The HPMA copolymer design feature, which allows control of the molecular weight

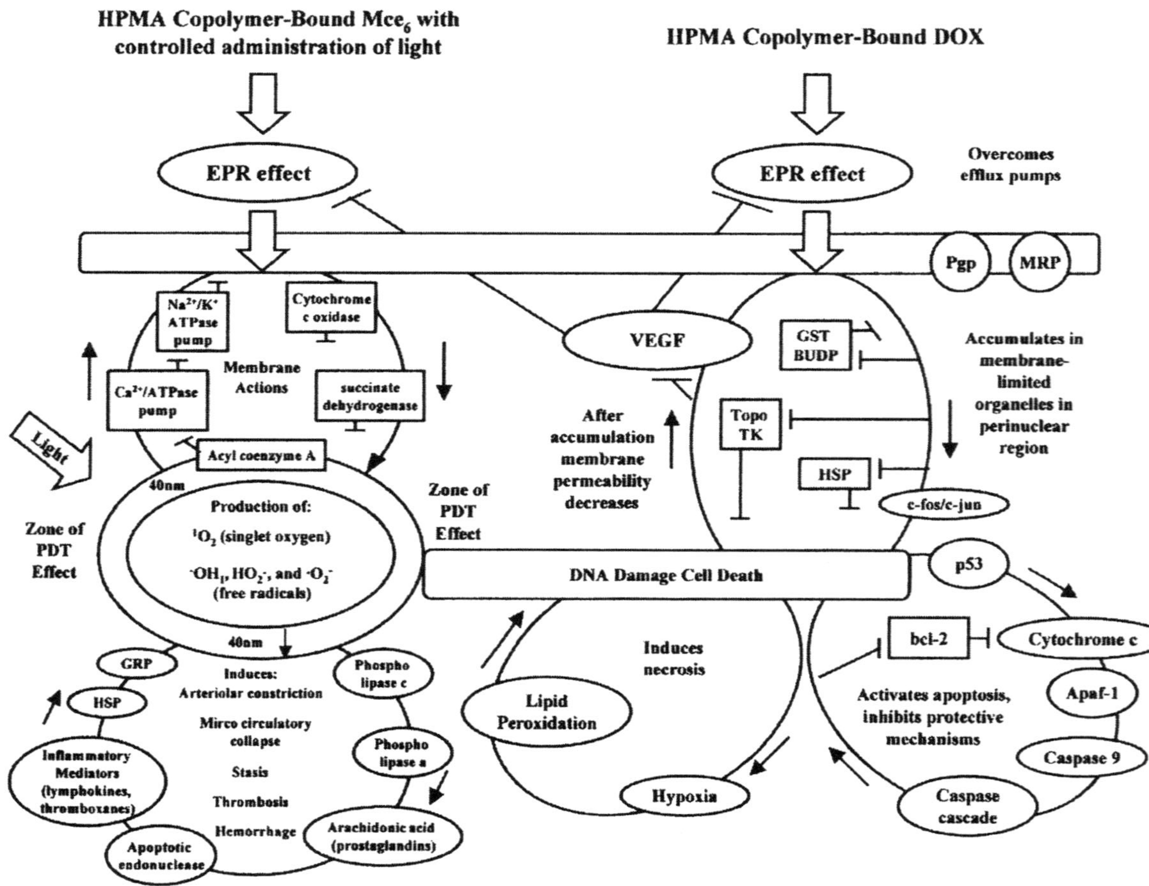
HPMA Copolymer-Bound Mce$_6$ with controlled administration of light
HPMA Copolymer-Bound DOX
EPR effect
EPR effect
Overcomes efflux pumps
Pgp
MRP
Na^{2+}/K^{+} ATPase pump
Cytochrome c oxidase
Membrane Actions
Ca^{2+}/ATPase pump
succinate dehydrogenase
Light
Acyl coenzyme A
40nm
Zone of PDT Effect
Production of:
$^1O_2$ (singlet oxygen)
$\cdot OH_1$, $HO_2\cdot$, and $\cdot O_2^-$ (free radicals)
40nm
Zone of PDT Effect
VEGF
After accumulation membrane permeability decreases
GST BUDP
Topo TK
HSP
Accumulates in membrane-limited organelles in perinuclear region
c-fos/c-jun
DNA Damage Cell Death
p53
bcl-2
Cytochrome c
Apaf-1
Caspase 9
Caspase cascade
Activates apoptosis, inhibits protective mechanisms
Induces necrosis
Lipid Peroxidation
Hypoxia
GRP
HSP
Inflammatory Mediators (lymphokines, thromboxanes)
Apoptotic endonuclease
Induces:
Arteriolar constriction
Mirco circulatory collapse
Stasis
Thrombosis
Hemorrhage
Phospho lipase c
Phospho lipase a
Arachidonic acid (prostaglandins)

to insure the size is less than the renal threshold as well as control of the degradability of the tetrapeptide (G-F-L-G) side chains, effectively avoids long term accumulation and reduces toxicity. These features are considered the primary level of selectivity- systemic in nature- which controls systemic biodistribution and reduces nonspecific toxicity. The abnormal vasculature of solid tumors, such as noted in ovarian cancer, results in an increased uptake of macromolecular drugs in tumor tissues compared to free drugs. This secondary level of selectivity or tissue selectivity is attributed to the "enhanced permeability and retention effect (EPR) of solid tumors" characterized by Maeda [23]. The EPR effect is caused by; a) abnormal vascular architecture and angiogenesis; b) increased vascular permeability due to vasoactive substances including VEGF, bFGF, bradykinin, nitric oxide, peroxynitrite, prostaglandins, cytokines, and uPA; and finally, poor lymphatic drainage.

The tetrapeptide attachment and release site (or spacer) represents the third or subcellular level of targeting. The peptide spacer (Gly- Phe- Leu- Gly-) or (G-F-L-G) has been designed to allow HPMA copolymer drug conjugates to maintain their stability in the circulation and yet maintain susceptibility to enzymatic hydrolysis in the lysozomal compartment. This subcellular delivery system overcomes the P-glycoprotein efflux pump found in multi-drug resistant ovarian carcinoma cell lines. The spacer also reduces the nonspecific toxicity of the HPMA copolymer bound doxorubicin by limiting its release to a subcellular location. While HPMA copolymer bound mesochlorin e6 is active whenever and wherever it is exposed to light the quantum yield of singlet oxygen is greater when bound to HPMA copolymer via the spacer. New approaches for enhanced targeting include the addition of antibodies or folic acid as targeting agents. These, and other molecules, will function as tissue and subcellular localizing properties of the drug delivery system.

Finally on a subcellular/molecular level, HPMA copolymer delivered agents demonstrate a unique selectivity for various structures, signaling pathways and genes. HPMA copolymer bound doxorubicin in comparison to free drug: overcomes the MDR 1 ATP driven efflux pump and down regulates the MRP gene; suppresses or activates to a lesser degree than free drug HSP-70, GST-π, BUDP, Topo II α and Topo II β genes; activates p53, Apaf-1, Caspase 9, c-fos, genes; and, inhibits the bcl-2 gene. In the case of HPMA copolymer bound mesochlorin e6, the administration of light results in the creation of singlet oxygen $^1O_2$, and the free radicals $^{\cdot}OH$, HO_2, and $O_2^{\cdot}$. Within a 40 nm radius of the photosensitizer complex, membrane structures and/or DNA may be damaged. Specifically, the following membrane activities are inactivated: cytochrome c oxidase, succinate dehydrogenase, respiration, acyl coenzyme A, Ca^{2+}/ATPase, Na^+/K^+ ATPase. A cascade of events leads to vascular endothelial damage resulting in hemorrhage, stasis-thrombosis, arteriolar constriction and microcirculatory collapse. Some of the pathways which participate in these processes include the phospholipase a and c, arachidonic acid and prostaglandin synthesis, apoptotic endonuclease, multiple inflammatory mediators, heat shock proteins, and glucose-regulated proteins. The combination of HPMA copolymer doxorubicin and mesochlorin e_6 thus results in a myriad of effects which result in the significant potentiation and unexpected biological activity of the combination compared to a simple combination of the effects of the HPMA copolymer bound agents alone.

REFERENCES

1. Oriel KA, Hartenbach EM, Remington PL. Trends in United States ovarian cancer mortality: 1979-1995. Obstet Gynecol 93:30-33 (1999).

2. NIH Consensus Development Panel. Ovarian cancer: Screening, treatment, and follow-up. JAMA 273:491-497 (1995).

3. Wolff BE, Sugarbaker RH. Intraperitoneal chemotherapy and immunotherapy. Recent Res Cancer Res 110:254-273 (1988).

4. Brenner DE. Intraperitoneal chemotherapy: A review. J Clin Oncol 4:1135-1147 (1986).

5. Yong RC, Decker DG, Wharton JT, et al. Staging laparotomy in early ovarian cancer. JAMA 250:3072 (1983).

6. Berek J. Epithelial ovarian cancer. In: Practical Gynecological Oncology, Berek JS, Hacker NS (eds), Williams and Wilkins, Philadelphia, PA, 366 (1994).

7. Advanced Ovarian Cancer Trialists Group. Chemotherapy in advanced ovarian cancer: An overview of randomized clinical trials. Br Med J 9:89 (1991).

8. Ovarian Cancer Meta-Analysis Project. Cyclophosphamide plus cisplatin versus cyclophosphamide, doxorubicin, and ciplatin chemotherapy of ovarian carcinoma: A meta-analysis. J Clin Oncol 9:1668 (1991).

9. Williams CJ. Implications of an Overview of Chemotherapy in Advanced Ovarian Carcinoma. Br J Cancer 66:225-6 (1992)

10. Putnam D, Kopecek J. Polymer conjugates with anticancer activity. Adv Polym Sci 122:55-123 (1995).

11. Reynolds T. Polymers Help Guide Cancer Drugs to Tumor Targets- Keep Them There. J Natl Cancer Inst 87:1582 (1995).

12. Matsumura Y, Maeda H. A new concept for macromolecular therapeutics in cancer chemotherpay: mechanisms of tumoritropic accumulation of proteins and antitumor agent SMANCS. Cancer Res 6: 6387 (1986).

13. Noguchi Y, Wu J, Duncan R, Strohalm J, Ulbrich K, Akaike T, Maeda H. Early phase tumor accumulation of macromolecules: A great difference in clearance rate between tumor and normal tissues. Jpn J Cancer Res 89:307-14 (1998).

14. Shiah J-G, Sun Y, Peterson CM, Kopeček J. Biodistribution of free and N-(2-hydroxypropyl)methacrylamide copolymer bound mesochlorin e_6 and adriamycin in nude Mice bearing human ovarian carcinoma OVCAR-3 xenografts. J Contr Rel 61:145-57 (1999)

15. Seymour LW, Ulbrich K, Strohalm J, Kopeček J. The pharmacokinetics of polymer-bound adriamycin, Biochem Pharmacol 39:1125-30 (1990)

16. Remanová P, Kopeček J, Duncan R, Lloyd JB. Stability in rat plasma and serum of lysosomally degradable oligopeptide sequences in N-(2-hydroxypropyl)methacrylamide) copolymers. Biomaterials 6:45-48 (1985).

17. Simekova J, Plocova, Říhová B, Kopeček J. Activation of complement in the presence of in N-(2-hydroxypropyl)methacrylamide) copolymers. J Bioact Comp Polym 1:20-31 (1986).

18. Lloyd JB, Duncan R, Kopeček J. Synthetic polymers as targetable carriers for drugs. Pure Appl Chem 56:1301-1304 (1984).

19. Kopeček J. Controlled degradability of polymers-a key to drug delivery systems. Biomaterials 5:19-25 (1984).

20. Omelyanenko V, Kopečeková P, Gentry C, Kopeček J. Targetable HPMA copolymer-adriamycin conjugates. Recognition, internalization, and subcellular fate. J Control Rel 53:25-37 (1998).

21. Slobbe R, Poels L, tenDam G, Boerman O, Nieland L, Leunissen J, Ramaekers F, VanEys G. Analysis of idiotype structure of ovarian cancer antibodies: Recognition of the

same epitope by two monoclonal antibodies differing mainly in their heavy chain variable sequences. Clin Exp Immunot 98:95-103 (1994).
22. Li S, Deshmukh HM, Huang L Folate-mediated targeting of antisense oligodeoxynucleotides to ovarian cancer cells. Pharm Res 15:1540-1545 (1998).
23. Maeda H, Seymour LM, Miyamoto Y. Conjugates of anticancer agents and polymers: Advantages of macromolecular therapeutics in vivo. Bioconjug Chem 3:351-362 (1992).
24. Duncan R. Drug-polymer conjugates:potential for improved chemotherapy. Anticancer Drugs 3:175-210 (1992).
25. Řihova R, Kopeček J, Ulbrich K, Chytry V. Immunogenicity of N-(2-hydroxypropyl)methacrylamide copolymers. Makromol Chem Suppi 9:13-24 (1985). .
26. Cuvier C, Robot-Treupel L, Millot JM, Lizard G, Chevillard S, Manfait M, Couvreur P, Poupon MF. Doxorubicin-loaded nanospheres bypass tumor cell multidrug resistance. Biochem Pharm 44:509-517 (1992).
27. Bodley AL, Liu LF. Topoisomerase as novel targets for cancer chemotherapy. Biotechnology 6:1315-1319 (1988).
28. Denny WA. DNA-intercalating ligands as anticancer drugs: prospects for future design. Anti-Cancer Drug Des 4:241-249 (1989).
29. Bristow MR, Billingham ME, Masson JW, Daniels JR. Clinical spectrum of anthracycline antibiotic cardiotoxicity. Cancer Treat Rep 62:873-878 (1978).
30. Lefrak EA, Pitha J, Rosenheim S, O'Bryan RM, Burgess MA, Gottlieb JA. Adriamycin (NSC 123127) cardiomyopathy. Cancer Chemother Rep 6:203-208 (1975).
31. Ogura R, Sugiyama M, Haramaki N, Hidaka T. Electron spin resonance studies on the mechanism of Adriamycin-induced heart mitochondrial damages. CancerRes 51:3555-3558 (1991).
32. Lu JM, Peterson CM Sun Y, Peterson CA, Shiah J-G, Straight RC, Kopeček J. Cooperativity between free and N-(2-hydroxypropyl)methacrylamide copolymer bound adriamycin and mesochlorin e6 monoethylene diamine induced photodynamic therapy in human epithelial ovarian carcinoma in vitro. Int J Oncol 15:5-16 (1999).
33. Peterson CM, Lu JM, Sun Y, Peterson CA, Shiah JG, Straight RC, Kopeček J. Combination chemotherapy and photodynamic therapy with N-(2-hydroxypropyl)methacrylamide copolymer-bound anticancer drugs inhibit human ovarian carcinoma heterotransplanted in nude mice. Clin Cancer Res 56:83-94 (1999).
34. Duncan R, Kopečeková P, Strohalm J, Hume IC, Lloyd JB, Kopeček J. Anticancer agents coupled to N-(2-hydroxyprophyl)methacrylamide copolymers 2. Evaluation of daunomycin conjugates in vivo against L1210 leukaemia. Brit J Cancer 57:147-156 (1988).
35. Vasey P, Twelves C, Kaye S, Wilson P, Morrison R, Duncan R, Thomson A, Hilditch T, Murray T, Burtles S, Cassidy J. Phase I clinical and pharmacokinetic study of PK1 (HPMA copolymer doxorubicin): first member of a new class of chemotherapeutic agents: drug-polymer conjugates. Clin Cancer Res 5: 83-94 (1999).
36. Minko T, Kopečeková P, Kopeček J. Comparison of the anticancer effect of free and HPMA copolymer-bound adriamycin in human ovarian carcinoma cells. Pharm Res 16:986-996 (1999).
37. Seymour LW, Duncan R, Strohalm J, Kopeček J. Effect of molecular weight (Mw) of of N-(2-hydroxypropyl) methacrylamide copolymers on body distribution and rate of excretion after subcutaneous, intraperitoneal and intravenous administration to rats. J J Biomed Mater Res 21:1341-58 (1987).
38. Řihová B, Ulbrich K, Kopeček J, Mančal P. The immunogenicty of N-(2-hydroxypropyl) methacrylamide copolymers-potential hapten or drug carriers. Folia Microbiol 28:217-27 (1983).

39. Řihová B, Kopeček J, Ulbrich K, Pospišil M, Mančal P. Effect of the chemical structure of N-(2-hydroxypropyl) methacrylamide copolymers on their ability to induce antibody formation in inbred strains of mice. Biomaterials 5: 143-8 (1984).
40. Řihová B, Kopeček J, Ulbrich K, Chytry V. Immunogenicity of N-(2-hydroxypropyl) methacrylamide copolymers. Makromol. Chem Supl 9:13-24 (1995).
41. Simeckova J, Řihová B, Plocová D, Kopeček J. Activity of complement in the presence of N-(2-hydroxypropyl) methacrylamide copolymers. J Bioact Compat Polymers 1:20-31 (1986).
42. Řihová B, Bilej M, Větvička V. Biocompatibility of N-(2-hydroxypropyl) methacrylamide copolymers containing doxorubicin. Biomaterials. 10:335-42 (1989).
43. Vasey PA, Duncan R, Kaye SB, Cassidy J. Phase 1 clinical and pharmacokinetic study of PK1 (N-(2-hydroxypropyl)methacrylamide copolymer doxorubicin): first member of a new class of chemotherapeutic agents-drug polymer conjugates. EROTC Abstract
44. Duncan R, Seymour LW, O'Hare KB, Flanagan PA, Wedge S, Ulbrich K, Strohalm J, Subr V, Spreafico F, Grandi M, Ripamonti M, Farao M, Suarato A. Preclinical evaluation of polymer bound doxorubicin. J Controlled Rel 19: 331-46 (1992).
45. Thomson AH, Vasey PA, Murray LS, Cassidy J, Fraier D, Frigerio E, Twleves C. Population pharmacokinetics in phase I drug development: a phase I study of PK1 in patients with solid tumors. Br J Ca 81:99-107 (1999).
46. Loadman PM, Bibby MC, Double JA, Al-Shakhaa WM, Duncan R. Pharmacokinetics of PK1 and doxorubicin in experimental colon tumor models with differing responses to PK1. Clin Cancer Res 5:3682-8 (1999)
47. Peterson CM , Reed R, Jolles CJ, Jones KP, Straight RC, Poulson AM. Photodynamic therapy of human ovarina epithelial carcinoma, OVCAR-3, heterotransplanted in the nude mouse. Am J Obstet Gynecol 167:1852-5 (1992).
48. Chaplin DJ. The effect of photodynamic therapy on tumor vascular function. Int J Radiat Biol 60:311-325 (1991).
49. Feyh J, Goetz A, Heiman A, Konigsberger R, Kastenbauer E. Microcirculatory effects of photodynamic therapy with hematoporphyrin derivative. Laryngo-Rhino-Otol 70:99-101 (1991).
50. Moan J. Porphyrin-sensitized photodynamic inactivation of cells: A review. Lasers Med Sci 1:5-12 (1986).
51. Kennedy JC, Nadeau P, Petryka ZJ, Pottier RH, Weagle G. Clearance times of photophyrin derivatives from mice as measured by in vivo fluorescence spectroscopy. Photochem Photobiol 55:729-734 (1992).
52. Shiah J-G, Koňák Č, Spikes JD, Kopeček J. Influence of pH on aggregation and photoproperties of N-(2-hydroxypropyl)methacrylamide copolymer-meso chlorin e6 conjugates. Drug Delivery 5:119-26 (1998)
53. Brophy PF, Keller SM. Adriamycin enhanced in vitro and in vivo photodynamic therapy of mesothelioma. J Surg Res 52:631-634 (1992).
54. Peterson CM, Lu JM, Gu ZW, Shiah JG, Lythgoe K, Peterson CA, Straight RC, Kopeček J. Isobolographic assessment between adriamycin and photodynamic therapy with meso-chlorin e_6 monoethylene diaamine in human ovarian carcinoma (OVCAR-3) in vivo. J Soc Gynecol Invest 2:772-777 (1995).
55. Shiah J-G, Sun Y, Peterson CM, Straight RC, Kopeček J. Antitumor activity of HPMA copolymer mesochlorin e_6 and adriamycin in combination treatments. Clin Cancer Res 6:1008-15 (2000).
56. Krinick NL, Sun Y, Joyner D, Spikes JD, Straight RC, Kopeček J. A polymeric drug delivery system for the simultaneous delivery of drugs activatable by enzymes and/or light. J Biomat Sci, Polym Ed 5:303-324 (1994).

57. Minko T, Kopečekova, Kopeček J. Efficacy of the chemotherapeutic action of HPMA copolymer-bound doxorubicin in a solid tumor model of ovarian carcinoma. Int J Cancer 86:108-17 (2000).
58. Minko T, Kopečeková P, Pozharov V, Jensen KD, Kopeček J. The influence of cytotoxicity of macromolecules and of VEGF gene modulated vascular permeability and retention effect in resistant solid tumor. Pharm Res 17:505-14 (2000).

Drug-HPMA-HuIg Conjugates Effective Against Human Solid Cancer

BLANKA ŘÍHOVÁ[*], JIŘÍ STROHALM[#], KATEŘINA KUBÁČKOVÁ[^], MARKÉTA JELÍNKOVÁ[*], LAĎKA ROZPRIMOVÁ[+], MILADA ŠÍROVÁ[*], DANA PLOCOVÁ[#], TOMÁŠ MRKVAN[*], MAREK KOVÁŘ[*], JINDŘIŠKA POKORNÁ[*], TOMÁŠ ETRYCH[#], KAREL ULBRICH[#]

**Institute of Microbiology, Academy of Sciences of the Czech Republic, Vídeňská 1083, 142 20 Prague 4, Czech Republic; # Institute of Macromolecular Chemistry, Academy of Sciences of the Czech Republic, Heyrovsky sq.2, 16206 Prague 6, Czech Republic; ^The University Hospital Motol, V úvalu 84, 150 18 Prague 5, Czech Republic, + AGILAB-Biochemical and Immunological Laboratory, Jeseniova 101, 130 00 Prague 3, Czech Republic*

1. INTRODUCTION

Patients whose tumors fail to respond to conventional therapy or whose tumors have become refractory to classical chemotherapy might be eligible for investigation protocols and/or for new approaches in the treatment of cancer. One of them is affinity therapy based on water-soluble synthetic polymeric carriers. In such macromolecular systems the drug is either complexed with a carrier or covalently bound to a carrier that is targeted or non-targeted. Targeting can be either active or passive. Active targeting means that the drug conjugate contains a ligand complementary to the receptor on the target cell. Passive targeting is due to the a) increased permeability of vascular discontinuous endothelium in tumors that allows extravasation of high-molecular weight material and to the b) poor lymphatic drainage that limits elimination of accumulated macromolecules from tumors. This phenomenon is called Enhanced Permeability and Retention effect (EPR effect) according to Maeda and Matsumura[1]. The advantages of polymer-bound drugs in affinity therapy are a) increased pharmacological efficacy, b) increased MTD, c) decreased non-specific toxicity, d) controlled biodistribution, e) long-lasting circulation in bloodstream, f) ability to partially overcome MDR and g) immunoprotection and immunomobilization. The demonstration that macromolecular systems based on synthetic polymers can be both a powerful anti-cancer agent and an inducer of anti-tumor immunity[2, 3] is extremely important as the immune system of cancer patients is usually exhausted by extensive growth of the malignant cells and by an intensive classical chemotherapy or radiotherapy.

1.1 Initial Comments

Water-soluble [*N*-(2-hydroxypropyl)methacrylamide] (PHPMA) copolymer represents an efficient synthetic polymeric carrier to which a drug and an actively/passively targeting moiety is conjugated through biodegradable peptidyl linker, mostly GlyPheLeuGly[4]. We and others[5-19] have demonstrated the efficacy of PHPMA-bound doxorubicin, daunomycin, farmorubicin, methotrexate, 5-fluorouracil and chlorin e_6 non-targeted or targeted with monoclonal and polyclonal antibodies, carbohydrates and lectins against numerous cancer cell lines *in vitro* and experimental tumors *in vivo*. The targeted or non-targeted water-soluble conjugate is non-active during transport in bloodstream and tissue fluids[20] as the drug is released and activated only intracellularly after enzymatic cleavage of the bond between the drug and the oligopeptidic side-chain by lysosomal cysteine proteinases[21]. It was shown that HPMA copolymer-bound doxorubicin partially overcomes energy-driven P-glycoprotein efflux pump found in some multi-drug resistant (MDR) cancer cell lines[22, 23] and has considerably reduced non-specific toxicity including hepatotoxicity[24], nephrotoxicity[25], cardiotoxicity[24, 26], myelotoxicity[24, 27] and toxicity against thymus[28, 29]. Recently, we have reported a new evidence that PHPMA-bound drugs, unlike free drugs, have both cytostatic and immunomobilizing activity (CIA)[3].

The reduction of circulating lymphocytes generally seen in patients with advanced cancer reflects their immunosuppressive conditions. There is evidence to suggest that immunosuppression favors the growth of at least some existing malignant cells[30]. Thus, in this study we first address the question of the targeting and/or immunostimulatory effect of human immunoglobulin (HuIg) bound to PHPMA carrier with doxorubicin. Intravenous Ig (IVIg; HuIg) is the human serum Ig that is mainly composed of IgG prepared from plasma pools of thousands of healthy blood donors. It was demonstrated[31] that administration of IVIg to mice inoculated with melanoma or sarcoma cells induced a statistically significant inhibition of metastatic lung foci and prolongation of survival time. *In vitro* studies revealed that IVIg stimulates the production of IL-12, a cytokine with significant effect on the tumor-specific immune response. Since IVIg has only minor side effects and it is used extensively in other clinical conditions, it may be considered as a potential therapy for the prevention of tumor spread in humans[31]. Proposed mechanisms for anti-metastatic effects of normal polyspecific immunoglobulin G (IVIg; HuIg) are a) the presence of natural antibodies in the serum directed to the cytoplasm, nuclear membrane and cell membrane of different malignant tumors and/or the presence of antinuclear antibodies (ANA)[32]. Both types of antibodies could be responsible for direct antibody-dependent cytotoxicity (ADCC) or for complement-dependent lysis of cancer cells, b) the ability to enhance defense mechanisms of the host by stimulation of IL-12 an other anti-tumor and anti-angiogenic cytokines, c) the potential to activate NK cells, and d) the increase of MW of the conjugates, i.e. the EPR effect.

2. SYNTHESIS OF DOXORUBICIN-PHPMA-HUIG CONJUGATE

N-(2-Hydroxypropyl)methacrylamide (HPMA) was prepared by methacryloylation of 1-aminopropan-2-ol in methylene chloride. Methacryloylglycyl-DL-phenylalanyl-L-leucylglycine 4-nitrophenyl ester (Ma-Gly-Phe(D,L)-Leu-Gly-ONp) was prepared by methacryloylation of glycylphenylalanine and conjugation with leucylglycine methyl ester followed by hydrolysis and esterification with 4-nitrophenol using a procedure described by Ulbrich at al.[33]. The product was chromatographically pure (HPLC, LDC Analytical, USA, a reversed-phase column Tessek SGX C18 (150 x 3 mm), UV detection, methanol-water, gradient 50-100 vol.-% methanol, flow rate 0.5mL/min). Amino acid analysis (LDC Analytical, USA; precolumn OPA derivatisation):Gly:L-Phe:D-Phe:L-Leu = 2.03:0.52:0.47:1.00.

The conjugate was prepared from polymer precursor I, a copolymer of HPMA with Ma-Gly-Phe(D,L)-Leu-Gly-ONp (prepared by radical precipitation copolymerisation in acetone, initiator AIBN, 0.6 wt%; concentration of monomers 12.5 wt%, 60 °C, 24 h)[33] containing 8.6 %mol ONp groups. 1,47g doxorubicin.HCl (2.53 . 10^{-3} mol) and 16,43 g polymer precursor I (M_w = 25 000; M_w/M_n = 1.4; ONp mol % = 8.6) was dissolved in 108 mL DMF under stirring. 0,643 g (6.35 . 10^{-3}) mol triethylamine dissolved in 10 mL DMF was added in 4 portions within 30 min. The reaction was carried out in the dark. The reaction mixture was stirred for 2 h at 25 °C, the polymer was precipitated into 4 L of acetone:diethylether mixture (2:1), isolated by filtration and reprecipitated from methanol (70 mL) into the same mixture of solvents. The product containing doxorubicin (Dox) and rest of reactive groups (polymer precursor II) was isolated by filtration, washed twice with acetone, diethylether and dried in vacuum.

13,1g of the doxorubicin-containing polymer precursor II (M_w = 26 000; M_w/M_n = 1.4; ONp mol % = 4.1; doxorubicin wt % = 5.8) was dissolved in 400 mL of distilled water at 5 °C, the pH of the solution was adjusted to 7 using end-point titrator (sodium tetraborate) and a solution of 4,73 g HuIg in 110 mL of water was added. In the patient D.H. (for all injections) and in patient E.G. (for first and half of the second injection) we used as HuIg autologous IgG isolated from the sera by precipitation with 40% ammonium sulfate followed by extensive dialysis against distilled water and PBS (pH 7.35). Isolated IgG was then centrifuged 15 min at 12 000 rpm and aggregate-free was used for a conjugation to polymer precursor II. Allogeneic human γ-globulin (HuIg) was Intraglobin F from Biotest Pharma. The mixture was stirred 1 h at 12 °C at pH 7.8, another 4 h at 20 °C and pH 8, and the reaction was completed within next 15 h at pH 8.3 and 15 °C. Aqueous solution of 1-amino-2-propanol was added and after 30 min, pH was adjusted to 6.8 by 0.1 M HCl. The product was purified on GPC column (5 x 80 cm) packed with Sephadex G-25 using water or saline (Infusia 1/1). Concentration of the polymer drug in a sterile, non-pyrogenic saline was adjusted to 0.5 mg Dox equivalent in 1 mL and after sterilization through Millipore filter (0.22 μ) used for infusion. Aqueous solution was freeze-dried and polymer drug stored as lyophilisate at 4 °C.

Polymer precursors I and II were characterized by UV spectrophotometry (the content of oligopeptide side chains terminating in 4-nitrophenoxy groups, λ = 274 nm, ε = 9 600 L $mol^{-1}.cm^{-1}$, DMSO), by amino acid analysis (LDC Analytical, USA; precolumn OPA derivatization) and by liquid chromatography (weight- and number-average molecular weights, M_w and M_n) after aminolysis of reactive groups with 1-aminopropan-2-ol. Polymer-Dox conjugate was characterized and tested for the content of free polymer, free drug or protein by FPLC Pharmacia equipped with Superose 6 column (RI and UV detectors) and by electrophoresis (Pharmacia-LKB Fast System, SDS PAGE, gels with gradient 4 – 15). Molecular weights of the final conjugate and polymer precursors were determined using LC AKTA-Pharmacia equipped with Superose 6 or TSK 5000 PW columns and RI (refractive index) and multiangle light scattering DAWN-DSP-F (Wyatt Technology Corp.) detectors. The protein content in the conjugate was estimated by amino acid analysis (LDC Analytical, USA; precolumn OPA derivatisation) and Dox content by UV spectrophotometry (water, ε = 11 500 L mol^{-1} cm^{-1}, λ = 488 nm). Neither GPC nor electrophoresis showed significant amounts of free protein in the conjugates and the content of free Dox in the conjugate was less than 0.05% of the total Dox content. Polymer conjugate characterization: M_w = 660 000; M_w/M_n approx. 4; Dox, wt % = 4.35; HuIg, wt % = 25. All conjugates were free of the endotoxin (proven by LAL Assay).

3. PATIENT CASES

One patient (D. H.) with biopsy-proven, generalized angiosarcoma and four patients (E. G., J. K., K. R. and K. H.) with biopsy-proven, generalized breast carcinoma were treated with drug-PHPMA-HuIg.

In August 1990 a 28-year-old female (D.H.) underwent orthotopic heart transplantation for angiosarcoma. After surgery she was treated with conventional combination adjuvant chemotherapy (vincristin, cyclophosphamid, actinomycin D, holoxan and uromitexan). In August 1991 she was found to have developed secondary tumors in lungs. Selected chemotherapy with farmorubicin, cosmegen and cyclophosphamid did not stop the progression of the disease (in October 1991 the progression of secondary tumors in lungs was noted and metastases in soft tissues were discovered) and she was given high-dose combination chemotherapy with ifosfamid, uromitexan, dacarbazin and farmorubicin. In June 1992 computer tomography confirmed multiple tumors in the brain and it was decided to start palliative experimental therapy with HPMA copolymer-bound farmorubicin containing targeting autologous IgG, where specific antibodies against biopsy from soft tissue metastases were proven by ELISA test. At the end of June 1992 the patient was infused three times with farmorubicin-PHPMA-HuIg conjugate (total dose of farmorubicin was 265mg /m^2).

A 36-year-old patient E. G. had found by self-examination a tumor that was later on diagnosed as a breast carcinoma and mastectomy was performed with exenteration of axilla. She received three cycles of adjuvant chemotherapy of FAC (5-FU, adriamycin, cyclophosphamide), followed by three cycles of CMF (cyclophosphamide, methotrexate, prednison). Four years later she developed solitary bone metastases for which she received tamoxifen. Later, due to the progressive disease and increase in serum tumor markers she was treated with aminoglutetimid and then with anastrazol. One year later, multiple metastases in liver and bone were diagnosed and systemic treatment was started with combination of docetaxel and vinorelbin. The response to the chemotherapy was modest and after four cycles ultrasound scan confirmed a new progression in the liver. From October 2000 she suffered from worsening of visus with progression to amaurosis. A month later a stereotactic irradiation was performed for metastases to gyri orbitales. In November 2000 she started palliative therapy with Dox-PHPMA-HuIg. She was infused five times (30/11/00; 19/12/00;

9/1/01; 3/4/01; 24/4/01) with 99 mg Dox/m^2/dose (total dose of doxorubicin was 495 mg/m^2). Due to technical problems, autologous IgG was used as a targeting moiety (HuIg) only for the first treatment and half of the second treatment. Conventional IVIg (Intraglobin F, Biotest Pharma) was used for the half of the second treatment and for the third, fourth and fifth treatment.

A 51-year-old female J. K. underwent mastectomy with exenteration of axilla for multifocal breast carcinoma infiltrating axillary lymph nodes. The patient received six cycles of adjuvant treatment with adriamycin, 5-fluorouracil and cyclophosphamide following with tamoxifen. A liver metastatic disease was diagnosed and confirmed by laparotomy one year latter and the patient was treated with three cycles of docetaxel and vinorelbine, then with capecitabine but without substantial effect on liver metastases. It was decided to start palliative therapy with Dox-PHPMA-HuIg. Patient was infused five times (3/4/01; 30/4/01; 5/6/01; 10/7/01; 14/8/01) with 148 mg Dox/m^2/dose (total dose of doxorubicin was 740 mg/m^2). For all courses was used as a targeting moiety conventional IVIg (HuIg; Intraglobin F, Biotest Pharma).

Similarly, a 36-year-old patient K. R. underwent mastectomy with exenteration of axilla for breast carcinoma infiltrating axillary lymph nodes. The patient was treated with four regular and one mobilizing cycle of adjuvant FAC chemotherapy (5-fluorouracil, adriamycin, cyclophosphamide). One month after the last cycle she was given a mobilizing dose of G-GSF with the aim of receiving graft for the tandem autologous stem cell transplantation (A-SCT). Six weeks after successful A-SCT she underwent aktinotherapy (total dose 50 Gy) and was treated with Tamoxifen and seventeen times with Herceptin (the total dose 2550 mg) without a significant effect on the progression of the disease, however. In February 2002 she started with palliative therapy with Dox-PHPMA-HuIg. She was infused four times (12/2/02; 12/3/02; 9/4/02; 9/7/02) with 148 mg Dox/m^2/dose (total dose of doxorubicin was 592 mg/m^2). Conventional IVIg (HuIg; Intraglobin F, Biotest Pharma) was used as a targeting moiety for 4 courses.

A 42-year-old patient K. H. underwent in 1995 radical mastectomy for infiltrating ductal breast carcinoma that was followed by adjuvant chemotherapy with FAC and aktinotherapy. In 2000 generalized breast carcinoma was diagnosed followed with the treatment with Taxol, Navelbin and Herceptin without a substantial effect on the progression of the disease. Thus, in April 2002 it was decided to start palliative therapy with Dox-PHPMA-HuIg (Intraglobin F was used as a targeting moiety). She has been as yet infused three times (9/4/02; 7/5/02; 4/6/02) with 148 mg Dox/m^2/dose (total dose of doxorubicin was 450 mg/m^2).

Patient E. G. was hospitalized only for the first course, receiving further courses of Dox-PHPMA-HuIg as an outpatient similarly as patients J. K., K.R. and K.H. No administration-related toxicity of tested conjugates was observed. Blood samples were drawn from all patients 24 h, 48 h, 72 h, 7 d, 14 d, 21 d, 28 d and eight weeks after the infusion and immediately checked for more than 116 biochemical and immunological parameters.

Before participating in experimental palliative therapy all patients gave written informed consent. The study was approved by the Ethics Committee of the Institute of Clinical and Experimental Medicine (patient D. H.) and by the Ministry of Health of the Czech Republic (patients E. G., J. K., K. R. and K. H).

4. CLINICAL PROTOCOL

4.1 The effect of treatment with farmorubicin-PHPMA-HuIg on patient with metastatic angiosarcoma

Patient D. H. was treated with the conjugate containing synthetic copolymer three times without any signs of intolerance. Ninety five percent reduction in the number of secondary lung tumors and disappearance of metastases in soft tissue indicated the therapeutic potential of the conjugate. In fact, at that progressive stage of the disease farmorubicin-PHPMA-HuIg was the only cytostatic with obvious anti-tumor effect. Moreover, an immunoprotective character of the conjugate was documented for the first time in a human being. Application of free farmorubicin caused in the patient, who was heavily immunosuppressed due to heart transplantation, a deep agranulocytosis and drop in peripheral blood reticulocytes. For the restoration of a normal blood count it was necessary to apply GM-CSF (Neupogen) as a growth factor stimulating bone marrow stem cells. On the other hand, the treatment with farmorubicin-PHPMA-HuIg did not show significant myelotoxicity. The drop in peripheral blood reticulocytes was very low and transient. In a few days the normal blood count was restored without any additional treatment with growth factors. The patient died as a consequence of brain metastases progression[3, 34].

4.2 The effect of treatment with doxorubicin-PHPMA-HuIg on patients with advanced breast cancer

4.2.1 Biochemical data; liver tests and tumor markers

ALP (alkaline phosphatase) as a marker for bone involvement decreased in the patient E. G. continuously, which correlated well with the findings on the bone scan. From the third cycle on we have detected also a considerable decrease in liver transaminases; ALT, alanine aminotransferase, GMT, glutamyl transpeptidase and AST, aspartate aminotransferase (Table 1)[34]. Only slightly elevated levels of AST and ALT and a normal level of ALP was seen in patient J. K. Similarly as in patient E.G., normal values were reached during the first and the second course of the treatment. The value of GMT (three times above the normal value at the beginning) decreased by 50%. In patients K. R. and K. H. the liver test were almost normal during the whole therapeutic follow-up with no significant changes.

Table 1. Plasma concentration of AST, ALT, GMT and ALP in the patient E.G.

		AST µkat/L	ALT µkat/L	GMT µkat/L	ALP µkat/L
Normal value		<0.50	<0.55	<0.60	<2.80
Patient E. G.					
Before the treatment		1.27	2.12	10.12	6.80
First application	72 h	0.99	1.90	11.44	8.31
Fifth application	72 h	1.15	0.99	3.42	4.24

C-reactive protein (CRP) is one of the acute phase plasma proteins that are adaptively regulated in response to most forms of inflammation, infection and tissue injury and represents a valuable objective marker of disease activity[35, 36]. In normal healthy subjects CRP is a trace plasma protein. In response to bacterial infection, trauma, tissue necrosis, most forms of inflammation and malignant neoplasia CRP production is rapidly and dramatically increased. Such an increase is often associated with dissemination of the disease and with a poor prognosis for cancer patients[37, 38]. Elevated serum level of CRP is also significantly related to the reduction of lymphocytes in peripheral blood and can be an indicator of impaired immunity[39] and there is also evidence that in particular circumstances CRP may have proinflammatory activity, but there is little to suggest that this is a general phenomenon. CRP concentration drops rapidly to the normal with remission of pathology, either spontaneous or in response to the treatment. However, as a result of controversial data, the function(s) of CRP in health and disease is still unknown. They may well be multiple, and include modulation of inflammation, participation in handling of damaged or dead cells and involvement in lipid metabolism.

In patient E. G. serum CRP level that was eight times higher that the normal value before application of Dox-PHPMA-HuIg decreased after the treatment very rapidly. Seventy two hours after the first administration the patient had in her serum only one third of the pre-treatment value of CRP and in one week this level reached a normal level and remained in the physiological rates during the whole therapeutic follow-up[34] (Table 2). On the other hand, we have seen quite normal values of CRP in the patient J. K. and only transiently elevated levels of CRP in the patient K. R. (9.4mg/L 28 days after the second treatment, 10.5 mg/L 28 days after the third treatment, 27.8 mg/L 28 days after the fourth treatment). Quite a different result was obtained in the patient K.H. Before the treatment, she had a physiological serum level of CRP (7. 8 mg/L). Three days after the first treatment, the level of CRP surged to a nearly ten times higher value (56.4 mg/L) that again dropped back to the normal level (7.4 mg/L) in the following weeks. The increase in the CRP level 72 h after the treatment was seen also after the second and after the third treatment where the elevation was not so dramatic (Table 2a).

Tumor markers have a diagnostic and prognostic value. Their appearance in the peripheral blood is useful for monitoring the treatment and cancer course. We have tested nine tumor markers, among them β_2-microglobulin, α-fetoprotein (AFP), CA 72-4, ferritin, CA 125, CA 15-3, CA 19-9, carcinoembryonic antigen (CEA) and neuron-specific enolase (NSE). AFP and CEA belong to the so-called "oncofetal" antigens, which are normally found in fetal tissues and plasma and are present only in very small quantities in normal adult subjects. CEA expression is most frequently associated with adenocarcinoma of colon, breast and lung. Estimation of CEA plasma level represents a good method for the detection of disseminated breast cancer cells as its decrease reflects partial remissions of the metastases[40]. Ferritin is a non-specific tumor marker that belongs, similarly as CRP, to the "positive acute phase proteins". It is particularly suitable for monitoring Hodgkin lymphoma and melanoma but pathologically increased levels are observed also in colorectal and breast cancer. In patient E.G., significantly elevated levels of five tumor markers, i.e. β_2-microglobulin, CA 72-4, ferritin, CA 125 and CEA decreased continuously during the treatment and either dropped to the normal value permanently (β_2-microglobulin 24 h after the first treatment, CA 72-4 and ferritin three weeks after the second treatment) or temporarily (the level of CA 125 was physiological before and three weeks after the fourth treatment, the level of CEA reached physiological level fourteen days after the third treatment and was almost normal six weeks after the fifth treatment) (Table

2, 3). CA 15-3 is a conventional serum marker sensitive for disseminated breast cancer cells and its decrease in the serum reflects partial remission of the disease[40-42].

Table 2. Plasma concentration of CRP, β_2-microglobulin, CA 72-4 and ferritin in the patient E.G.

	CRP mg/L	β_2-microglobulin mg/L	CA 72-4 KIU/L	ferritin g/mL
Normal value	<8.0	0.80-1.90	<2.5	24-160
Patient E. G.				
Before the treatment	63.0	2.09	3.4	247
First application 72 h	21.0	1.48	3.7	309
Fifth application 72 h	2.0	1.48	0.6	55

Table 2a. Plasma concentration of CRP (mg/L) in the patient K.H.

application	Ist			IInd			IIIrd		
	72h	7d	28d	72h	7d	28d	72h	7d	28d
	56.4*	13.6	7.4	50.0	10.3	5.9	15.9	13.0	5.4

*normal value = < 8.0 mg/L

Serum levels of CA 15-3, NSE and AFP were not normalized during the treatment but their movement towards physiological values was quite obvious (Table 3). The only tumor marker whose level increased during the treatment with polymeric conjugate was CA 19-9[34].

Comparison of the effect of free and polymer-bound drug on some biochemical and immunological data was possible in the patient J. K. who experienced one course of free doxorubicin given in January 2001. Before the treatment, ALP and all liver transaminases, i.e. AST, ALT and GMT, were slightly above the normal values. AST reached physiological value 72 h up to seven days after the treatment with free drug and ALT reached physiological value 72 h after the treatment with free drug and beginning with the second treatment with polymer-bound drug during the whole therapeutic follow-up. After the treatment with free drug the physiological level of ALP increased and was still high before the treatment with polymer-bound drug. Physiological values were recorded only in samples taken during the second and third course with Dox-PHPMA-HuIg[34].

In contrast to patient E.G., serum levels of β_2-microglobulin, AFP, CA 72-4, ferritin, CA 125, CA 19-9 and CEA were and stayed physiological. Elevated serum levels of CA 15-3 and NSE decreased both after the treatment with free doxorubicin and after the treatment with Dox-PHPMA-

HuIg and the decrease was substantial. The value of CA 15-3 reached half of the pre-treatment value already after the third treatment with polymeric drug and continuous decrease was recorded until the end of the therapeutic follow-up, i.e. one month after the fifth treatment. The decrease of serum level of NSE was quite obvious already in the sample taken before the second treatment with polymer-bound drug and, similarly as with CA 15-3, continuous decrease was recorded until the end of the therapeutic follow-up. Only transient drop to the normal value was seen one month after the third treatment[34]. In the patient K. R., only CEA, CA 15-3 and ferritin had pathological values before application of the polymeric drug and no significant response to the treatment was seen. Pathological values of β_2-microglobulin, AFP, CEA, CA 125, CA 15-3, ferritin and NSE were detected before the treatment in patient K. H., with a substantial decrease (by at least 50%) during the treatment in β_2-microglobulin, CEA, CA 125 and CA 15-3. AFP, ferritin and NSE reached a normal value four weeks after the third treatment.

Table 3. Plasma concentration of CA 15-3, CEA and NSE in the patient E.G.

		CA 15-3 KIU/L	CEA µg/L	NSE µg/L
Normal value		<22.0	<5.0	1.0-13.0
Patient E. G.				
Before the treatment		660.0	11.6	N. D.
First application	72 h	790.0	11.8	N. D.
	14 d	840.0	8.9	124.6
Fifth application	72 h	554.0	6.4	84.2
	48 d	380.3	5.0	48.9

4.2.2 Hematological and immunological data

In the blood count a light anemia and leukopenia was apparent in all patients throughout the treatment courses. We have detected a lower absolute number of T lymphocytes and cytotoxic T cells ($CD8^+$ cells) in patients E. G. and J. K. and normal number in patients K. R. and K. H. A slightly increased number of T helper cells ($CD4^+$ cells) and a significant increase of $CD16^+56^+$ cells representing natural killer (NK) cells were seen in all patients. In the patient J. K. such an increase of $CD16^+56^+$ cells was recorded only after the treatment with polymer-bound drug. On the other hand, before and during the treatment the number of $CD19^+$ cells (B lymphocytes) was low in all patients, without a significant response to the application of free or polymer-bound form of doxorubicin. Reticulocytes in the peripheral blood reflect the status of patient's bone marrow. In the patient J.K. who received both forms of the drug, i.e. free and polymer-bound doxorubicin, it was possible to directly compare their effect on reticulocytes. While the treatment with free drug resulted in a significant decrease detectable already 24 h after the treatment and decreased reticulocyte count was recorded at least three weeks, the number of reticulocytes was stable throughout the five treatments with Dox-PHPMA-HuIg. Surprisingly, an increase of peripheral blood reticulocytes was observed in patients E. G., K. R. and K. H. (Table 4)[34].

Table 4. Reticulocytes in peripheral blood*

		patient			
Normal value		E. G.	J. K.	K. R.	K. H.
5-15					
Before the treatment with free drug		ND	16	ND	ND
First treatment	24 h	ND	3	ND	ND
	48 h	ND	5	ND	ND
	72 h	ND	7	ND	ND
	7 d	ND	12	ND	ND
	14 d	ND	8	ND	ND
	21 d	ND	10	ND	ND
Before the first treatment with polymer-bound drug		8	13	2	3
First treatment	72 h	9	16	7	3
	7 d	4	14	4	4
	14 d	10	17	ND	ND
Before the last treatment with polymer-bound drug		15	11	9	5
Last treatment	72 h	16	13	4	5
	7 d	14	12	4	5
	14 d	14	16	7	18

* ‰ of total erythrocytes

4.2.3 Activity of NK and LAK cells

Natural killer (NK) cells are spontaneously cytotoxic immune effector cells with the ability to selectively destroy tumor cells and virus-infected cells without harming normal cells. Chronically low levels of NK activity are seen in cancer, acquired or congenital immunodeficiency disease (AIDS) and in severe life-threatening viral infections (HSV, EBV, CMV). LAK cells are either T or NK cells that have been activated by interleukin 2 or other cytokines to enhance cell-mediated cytolysis of tumors. Persistently low levels of the NK cell number or activity in patients with advanced cancer may be associated with increased risk of disease progression[43, 44]. Therefore, it may be advantageous for patients to receive therapy designed to augment NK cell function.

In both patients, activity of NK and LAK cells in the peripheral blood before the treatment was comparable with healthy donors. In the patient E. G., a substantial increase of NK activity has been observed 72 h after the first, second and third treatments and such an increase persisted until day 84 after the third treatment (Table 5). No comparable activation of NK cells was detected after the fourth and fifth treatment when even depressed natural killer activity had been seen in the peripheral blood. Similarly, while an increase in LAK activity had been obvious after the second and third treatment (Table 5; data after the first treatment are not available) no such an increase was recorded after the fourth and fifth administration of Dox-PHPMA-HuIg. In the patient J. K., only a slight increase in NK activity was observed three weeks after the second treatment and three days after the third treatment. The activity of LAK cells was slightly depressed immediately after the first and second treatment and only a slight increase was observed in the third week after the second course of the polymeric drug. No activation was detected after the fourth and fifth treatment. In patient K. R. a substantial increase in NK and LAK cell activity was seen three days after the first and second injection of polymeric drug and in patient K. H. three days after all three injections. The experiments are in progress and data after fourth and fifth injection are not yet available. There are at least two explanations for such a result. First, that activated NK cells cannot be detected in the peripheral blood at later dates after the application of the polymeric drug as they move to the tumor site[34], or that the activation of such effector cells is only transient.

Table 5. Activity of NK and LAK cells in peripheral blood of patient E. G.

		K562 killing (%)	Daudi killing (%)
Healthy donor		20.65	25.61
Patient E. G.			
Before the treatment		<23.65	ND
First application	24 h	18.50	ND
	72 h	44.86	ND
	7d	38.53	ND
	21 d	31.32	17.83
Second application	72 h	38.92	39.50
	7 d	31.39	14.12
Third application	72 h	41.9	49.79
	7 d	19.26	22.75

4.2.4 HPLC analysis of serum samples

Analysis of plasma samples by gradient-based HPLC confirmed a long-term persistence of macromolecular therapeutics in the peripheral blood; this is in agreement with the data from clinical trials obtained after the treatment of cancer patients with non-targeted doxorubicin-PHPMA conjugate (PK1)[45, 46]and with the data obtained in experimental animals after injection with targeted and non-targeted HPMA copolymer-based drug conjugates[47]. Twenty four hours after the application the amount of doxorubicin in the blood of patient E. G. represented 24 h after the application 70% of injected dose, 72 h 11% of the injected dose and 21 days still of about 1 – 2 % of the injected dose. Similarly as others[20, 45, 46] we have seen that doxorubicin-PHPMA conjugate is stable in the bloodstream and the drug remains in the peripheral blood and urine mostly in its polymer-bound form[34].

4.2.5 Antibody response against the protein moiety of Dox-PHPMA-HuIg conjugate

Serious complication of immunotoxin therapy in human patients is the formation of human (HAMA) antibodies directed against a targeting moiety, i.e., against mouse or rat monoclonal antibodies. Decrease of immunogenicity of the proteins after their conjugation to PHPMA synthetic carrier was repeatedly shown in experimental animals[5, 48]. Thus, serum samples taken from patients E.G. and J.K. were analyzed by ELISA assay, non-modified as well as HPMA copolymer-bound human Ig being used as an antigen. Up to three weeks after the fifth application of the conjugate i.e., seven months after the first treatment of patient E. G. and up to three weeks after the fifth application of the conjugate, i.e., more than five months after the first treatment of patient J. K., the ELISA test did not reveal the presence of anti-human Ig antibodies in analyzed sera[34].

4.2.6 Functional activity of immunocompetent cells from the peripheral blood of the patients

Spontaneous as well as mitogen-induced proliferation of patient's blood mononuclear cells was monitored throughout the treatment courses. Concanavalin A (ConA) has been used as a T cell mitogen, lipopolysaccharide as a B cell mitogen and a combination of PMA and A23187 as a mitogen/antigen-independent activation signal. PMA is an activator of protein kinase C (PKC) and A23187 is an inducer of Ca^{2+} influx. During and after the treatment we did not detect any significant changes in the ability of patient's peripheral blood mononuclear cells to proliferate spontaneously, to react to T- and B-mitogens or to respond to mitogen/antigen-independent activation signal[34].

5. CLINICAL RESPONSE

According to the liver ultrasound scan and bone marrow computer tomography (CT), stabilization of the disease with a very good quality of life was achieved in patient E. G. for more than 18 months, in patient J. K. for more than one year, and in patients K.R. and K.H for more than eight and six months, respectively.[34].

6. CONCLUSION

N-(2-hydroxypropyl)methacrylamide copolymer (PHPMA)-bound doxorubicin conjugated with human Ig as a targeting moiety was used for the first time in the setting of metastatic breast cancer (patients E. G., J. K., K. R. and K.H.) and angiosarcoma (patient D. H) resistant to conventional cytotoxic chemotherapy. It was confirmed that Dox-PHPMA-HuIg conjugate is stable and doxorubicin remains in the peripheral blood mostly in its polymer-bound form. In patients E. G., J. K., K.R. and K.H. more than 116 biochemical and immunological parameters were tested in blood samples taken from the patients 24 h, 48 h, 72 h, 7 d, 14 d and 21, 28 and eight weeks after the treatment. In the patient E. G., 15 parameters had pathological values before the treatment. During the treatment, seven parameters dropped permanently or temporarily to a normal level and seven moved markedly towards the physiological value. While the number of peripheral blood reticulocytes was significantly decreased after the treatment with free doxorubicin, their number was stable or elevated after the treatment with Dox-PHPMA-HuIg conjugate. Increased absolute number of $CD16^{+}56^{+}$ and $CD4^{+}$ cells in the peripheral blood and activation of NK and LAK cells in a human patients support the data previously obtained in experimental animals pointing to a dual role, i.e. the cytotoxic and immunomobilizing character of doxorubicin-PHPMA conjugates containing a targeting immunoglobulin moiety.

ACKNOWLEDGEMENTS

This research was supported by the Grant Agency of the Czech Republic (grant 305/02/1425), by AS CR (grant S5020101), by IGA AV CR (A

4050201) and by Institutional Research Concept (AV0Z5020903). We would like to acknowledge the significant clinical collaboration of František Straka, M. D. from the Institute of Clinical and Experimental Medicine, Prague, Czech Republic in the case of the patient D. H. and excellent technical assistance of Hana Semorádová and Helena Mišurcová.

REFERENCES

1. Maeda, H., and Matsumura, Y., 1987, Tumouritropic and lymphotropic principles of macromolecular drugs. *CRC Crit. Rev. Ther. Drug Carrier Syst.* **6**: 193-210.
2. Suzuki, F., Pollard, R. B., Uchimura, S., Munakata, T., and Maeda, H., 1990, Role of natural killer cells and macrophages in the nonspecific resistance to tumors in mice stimulated with SMANCS, a polymer-conjugated derivative of neocarzinostatin. *Cancer Res.* **50**: 3897-3904.
3. Říhová, B., Strohalm, J., Kubáčková, K., Jelínková, M., Hovorka, O., Kovář, M., Plocová, D., Šírová, M., Šťastný, M., Rozprimová, L., and Ulbrich, K., 2002, Acquired and specific immunological mechanisms co-responsible for efficacy of polymer-bound drugs. *J. Control. Rel.* **78**: 97-114.
4. Kopeček, J., Rejmanová, P., Strohalm, J., Ulbrich, K., Říhová, B., Chytrý, V., Lloyd, J.B., and Duncan, R., 1991, Synthetic polymeric drugs, US patent 5,037,883.
5. Říhová, B., and Kopeček, J., 1985, Biological properties of targetable poly N-(2-hydroxypropyl) methacrylamide - antibody conjugates. *J. Control. Rel.* **2**: 289-310.
6. Duncan, R., Kopečková-Rejmanová, P., Strohalm, J., Hume, I., Cable, H. C., Pohl, J., Lloyd, J. B., and Kopeček, J., 1987, Anticancer agents coupled to N-(2-hydroxypropyl)methacrylamide copolymers. 1. Evaluation of daunomycin and puromycin conjugates *in vitro*. *Brit. J. Cancer* **55**: 165-174.
7. Říhová, B., Kopečková, P., Strohalm, J., Rossmann, P., Větvička, V., and Kopeček, J., 1988, Antibody-directed affinity therapy applied to the immune system: *In vivo* effectiveness and limited toxicity of daunomycin conjugated to HPMA copolymers and targeting antibody. *Clin. Immunol. Immunopathol.* **46**: 100-114.
8. Duncan, R., Kopečková, P., Strohalm, J., Hume, I. C., Lloyd, J. B., and Kopeček, J., 1988, Anticancer agents coupled to N-(2-hydroxypropyl)methacrylamide copolymers. II. Evaluation of daunomycin conjugates *in vivo* against L1210 leukaemia. *Brit. J. Cancer* **57**: 147-156.
9. Duncan, R., Hume, I. C., Kopečková, P., Ulbrich, K., Strohalm, J., and Kopeček, J., 1989, Anticancer agents coupled to *N*-(2-hydroxypropyl)methacylamide copolymers. 3. Evaluation of adriamycin conjugates against mouse leukaemia L1210 *in vivo*. *J. Contr. Rel.* **10**: 51-63.
10. Cassidy, J., Duncan, R., Morrison, G. J., Strohalm, J., Plocová, D., Kopeček, J., and Kaye, S.B., 1989, Activity of N-(2-hydroxypropyl)methacrylamide copolymers containing daunomycin against a rat tumour model. *Biochem. Pharmacol.* **38**: 875-879.
11. Duncan, R., 1992, Drug-polymer conjugates: potential for improved chemotherapy. *Anticancer Drugs* **3**: 175-210.
12. Říhová, B., Krinick, N. L., and Kopeček, J., 1993, Targetable photoactivatable drugs. 3. In vitro efficacy of polymer bound chlorin e_6 toward human hepatocarcinoma cell line (PLC/PRF/5) targeted with galactosamine and to mouse splenocytes targeted with anti-Thy 1.2 antibodies. *J. Contr. Rel.* **25**: 71-87.
13. Seymour, L.W., 1994, Soluble polymers for lectin-mediated drug targeting. *Adv. Drug Delivery Rev.* **14**: 89-111.

14. Říhová, B., 1996, Biocompatibility of biomaterials: hemocompatibility, immunocompatibility and biocompatibility of solid polymeric materials and soluble targetable polymeric carriers. *Adv. Drug Delivery Reviews* **21**:157-176.
15. Říhová, B., Strohalm, J., Plocová, D., Šubr, V., Šrogl, J., Jelínková, M., Šírová, M., and Ulbrich, K.,1996, Cytotoxic and cytostatic effects of anti-Thy 1.2 targeted doxorubicin and cyclosporin A. *J. Control. Rel*.**40**: 303-319.
16. Peterson, C. M., Lu, J. M., Sun, Y., Peterson, C.A., Shiah, J.-G., Straight, R. C., and Kopeček, J., 1996, Combination chemotherapy and photodynamic therapy with *N*-(2-hydroxypropyl)methacrylamide copolymer-bound anticancer drugs inhibit human ovarian carcinoma heterotransplanted in nude mice. *Cancer Res.* **56**: 3980-3985.
17. Minko, T., Kopečková, P., and Kopeček, J., 2000, Efficacy of chemotherapeutic action of HPMA copolymer-bound doxorubicin in a solid tumor model of ovarian carcinoma. *Int. J. Cancer* **86**: 108-117.
18. Říhová, B., Jelínková, M., Strohalm, J., Šubr, V., Plocová, D., Hovorka, O., Novák, M., Plundrová, D., Germano, Y., and Ulbrich, K., 2000, Polymeric drugs based on conjugates of synthetic and natural macromolecules. II. Anti-cancer activity of antibody or $(Fab')_2$-targeted conjugates and combined therapy with immunomodulators. *J. Control. Rel.* **64**: 241-26.
19. Říhová, B., Jelínková, M., Strohalm, J., Šťastný, M., Hovorka, O., Plocová, D., Kovář, M., Dráberová, L., and Ulbrich, K., 2000, Antiproliferative effect of a lectin-and anti-Thy-1.2 antibody-targeted HPMA copolymer-bound doxorubicin on primary and metastatic human colorectal carcinoma and on human colorectal carcinoma transfected with mouse *Thy-1.2* gene. *Bioconjugate Chemistry* **11**: 664-673.
20. Rejmanová, P., Kopeček, J., Duncan, R., and Lloyd, J.B., 1985, Stability in rat plasma and serum of lysosomally degradable oligopeptide sequences in *N*-(2-hydroxypropyl)methacrylamide copolymers. *Biomaterials* **6**: 45-48.
21. Kopeček, J., 1984, Controlled biodegradability of polymers - a key to drug delivery systems. *Biomaterials* **5**: 19-25.
22. Minko, T., Kopečková, P., Pozharov, V., and Kopeček, J., 1998, HPMA copolymer bound adriamycin overcomes *MDR1* gene encoded resistance in a human ovarian carcinoma cell line. *J. Contr. Rel.* **54**: 223-233.
23. Šťastný, M., Strohalm, J., Plocová, D., Ulbrich, K., and Říhová, B., 1999, A possibility to overcome P-glycoprotein (PGP)-mediated multidrug resistance by antibody-targeted drugs conjugated to *N*-(2-hydroxypropyl)methacrylamide (HPMA) copolymer carrier. *Eur. J. Cancer* **35**: 459-466.
24. Říhová, B., Kopečková, P., Strohalm, J., Rossmann, P., Větvička, V., and Kopeček, J., 1988, Antibody-directed affinity therapy applied to the immune system: *In vivo* effectiveness and limited toxicity of daunomycin conjugated to HPMA copolymers and targeting antibody. *Clin. Immunol. Immunopathol.* **46**: 100-114.
25. Říhová, B., Jegorov, A., Strohalm, J., Maťha, V., Rossmann, P., Fornůsek, L., and Ulbrich, K., 1992, Antibody-targeted cyclosporin A. *J. Control. Rel.* **19**: 25-39.
26. Yeung, T. K., Hopewell, J. W., Simmonds, R. H., Seymour, L. W., Duncan, R., Bellini, O., Grandi, M., Spreafico, F., Strohalm, J., and Ulbrich, K., 1991, Reduced cardiotoxicity of doxorubicin administered in the form of N-(2-hydroxypropyl)methacrylamide copolymer conjugates: an experimental study in the rat. *Cancer Chemother. Pharmacol.* **29**: 105 – 111.
27. Říhová, B., Bilej, M., Větvička, V., Ulbrich, K., Strohalm, J., Kopeček, J., and Duncan, R., 1989, Biocompatibility of N-(2-hydroxypropyl)methacrylamide copolymers containing adriamycin. *Biomaterials* **10**: 335 – 342.
28. Rossmann, P., Říhová, B., Strohalm, J., and Ulbrich, K., 1997, Morphology of rat kidney and thymus after native and antibody-coupled cyclosporin A application (Reduced toxicity of targeted drug). *Folia Microbiol.* **42**: 277-287.

29. Šťastný, M., Ulbrich, K., Strohalm, J., Rossmann, P., and Říhová, B., 1997, Abnormal differentiation of thymocytes induced by free cyclosporine is avoided when cyclosporine bound to N-(2-hydroxypropyl)methacrylamide copolymer carrier is used. *Transplantation* **63**: 1818-1827.
30. Penn, I., 1993, The effect of immunosuppression on preexisting cancers. *Transplant. Proc.* **25,** 1380-1382.
31. Shoenfeld, Y., and Fishman, P., 1999, Gamma-globulin inhibits tumor spread in mice. *Int. Immunology* **11**: 1247 – 1251.
32. Torchilin, V.P., Iakounbov, L.Z., Samokhin, G. P., Rammohan, R., Mongayat, D. A., and Lukyanov, A. L., 2001, Tumor cell surface-bound nucleosomes: universal molecular targets for tumoricidal autoantibodies. *J.Control. Rel.* **74**: 373-375.
33. Ulbrich, K., Šubr, V., Strohalm,J., Plocová,D., Jelínková,M., and Říhová, B., 2000, Polymeric drugs based on conjugates of synthetic and natural macromolecules. I.Synthesis and physicochemical characterization. *J. Control. Rel.* **64**: *63-79.*
34. Říhová, B., Strohalm, J., Kubáčková, K., Jelínková, M., Rozprimová, L., Šírová, M., Plocová, D., Etrych, T., Mrkvan, T., Kovář, M., Pokorná, J., Šťastný, M., and Ulbrich, K., Dual activity of PHPMA-based doxorubicin containing human Ig in four patients with disseminated breast cancer, submitted
35. Steel, D., and Whitehead, A.S., 1994, The major acute phase reactants: C-reactive protein, serum amyloid P component and serum amyloid A protein, *Immunology Today* **15**: 81-88.
36. Zach, O., Kasparu, H., Krieger, O., Hehenwarter, W., Girschikofsky, M., and Lutz, D., 1999, Detection of circulating mammary carcinoma cells in the peripheral blood of breast cancer patients via a nested reverse transcriptase polymerase chain reaction assay for mammaglobin mRNA, *J. Clin. Oncol.* **17**: 2015-2019.
37. Barber, M. D., Ross, J.A., and Fearon, K.C., 1999, Changes in nutritional, functional, and inflammatory markers in advanced pancreatic cancer, *Nutr. Cancer* **35**:106-110.
38. Lauerová, L., Dušek, L., Šimíčková, M., Rovný, F., Spurný, V., Rovný, F., Slampa, P., Žaloudík, J., Rejthar, A., Wotke, J., and Kovařík, J., 1999, Renal cell carcinoma-associated immune impairment that may interfere with the response to cytokine therapy. *Neoplasma* **46**:141-149.
39. Nozoe, T., Matsumata, T., and Sugimachi, K., 2000, Preoperative elevation of serum C-reactive protein is related to impaired immunity in patients with colorectal cancer. *Am. J. Clin. Oncol.* **23**: 263-266.
40. Berois, N., Varangot, M., Aizen, B., Estrugo, R., Zarantonelli, L., Fernandez, P., Krygier, G., Simonet, F., Barrois, E., Muse, I., and Osinaga, E., 2000, Molecular detection of cancer cells in bone marrow and peripheral blood of patients with operable breast cancer. Comparison of CD19, MUC1 and CEA using RT-PCR. *Eur. J. Cancer* **36**:717-723.
41. Lumachi, F., Brandes, A. A., Boccagni, P., Polistina, F., Favia, G., and D' Amico, D. F., 1999, Long-term follow up study in breast cancer patients using serum tumor markers CEA and CA 15-3. *Anticancer Res.* **19**: 4485-4489.
42. Huang, J., Hardy, J. D., Sun, Y., and Shively, J. E., 1999, Essential role of biliary glycoprotein (CD66a) in morphogenesis of the human mammary epithelial cell line MCF10F. *J.Cell Sci.* **112 (Pt 23***): 4193 – 4205.*
43. Montelli, T. C., Peracoli, M. T., Gabarra, R. C., Soares, A. M., and Kurokawa, C. S., 2001, Familial cancer: depressed NK-cell cytotoxicity in healthy and cancer affected members. *Arq. Neuropsiquiatr.* **59**:6-10.
44. Sephton, S.E., Sapolsky, R.M., Kraemer, H.C., and Spiegel, D., 2000, Diurnal cortisol rhythm as a predictor of breast cancer survival, *J. Natl. Cancer Inst.* **92**: 994-1000.
45. Julyan, P. J., Seymour, L. W., Ferry, D. R., Daryani, S., Boivin, Ch. M., Doran, J., David, M., Anderson, D., Christodoulou, Ch., Young, A. M., Hesselwood, S., and Kerr,

D.J., 1999, Preliminary clinical study of the distribution of HPMA copolymers bearing doxorubicin and galactosamine. *J.Control. Rel.* **57**: 281- 290.

46. Thomson, A. H., Vasey, P. A., Murray, L. S., Cassidy, J., Fraier, D., Frigerio, E., and Twelves, C., 1999, Population pharmacokinetics in phase I drug development: a phase I study of PK1 in patients with solid tumors. *British J.Cancer* **81**: 99 – 107.
47. Říhová, B., Vereš, K., Fornůsek, L., Ulbrich, K., Strohalm, J., Větvička, V., Bilej, M., and Kopeček, J., 1989, Action of the polymeric prodrugs based on N-(2-hydroxypropyl)methacrylamide. 2. Body distribution and T cell accumulation of ^{125}DNM. *J. Control. Rel.* **10**: 37-49.
48. Flanagan, P. A., Duncan, R., Říhová, B., Šubr, V., and Kopeček, J., 1990, Immunogenicity of protein-N-(2-hydroxypropyl)methacrylamide conjugates in A/J and B10 mice. *J. Bioact. Compat. Polymers* **5**: 151-166.

CM-Dextran-Polyalcohol-Camptothecin Conjugate

DE-310 with A Novel Carrier System and Its Preclinical Data

KAZUHIRO INOUE*, EIJI KUMAZAWA*, HIROSHI KUGA*, HIROSHI SUSAKI**, NORIKO MASUBUCHI#, and TETSUYO KAJIMURA##

**New Product Res. Lab. III, **Medicinal Chem. Res. Lab., #Drug Metabolism and Physico-chem. Res. Lab., ##Drug Safety Res. Lab., Daiichi Pharmaceutical Co., Ltd., 16-13, Kita-kasai 1, Edogawa-ku, Tokyo 134-8630, Japan*

1. INTRODUCTION

Macromolecular antitumor prodrugs have been studied and developed actively for these two to three decades, since Ringsdorf reported[1] on the basic design for polymeric drugs. Most of them could accumulate in tumor tissue, based on EPR (Enhanced Permeability and Retention) effect demonstrated and named by Maeda et al.[2-4]. The recent clinical results of macromolecular prodrugs such as PK1[5, 6] have indicated that the polymer therapeutics are now promising for treatment of cancer.

For the construction of (macromolecular carrier)-(peptidyl spacer)-(antitumor drug) conjugate system[7-9], we first evaluated the usefulness as carriers of some naturally-occurring polysaccharides and their derivatives, and then studied on drug-release profiles of some peptidyl spacers through which a parent drug was covalently linked to a carrier. It was suggested that carboxymethyldextran polyalcohol (CM-Dex-PA), one of polyhydroxylated carboxymethylpolysaccharides, could be an excellent carrier for passive tumor-targeting by EPR effect, based on the following rationale: a) CM-Dex-PA shows a high water-solubility enabling its conjugate with a drug to be water-soluble; b) its main chain, dextran polyalcohol (Dex-PA), has a structural flexibility and similarity to polyethylene glycol (PEG) with a stealthy efficacy; and c) its main chain (Dex-PA) is acid-labile, as well known[10] as "Controlled Smith Degradation" of polysaccharides, which

Polymer Drugs in the Clinical Stage, Edited by Maeda et al.
Kluwer Academic/Plenum Publishers, New York, 2003

strongly suggests that CM-Dex-PA is a biodegradable carrier slowly depolymerized in the lysosomal acidic-environment after endocytosis such as phagocytosis. Thus for the application of a camptothecin analog DX-8951f[11], methanesulfonic acid salt of DX-8951, to the conjugate system, we utilized the CM-Dex-PA carrier with molecular sizes higher than renal filtration threshold to avoid a rapid renal excretion and thereby to maintain a high plasma level of the drug conjugate. In preclinical studies, DE-310, which was obtained by optimising the conjugate system CM-Dex-PA-GGFG-DX-8951, showed a long retention of high conjugate-levels in blood, a preferential tumor-accumulation and sustained releases of both DX-8951 and glycyl DX-8951 (G-DX-8951) in tumor tissue, and resulted in exhibition of a superior antitumor efficacy with a high therapeutic index by single iv dose. In addition, the carrier moiety of DE-310 was shown to be gradually depolymerized and excreted mainly into urine after iv dose of DE-310. Phase I trials of DE-310 have been going in US and Europe, while DX-8951f is now in phase III.

We here describe the concept and design for the construction of DE-310 and then the outlines of its preclinical results.

2. CONCEPT AND DESIGN

We designed a macromolecular carrier system so that the macromolecular conjugate could utilize EPR effect efficiently by an extremely long retention of its high plasma-levels (Fig. 1), and so that it could show a drug-release rate appropriate to a parent drug applied to the system in tumor tissue without releasing the drug in bloodstream.

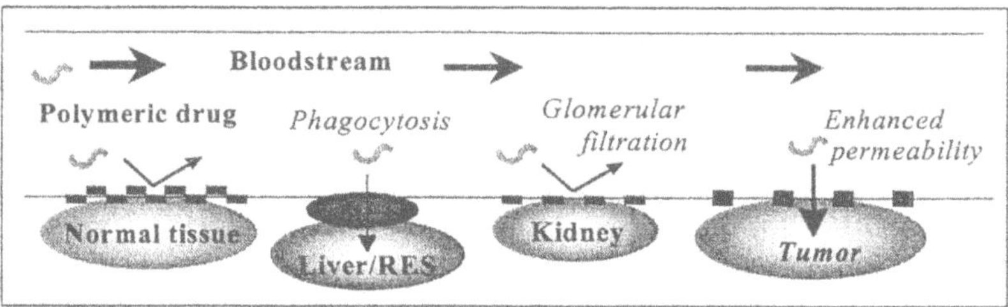

Figure 1. Passive tumor-targeting based on EPR effect.

Peptidyl spacer was used for releasing the parent drug from the conjugate by lysosomal enzymes of cathepsins after its uptake into cells. The longer retention of the conjugate in bloodstream should lead it to a more preferential tumor-accumulation, in proportion to its levels of tumor vascular permeability, and the control of drug-release should bring out the best in the parent drug applied to the system. For this DDS concept, as described in section 1, we selected a stealthy and biodegradable carrier, CM-Dex-PA, with molecular sizes larger than the renal threshold, and a peptidyl spacer, GGFG, to provide a slow release of the parent drug DX-8951 with a time-dependent cytocidal activity. The PA carrier with a high structural-flexibility and hydrophilicity was also suggested to have some capability of maintaining its stealthy property even after conjugation with the hydrophobic drug, differing from non-PA-polysaccharide carriers.

3. OPTIMISATION OF CM-DEX-PA-GGFG-DX-8951

CM-Dex-PA used as the carrier of the conjugate had a long retention of high plasma-levels in Meth A tumor-bearing mice. The carrier with a degree of carboxymethylation of 0.4 showed the highest plasma AUC and the most preferential tumor-accumulation, being in inverse ratio to its degrees (Table 1).

Table 1. Plasma $AUC_{1\text{-}168hr}$ and $AUC_{1\text{-}168hr}$ ratios of tumor to liver of CM-Dex-PA[a] (MW ca. 300K) with different degrees of carboxymethylation after a single iv dose to Meth A tumor-bearing mice.

Degrees of carboxymethylation (per sugar residue)	AUC_{plasma} (μg hr/ml)	AUC_{tumor}/AUC_{liver}
0.4	33845 (1.0)[b]	1.8
0.8	25823 (0.76)	1.5
1.2	16493 (0.45)	1.2

[a] CM-Dex-PA was labelled with ^{3}H-glycine. [b] Parentheses represent AUC ratios.

The peptidyl spacer (GGFG) provided slow releases of both DX-8951 and G-DX-8951 *in vitro* (tumor homogenates and cathepsins) and *in vivo*; the slow drug-release in tumor tissue is extremely advantageous to cytotoxicity of the time-dependent antitumor drug, DX-8951. A high steric hindrance of the bulky DX-8951 moiety was found to be responsible for the slow releases of both drugs from CM-Dex-PA-GGFG-DX-8951, while the GGFG spacer showed a fast drug-release with such a less bulky drug as doxorubicin.

The CM-Dex-PA-GGFG-DX-8951 conjugate was optimised on molecular sizes, degrees of carboxymethylation and loadings of DX-8951 to obtain DE-310, as follows. CM-Dex-PA was synthesized by carboxymethylation of Dex-PA which was obtained by periodate oxidation of dextran followed by borohydride reduction. Tetra-peptidyl DX-8951 (GGFG-DX-8951) was covalently linked to CM groups of CM-Dex-PA through acid amide bonds to give CM-Dex-PA-GGFG-DX-8951. The conjugates with various ranges of molecular size, degrees of carboxymethylation and contents of DX-8951 were synthesized, and their antitumor activities and therapeutic indexes were evaluated with murine Meth A fibrosarcoma solid tumor-bearing mice.

As the results, the conjugates with MWs (ca.100K~ca.500K), degrees of carboxymethylation (ca.0.3~ca.0.4 per sugar residue) and DX-8951 contents (less than 8%), although these values depend on analytical methods used, showed the equivalency. Thus, based on these results, DE-310 was specified. The structural feature of DE-310 is shown in Fig. 2, which was determined by the analytical methods such as Controlled Smith Degradation[10] (analyses of mild-acid degradation products of DE-310) and NMR spectroscopy.

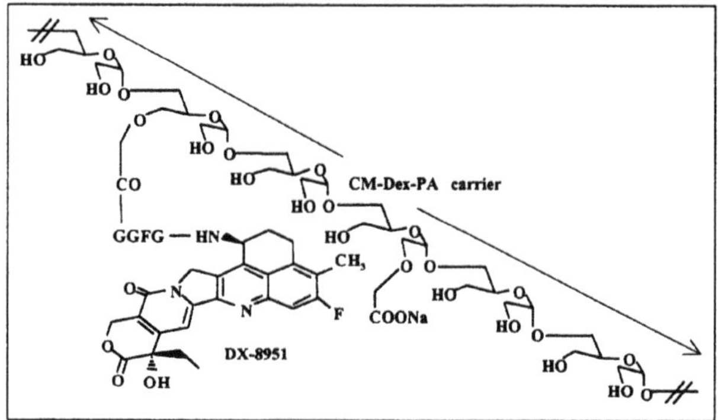

Figure 2. Partial structural feature of DE-310

4. PRECLINICAL RESULTS OF DE-310

DE-310 was studied[12-14] on its pharmacokinetics, antitumor effects and toxicities, compared with the parent drug DX-8951f.

4.1 Tissue Distribution in Tumor-Bearing Mice

As shown in Table 2, after a single iv dose of DE-310 to Meth A solid tumor-bearing mice, conjugated DX-8951 (carrier-bound DX-8951), free DX-8951 and G-DX-8951, detected in tumor and normal tissues, were determined by HPLC.

Table 2. $AUC_{0\text{-}inf}$ ratios of conjugated DX-8951, free DX-8951 and G-DX-8951 after a single iv dose of DE-310 to Meth A tumor-bearing mice (5.7 mg eq. DX-8951/kg).

Tissue	Conjugated DX-8951	Free DX-8951	Free G-DX-8951
Plasma	6.3	0.03	0.06
Tumor	1.0	1.0	1.0
Liver	0.34	0.34	1.1
Lung	0.61	0.04	0.14

As for conjugated DX-8951, its plasma level ($AUC_{0\text{-}inf}$) was 6-times higher than its tumor level, the tumor level being 3-times higher than its liver level. On the other hand, $AUC_{0\text{-}inf}$ of free DX-8951 in tumor was 30-times higher than that in plasma, and 3- and 28-times higher than that in liver and in lung, respectively. $AUC_{0\text{-}inf}$ of free G-DX-8951 in tumor was also 16-times higher than that in plasma, and close to that in liver. *In vitro* cytotoxicity of DX-8951, 26 to 190-times higher than that of G-DX-8951, suggested that the released DX-8951 could principally contribute to efficacy and toxicity of DE-310. Conjugated DX-8951, free DX-8951 and G-DX-8951 in tumor tissue showed a similar half life ($t_{1/2}$) of 2~3 days, while DX-8951f had a $t_{1/2}$ of 0.3hr in plasma and its AUC ratio of liver to tumor was 7.

In addition, whole body autoradiography of Meth A-bearing mice showed that radioactivity in tumor was higher than that in normal tissues tested, 168hr after a single iv dose of either ^{14}C-DX-8951-labeled DE-310 or ^{14}C-carrier-labeled DE-310.

These results demonstrate that DE-310 has a high potency for the effective and preferential tumor-targeting and for the slow and sustained release suitable for the time-dependent antitumor drug DX-8951f, probably without releasing the drugs in bloodstream, in agreement with the DDS concept described in section 2.

4.2 Cumulative Excretion after A Single IV Dose

Either ^{14}C-DX-8951-labeled DE-310 or ^{14}C-carrier-labeled DE-310 was intravenously administered to normal mice.

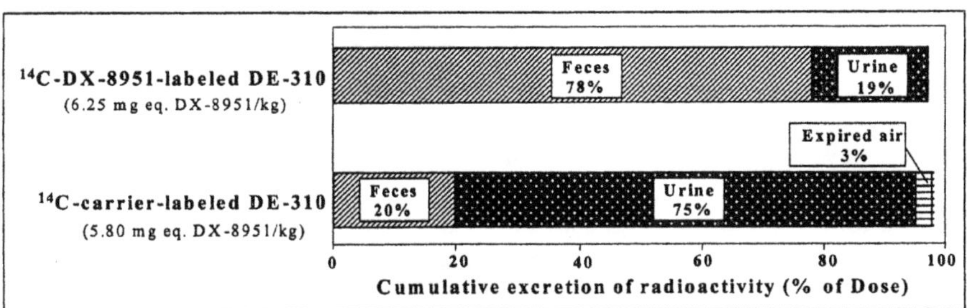

Figure 3. Cumulative excretion of radioactivity 42 days after a single iv dose of ^{14}C-DX-8951-labeled DE-310 and ^{14}C-carrier-labeled DE-310 to mice.

The plasma levels of radioactivity decreased with almost the same $t_{1/2}$ of 2.6 days for both of ^{14}C-labeled DE-310s. ^{14}C-DX-8951-labeled DE-310 and ^{14}C-carrier-labeled DE-310 were excreted primarily into the feces and the urine, respectively, and the elimination of radioactivity within 42 days was 97% for the former and 98% for the latter (Fig. 3), while the elimination of 95% of radioactivity was completed within 18 days for the former. These results indicate that the carrier moiety of DE-310 is gradually degraded to molecular sizes susceptible of glomerular filtration.

4.3 Antitumor Efficacy

Antitumor effects by a single iv dose of DE-310 were compared with those by a single dose or multiple doses of the parent drug DX-8951f, using the Meth A solid tumor model.

In a short-term assay (Fig. 4), DE-310 shrank the tumor by a single treatment (qdx1) at maximum tolerated dose (MTD) and at 1/4 MTD, occurring with no body weight loss at 1/4 MTD, and inhibited tumor growth even at 1/16 MTD. In contrast, DX-8951f (qdx1) showed only an inhibition of tumor growth even at MTD, and daily 5 treatments (qdx5) of DX-8951f at MTD were required to shrink the tumor, while the treatments of DX-8951f (qdx5) at 1/4 MTD inhibited tumor growth with a body weight loss.

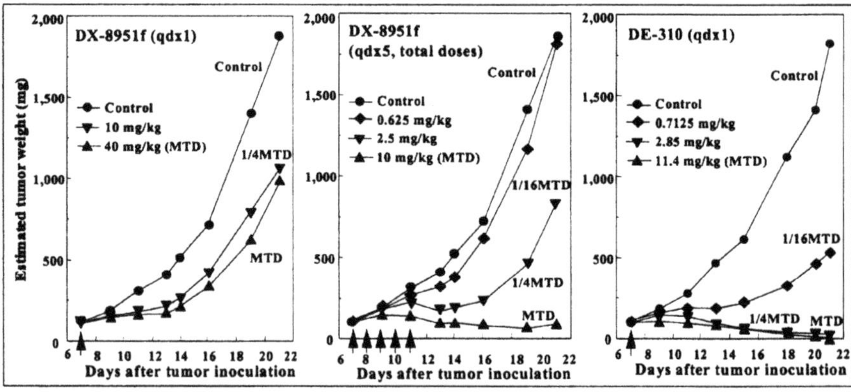

Figure 4. Antitumor effects of DE-310 (a single dose) compared with those of the parent drug DX-8951f (a single dose or daily 5 doses) with Meth A solid tumor model (short-term assay). Dose levels of DE-310 and DX-8951f are expressed as DX-8951.

In a long-term assay (Fig. 5), tumors in mice treated with DE-310 (qdx1) at MTD and at 1/2 MTD had disappeared from the 15th day after the dose, and all 6 mice were tumor-free even on the 60th day, and also DE-310 (qdx1) at 1/4 MTD and at 1/8 MTD resulted in the complete disappearance of tumor masses in 4 out of 6 mice for each dose on the 60th day.

In addition, DE-310 (qdx1) exhibited potent antitumor effects against human tumor xenografts in mice, and also significantly prolonged survival in the lung metastasis model (3LL) and in the liver metastasis model (M5076).

As shown in Fig. 6, DE-310 induced far less myelotoxicity than DX-8951f at doses giving similar degrees of antitumor effect with inhibition ratios (IR) over 90%.

From the results of toxicological studies with mice and dogs, it was also suggested that DE-310 has no critical toxicity other than DX-8951f alone, which might be newly produced by the conjugation.

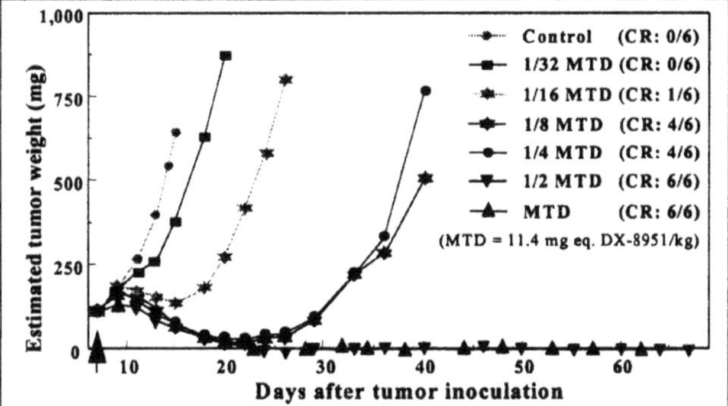

Figure 5. Tumor growth curves and complete response ratios (CR) after a single dose of DE-310 with Meth A solid tumor model (long-term assay).

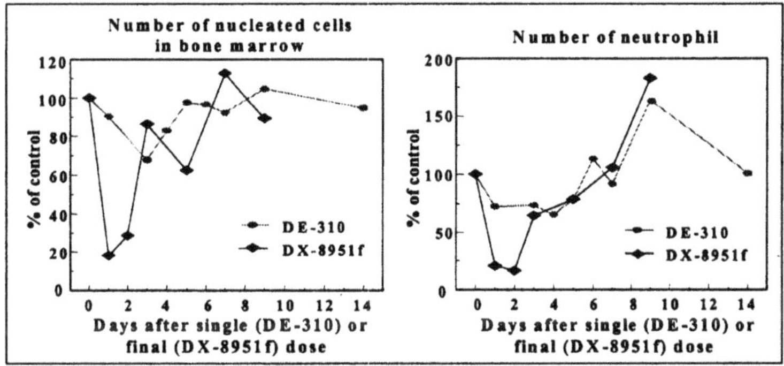

Figure 6. Hematological changes by DE-310 and DX-8951f at doses showing similar degrees of antitumor effect. DE-310: a single dose (qdx1; 2.5 mg eq. DX-8951/kg, IR 92-95%); DX-8951f: multiple doses (qdx2/q4dx4; 0.94 mg/kg x 8, IR 91%)

5. CONCLUSION

The pharmacokinetics of DX-8951f were greatly improved by DE-310 with the extremely longer retention in bloodstream, resulting in the preferential tumor-targeting, and with the slow release appropriate to camptothecin analog DX-8951f in tumor tissue. On the basis of the pharmacokinetic improvement, DE-310 exhibited enhanced antitumor effects with reduced toxicities by a single and low dose, compared with DX-8951f. These preclinical results suggest that DE-310 is a promising agent for cancer treatment. The phase I trials are still ongoing and recently, the interim clinical data have been reported[15, 16].

ACKNOWLEDGMENTS

This DDS technology has been developed with the support of Drug Delivery System Institute, Ltd., which was funded by the Japanese Government (the Organization for Pharmaceutical Safety and Research).

We would like to thank Prof. M. Hashida and Prof. R. Duncan for invaluable advices and discussions. We would also like to thank Prof. H. Maeda for the opportunity to contribute this chapter on polymeric drugs.

REFERENCES

1. Ringsdorf, H., 1975, Structure and properties of pharmacologically active polymers. J. Polym. Sci. Polym. Symp. **20**: 135-153.
2. Matsumura, Y., and Maeda, H., 1986, A new concept for macromolecular therapeutics in cancer chemotherapy: mechanism and antitumor agent smancs. Cancer Res. **46**: 6387-6392.
3. Maeda, H., Wu, J., Sawa, T., Matsumura, Y., and Hori, K., 2000, Tumor vascular permeability and EPR effect in macromolecular therapeutics: a review. J. Control. Release **65**: 271-284.
4. Maeda, H., 2001, The enhanced permeability and retention (EPR) effect in tumor vasculature: the key role of tumor-selective macromolecular drug targeting. Advan. Enzyme Regul. **41**: 189-207.
5. Duncan, R., Seymour, L.W., O'Hare, K.B., Flanagan, P.A., Wedge, S., Hume, I.C., Ulbrich, K., Strohalm, J., Subr, V., Spareafico, F., Grandi, M., Ripamonti, M., Farao, M., and Suarato, A., 1992, Preclinical evaluation of polymer-bound doxorubicin. J. Control. Release **19**: 331-346.
6. Vasey, P.A., Twelves, C., Kaye, S.B., Wilson, P., Morrison, R., Duncan, R., Thomson, A., Murray, L., Hilditch, T.E., Murray, T., Burtles, S., Frigerio, E., Fraier, D., and Cassidy, J., 1998, Phase I clinical and pharmacokinetic study of PK1. Abstructs of 3rd International Symposium on Polymer Therapeutics, p. 21.
7. Inoue, K., Okuno, S., Hamana, H., and Ito, T., 1993, Glyco-technology and DDS. FARUMASHIA **29**: 1256-1260.
8. Nogusa, H., Yano, T., Okuno, S., Hamana, H., and Inoue, K., 1995, Synthesis of carboxymethylpullulan-peptide-doxorubicin conjugates and their properties. Chem. Pharm. Bull. **43**: 1931-1938.
9. Sugawara, S., Okuno, S., Yano, T., Hamana, H., and Inoue, K., 2001, Characteristics of tissue distribution of various polysaccharides as drug carriers: influences of molecular weight and anionic charge on tumor targeting. Biol. Pharm. Bull. **24**: 535-543.
10. Goldstein, I.J., Hay, G.W., Lewis, A., and Smith, F., 1965, Controlled degradation of polysaccharides by periodate oxidation, reduction, and hydrolysis. Methods in Carbohydr. Chem. **5**: 361-370.
11. Kumazawa, E., and Tohgo, A., 1998, Antitumor activity of DX-8951f: a new camptothecin derivative. Exp. Opin. Invest. Drugs. **7**: 625-632.

12. Kumazawa, E., Ochi, Y., Tanaka, N., Kajimura, T., and Inoue, K., 2001, A novel macromolecular carrier system for the camptothecin analog DX-8951f [I]: its antitumor activities in the murine Meth A solid tumor model. Proc. Am. Assoc. for Cancer Res. **42**: 139.
13. Ochi, Y., Kumazawa, E., Nakata, M., Tanaka, N., and Inoue, K., 2001, A novel macromolecular carrier system for the camptothecin analog DX-8951f [II]: its antitumor activities in several model systems of human and murine tumors. Proc. Am. Assoc. for Cancer Res. **42**: 376.
14. Masubuchi, N., Gohda, R., Seki, H., Hayashi, K., Atsumi, R., and Inoue, K., 2001, A novel macromolecular carrier system for the camptothecin analog DX-8951f [III]: pharmacokinetic evaluation in normal and tumor-bearing mice. Proc. Am. Assoc. for Cancer Res. **42**: 376.
15. Soepenberg, O., De Jonge, M.J.A., Loos, W.J., Sparreboom, A., Eskens, F.A.L.M., De Heus, G., Elliott, S., Cheverton, P., Bastien, L., and Verweij, J., 2002, Phase I and pharmacologic study of the macromolecular topoisomerase-I-inhibitor DE-310 given once every 2 or 6 weeks in patients with solid tumors. Eur. J. Cancer (Suppl. 7) **38**: S45.
16. Takimoto, C.H., Forero, F., Schwartz, G.H., Tolcher, A.W., Hammond, L.A., Patnaik, A., Ducharme, M., Cooke, B., De Jager, R., and Rowinsky, E.K., 2002, A phase I and pharmacokinetic study of DE-310 administered as a 3 hour infusion every 4 weeks (wks) to patients (pts) with advanced solid tumors or lymphomas. Eur. J. Cancer (Suppl. 7) **38**: S46.

Polymeric Micelle Drug Carrier Systems: PEG-PAsp(Dox) and Second Generation of Micellar Drugs

NOBUHIRO NISHIYAMA[*], KAZUNORI KATAOKA[#]
[*]*Department of Pharmaceutics and Pharmaceutical Chemistry, University of Utah, UT, USA;*
[#]*Department of Materials Science, Graduate School of Engineering, The University of Tokyo, JAPAN*

1. INTRODUCTION

Polymeric micelles are one of the most refined and promising modalities of macromolecular drug delivery systems [1-6], and show unique disposition characteristics in the body suitable for the drug targeting (e.g., prolonged blood circulation and significant tumor accumulation as described in earlier chapter) [7-10]. Like the other promising modalities (i.e., water-soluble polymers and long-circulating liposomes), the polymeric micelle carrier systems might possess several advantages such as (1) the applicability to a variety of therapeutic agents (e.g., hydrophobic compounds, metal complexes and charged macromolecules such as polypeptides and nucleic acids), (2) unnecessariness of chemical structure

Abbreviations: enhanced permeability and retention effect (EPR effect); poly(ethylene glycol) (PEG); PEG-b-poly(α,β-aspartic acid) (PEG-PAsp); PEG-b-poly(β-benzyl L-aspartate) (PEG-PBLA); PEG-b-poly(α-glutamic acid) (PEG-PGlu); doxorubicin-conjugated PEG-b-PAsp (PEG-PAsp(Dox)); cisplatin-complexed PEG-b-PAsp (PEG-PAsp(CDDP)); cisplatin-complexed PEG-b-PGlu (PEG-PGlu(CDDP)); PEG-poly(D,L-lactide) (PEG-PDLLA); polyion complex micelle (PIC micelle); doxorubicin (Dox); cisplatin (*cis*-dichlorodiammineplatinum (II)) (CDDP); photodynamic therapy (PDT); photosensitiser (PS); protoporphyrin IX (PIX); dendrimer porphyrins (DP); positively-charged DP (32(+)DPZn); negatively-charged DP (32(-)DPZn); murine colon adenocarcinoma (C-26); Lewis lung carcinoma (LLC)

Polymer Drugs in the Clinical Stage, Edited by Maeda et al.
Kluwer Academic/Plenum Publishers, New York, 2003

modification of the drugs, (3) simplicity of micelle preparation, (4) high drug loading capacity, and (5) controlled drug release. These properties can be optimized by modulating the micelle core-forming blocks depending on the chemical and physicochemical properties of the drugs. Furthermore, recent advance in synthetic chemistry (especially, PEGylation chemistry) has allowed us to design the functional polymeric micelles with such functions as a target molecule-specific binding [11-14], stimuli-responsive [15-17] or environment-sensitive [18, 19] structural change, and so on. Thus, polymeric micelle carrier systems may potentially provide wealth of technology in the drug delivery or targeting. In this chapter, we review recent progress in research on polymeric micelles for cancer therapy, which has been accomplished mainly in our laboratory.

2. GENERAL COMMENTARY

2.1 Biodistribution of Macromolecular Carriers

A major purpose of using macromolecular carriers is to modulate the drug disposition in the body. It is well accepted that macromolecular carriers or drugs need to be biocompatible and possess certain characteristics to exhibit prolonged blood circulation [20] and exhibit tumor targeting EPR effect established since 1986 [21-23]. The prolonged blood circulation can reduce accumulation of drugs in undesirable sites causing serious side effects and also improve the bioavailability. Furthermore, the long-circulating nature of macromolecular carriers is of primary importance for the effective tumor accumulation based on the EPR effect (*Section 2.2.*). The main obstacles to long-circulation of macromolecular carriers are considered to be glomerular excretion in the kidney and recognition by the reticuloendothelial system (RES) located at the liver, spleen and lung. Since the threshold molecular weight exists for glomerular filtration (42,000 - 50,000 for water-soluble synthetic polymers [24]), it can be avoided by increasing the molecular weight of carriers. On the other hand, macromolecular carriers (especially, colloidal carriers) with low biocompatibility can be recognized by RES via complement activation and other mechanisms, and then eliminated from blood circulation. However, a surface modification of carriers with biocompatible polymers is able to impair or even avoid the recognition by RES [25, 26]. Among such water-soluble polymers, PEG is probably the most effective one due to the structure with high flexibility and a high degree of hydration [27]. Especially,

PEG chains of which one end is attached to surfaces effectively exhibit protein-resistant properties by a high steric repulsion effect [28].

2.2 Preferential Tumor Accumulation of Macromolecules

Preferential tumor accumulation of macromolecules is one of the most advantageous strategic bases of tumor-specific drug targeting using macromolecular carriers. Such enhanced tumor accumulation of macromolecules is mainly explained by microvascular hyperpermeability to circulating macromolecules and their impaired lymphatic drainage in tumor tissues. This phenomenon was termed the EPR effect by Maeda et al [21-23, 29]. It has been suggested that tumor microvascular hyperpermeability is due to overexpression of the vascular permeability factor (VPF) / vascular endothelial growth factor (VEGF) gene [30-32] as well as secretion of other factors such as basic fibroblast growth factor (bFGF) [32], bradykinin, nitric oxide, peroxynitrate, matrix metalloproteinases (MMP) and prostaglandins in tumor tissues [22, 29, 33-36]. To date, there is increasing evidence that synthetic polymers, liposomes and micelles accumulate in various types of tumors, which is most probably due to the above-mentioned EPR effect. This issue has been discussed fully in earlier chapter of this monograph.

3. ADVANTAGES OF POLYMERIC MICELLES AS A TUMOR-DIRECTED DRUG CARRIER SYSTEM

3.1 Micellar Forming Properties

Amphiphilic AB-type block copolymers spontaneously form polymeric micelles characterized by a size of decananometers, fairly narrow size distribution and segregated core-shell structure in aqueous solutions (Fig. 1) [2, 4, 5]. In our laboratory, polymeric micelles have been formed from a variety of diblock copolymers with a well-defined structure and a considerably narrow molecular weight distribution ($M_w/M_n \sim 1.10$). An inner core, which is surrounded by a palisade of hydrophilic polymers, serves as a nanoreservoir of various hydrophobic drugs. Due to the segregated core-shell structure and compacted inner core, a high loading of drugs might have less effect on the size and surface properties of the micelles, which may be the most critical factor in the disposition of the micelles in the body. Furthermore, since polymeric micelles generally have a remarkably low critical association concentration (c.a.c.) compared with low molecular surfactant micelles [4, 37], they function as a drug depot with controllable drug release in the body while exhibiting prolonged blood circulation.

3.2 Biodistribution of Polymeric Micelles

The blood circulating nature of polymeric micelles could be affected by a number of factors such as the sizes, size distribution, core-shell segregation, length of core- and shell-forming blocks, aggregation number, and critical association concentration (c.a.c). We have so far demonstrated that polymeric micelles with a diameter of several tens nanometer, a fairly narrow size distribution and a segregated core-shell structure were able to circulate stably in bloodstream. For example, remarkably prolonged blood circulation was observed for the micelles formed from PEG-PAsp(Dox) [7, 8], PEG-PBLA [38] and PEG-PAsp(CDDP) block copolymers [9]. Since tumor accumulation of macromolecules based on the EPR effect occurs in a passive manner (passive targeting), such prolonged blood circulation of polymeric micelles should be primarily needed for successful tumor targeting.

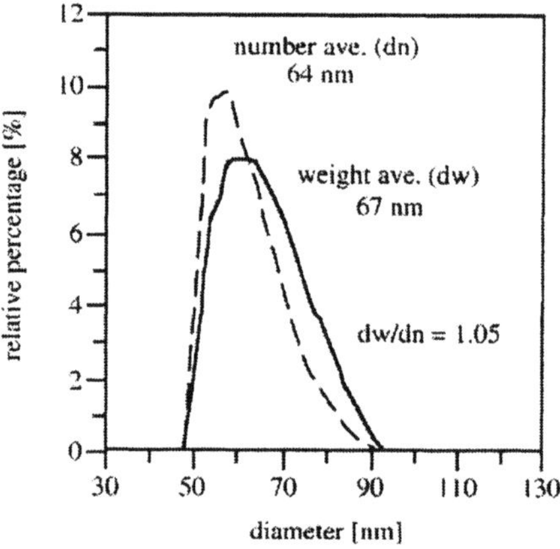

Figure 1. Weight and number-averaged distribution of Dox-loaded PEG-PBLA micelle measured by dynamic light scattering (DLS) in histogram mode (in distilled water, 25°C, polymer concentration: 0.1wt%). Solid line: weight-averaged distribution; dashed-line: number-averaged distribution. (Reprinted with permission from Ref. [38]. Copyright 2000 Elsevier Science.)

Regarding basic biodistribution study of polymeric micelles, we recently reported long-circulating polymeric micelles formed from PEG-PDLLA block copolymers [39]. In this study, small neutral and negatively-charged peptides (Tyr and Tyr-Glu) were installed on the distal end of PEG chains by utilizing a reactive aldehyde group, resulting in a preparation of neutral and negatively-charged polymeric micelles with zeta potentials of 1.3 mV and -10.6 mV, respectively [40]. Both polymeric micelles showed remarkably long blood circulation ($t_{1/2}$ ~ 18 h) in mice compared with similar systems reported by others (($t_{1/2}$ ~ 3 - 8 h) [41-44], and 25 % of the injected dose remained in blood circulation after 24 h post injection in spite of degradation of PDLLA chains in the reaction of micellar surface modification and during storage. Further, both micelles showed a distribution volume in the central compartment (V_0) nearly equivalent to the blood volume and a plasma-to-blood ratio nearly equal to the plasma space value (= 1 - hematocrit), suggesting that polymeric micelles distribute only in the blood compartment immediately after i.v. administration without interaction with blood cells. Actually, stable blood circulation of polymeric micelles was confirmed by a gel filtration assay [39].

In tissue distribution, both micelles showed the tissue-to-blood concentration ratios (K_b) comparable to the vascular space volumes (~ 0.2) in normal organs (lung, kidney, liver and spleen) up to 24 h except for small increase in the liver and spleen after 24 h, corresponding to the extracellular space volumes (~ 0.3) [39]. Such low K_b values in the liver and spleen were comparable to those obtained from long-circulating liposomes [45, 46]. Therefore, PEG-PDLLA micelles may avoid not only recognition by RES but also entrapment by hepatic sinusoidal capillaries characterized by large interendothelial cell junctions (~ 100 nm) and an absence of basement membranes in spite of the relatively small size of the micelles (~ 30nm). These data suggest that PEG-PDLLA micelles possess ideal long-circulating properties. The discrepancy between our observation and the others [41-44] may be due to the difference in the micellar size, size distribution and a degree of core-shell segregation. Note that similar prolonged blood circulation and reduced uptake by normal tissues were observed for the other polymeric micelle carrier systems by us (*Section 4.*). Further, in this study, it was observed that PEG-PDLLA micelles were slowly excreted into urine (24 % injected dose at 24 h) [39]. This phenomenon appears to be consistent with the lower molecular weight of PEG-PDLLA block copolymers than a threshold value for a glomerular excretion. Therefore, PEG-PDLLA micelles can provide quite safe drug delivery systems with the least risk of chronic nonspecific accumulation of polymers in the body. Another interesting aspect is that the surface charge modulation had a negligible effect on their long-circulating properties. Our observations seem to be inconsistent with the notion that the charges on the macromolecules greatly affect their disposition in the body [47, 48]. Probably, surface modification of polymeric micelles with small pilot molecules hardly change their disposition in the body if they already possess long-circulating properties. In fact, this may be quite important to achieve successful active drug targeting to solid tumors by using tumor cell-targeted molecules. In general, the tumor mass is located outside of the microvasculature, so that the extravasation of macromolecular carriers is a prerequisite for specific interaction of the targeted molecules with tumor cells at the local site. However, the extravasation of macromolecules is a non-specific passive process governed by the EPR effect as discussed previously. Therefore, long-circulating properties of polymeric micelles, which are not compromised by installing small pilot molecules on them, may be a good feature for successful active targeting. Importantly, although surface modification of polymeric micelles did not impair the long-circulating properties, it was confirmed that sugar-installed polymeric micelles still exhibit selective binding to RCA-1 lectin [13, 49].

4. RECENT PROGRESS IN POLYMERIC MICELLES FOR CANCER THERAPY

4.1 PEG-PAsp(Dox) Micelles

PEG-PAsp(Dox) micelles are a first generation of polymeric micellar drug developed in our laboratory (Fig. 2) [8, 50]. In this formulation, Dox was covalently linked to the side chain of the PAsp segment via an amide bond between the carboxylic group in PAsp and the primary amino group of the glycosidyl residue in Dox. Chemical conjugation of Dox into the PAsp segment with substitution ratio of approximately 50 % provided the PAsp segment with sufficient hydrophobicity to form a stable inner core of polymeric micelles [51].

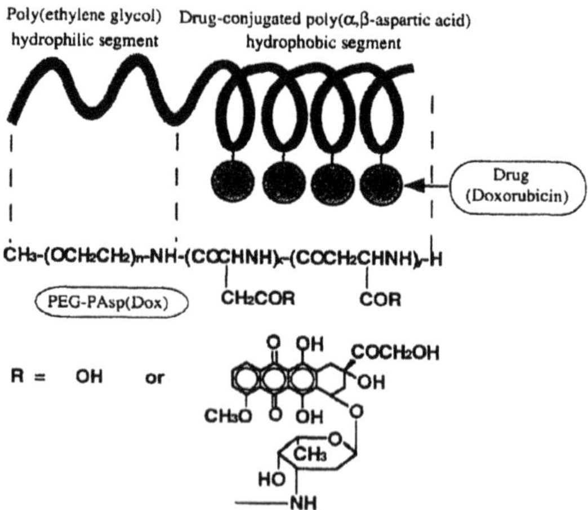

Figure 2. Chemical structure of doxorubicin-conjugated PEG-PAsp (PEG-PAsp(Dox)) block copolymers. This micelle also can entrappes non-covalently free Dox.

Indeed, PEG-PAsp(Dox) formed polymeric micelles with a diameter of 15 to 60 nm, which depended on the composition of block copolymers and drug contents [51, 52]. The dissociation rate of PEG-PAsp(Dox) micelles into unimers was estimated to be on the order of days in phosphate buffer saline, and it was slow even in the presence of 50% rabbit serum [53]. As a result, PEG-PAsp(Dox) micelles, where M_w of PEG and PAsp segments were 12,000 and 2,100 g mol^{-1}, respectively, showed prolonged blood circulation and significant tumor accumulation [7]. An inner core of PEG-PAsp(Dox) micelles can accommodate free Dox [52]. In fact, the physically entrapped Dox was responsible for the cytotoxic activity rather than the chemically conjugated one [54]. Nevertheless, it was found that the chemically conjugated Dox contributes to the stable physical entrapment of unconjugated drugs through a π-π interaction of the anthracycline structure in Dox between conjugated and unconjugated drugs [54]. Indeed, the entrapment efficiency of unbound Dox into the micelles increased with the proportion of chemically conjugated Dox to the PAsp segments [54], and the increased amount of both physically entrapped and chemically conjugated Dox was shown to improve the micellar structure in the column chromatography assay [54]. Recently, it was suggested that a dimer derivative of Dox molecules via an azomethine bond was formed in the micellar core when the physically entrapped Dox increased, and this species may contribute to stabilization of the micellar structure and retention of the loaded drugs as well [8, 54].

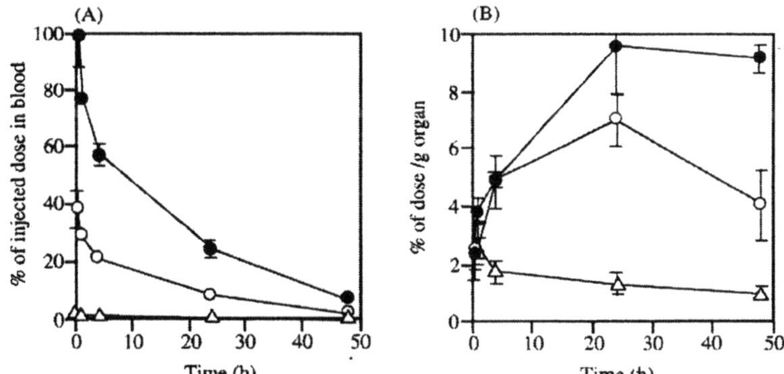

Figure 3. Time profiles of ^{14}C-labeled Dox in blood (A) or in the tumor (C-26) (B) in CDF_1 mice after i.v. drug administration (Δ:free Dox; O:PEG-PAsp(Dox) micelle Run 1: ●:Run 2). Dose was either 10 mg/kg for free Dox and 10 mg of physically entrapped Dox (including a dimer of Dox) per kg for PEG-PAsp(Dox) micelle. PEG-PAsp(Dox) micelle Run 1 and 2 were prepared at the ratio of chemically conjugated to physically entrapped Dox of 1.0 to 0.39 and 1.0 to 0.98, respectively. (Reprinted with permission from Ref. [8]. Copyright 1999 Taylor & Francis.)

In biodistribution assay where only the physically entrapped Dox in the micelles was radio-labeled with ^{14}C, PEG-PAsp(Dox) micelles showed remarkably prolonged blood circulation (24.6 % of injected dose was found at 24 h), while free Dox disappeared very quickly from the circulation (1.6 % of injected dose at 15 min) (Fig. 3 A) [8]. The plasma-to-blood partitioning ratio demonstrated that PEG-PAsp(Dox) micelles existed predominantly in the plasma fraction during the circulation (up to 48 h) while free Dox distributed to the blood cells. As for tissue accumulation, there was no notable difference for accumulation in the liver, spleen, kidney and heart between PEG-PAsp(Dox) micelles and free Dox [8]. In contrast to normal organs, PEG-PAsp(Dox) micelles accumulated effectively in the subcutaneously inoculated tumor (murine colon adenocarcinoma (C-26)) over 24 h, and eventually exhibited 7.4-fold higher tumor accumulation than free Dox at 24 h (Fig. 3 B) [8]. Such effective tumor accumulation of PEG-PAsp(Dox) micelles is most probably due to the EPR effect described in *Section 2.2.* of this chapter and elsewhere in this book. Consequently, PEG-PAsp(Dox) micelles showed higher tumor-to-normal tissue accumulation ratios (i.e., targeting efficiency) than free Dox (Table 1), suggesting improved therapeutic indices of the micellar formulation. Indeed, PEG-PAsp(Dox) micelles showed such significant in vivo antitumor activity as to lead to a complete tumor regression against C-26 [8]. It is worth noting that longer blood circulation, higher tumor accumulation and slower in vivo drug release were observed for the micelles with a higher loading amount of physically entrapped Dox (Fig. 3 and Table 1) [8], suggesting that the micellar stability and drug release rate in vivo can be controlled by the proportion of chemically conjugated Dox to the PAsp segments as well as loading amount of physically entrapped Dox and dimer of Dox. Therefore, it may be feasible to design the polymeric micelle formulation with preferable

Table 1. Accumulation ratios between tumor (C-26) and normal organs (Dose: 10 mg/kg for free Dox and 10 mg of physically entrapped Dox per kg for PEG-PAsp(Dox) micelle). (Reprinted with permission from Ref. [8]. Copyright 1999 Taylor & Francis.)

		Accumulation ratio#		
		Tumor/Muscle	Tumor/Heart	Tumor/Spleen
PEG-Asp(Dox) Run 1 *	24 h	10.0 ± 1.0	4.9 ± 0.3	0.65 ± 0.09
	48 h	8.9 ± 3.7	5.5 ± 1.9	0.39 ± 0.14
PEG-Asp(Dox) Run 2 *	24 h	13.0 ± 7.1	6.2 ± 1.1	0.80 ± 0.09
	48 h	19.0 ± 5.1	9.0 ± 0.6	0.77 ± 0.04
free Dox	24 h	1.4 ± 0.3	1.3 ± 0.2	0.13 ± 0.03
	48 h	1.8 ± 0.4	2.0 ± 0.4	0.13 ± 0.02

values are shown by mean ± SD (n= 3 or 4)

* PEG-PAsp(Dox) micelle Run 1 and 2 were prepared at the ratio of chemically conjugated to physically entrapped Dox of 1.0 to 0.39 and 1.0 to 0.98, respectively.

properties depending on the purposes (i.e., the stable micallar formulation with significant tumor accumulation or the depot formulation with sustained drug release). The optimized formulation of PEG-PAsp(Dox) is now being studied in a phase I clinical trial in Japan.

4.2 Versatile Polymeric Micelles for Hydrophobic Drugs

From the standpoint of versatile drug carrier systems, the development of polymeric micelles, which can physically entrap various drugs without their chemical structure modification, must be attractive. In our laboratory, amphiphilic PEG-PBLA block copolymers have been intensively studied as such versatile drug carrier systems [37, 38, 55-59]. PEG-PBLA spontaneously form polymeric micelles with a diameter of 20 nm, narrow size distribution and spherical shape due to a strong cohesive force of benzyl groups in the PBLA segments (Fig. 1) [37, 59]. PEG-PBLA micelles possessed a low critical association concentration (0.5 - 1.5 * 10^{-6} M) and solid-like inner core, which are in contrast to low molecular surfactant or Pluronic® micelles [37], and hence may serve as a potent nanocontainer of hydrophobic compounds. Indeed, Dox, indomethacin and pyrene were physically and stably encapsulated into the micelles through dialysis or O/W emulsion methods [58], and the encapsulated drugs showed remarkably high stability against chemical degradation during long time storage [57]. Dox-loaded PEG-PBLA micelles showed a high loading capacity (15 - 20 wt%) and pH-dependent sustained drug release over several days [38]. The release rate of the encapsulated drugs from the micelles appears to be controlled by the partition coefficient based on the pH of the medium, interaction between drugs and micellar core-forming blocks, and interaction between drugs themselves [38, 58, 59]. It was recently demonstrated that Dox encapsulated in PEG-PBLA micelles showed prolonged blood residence time in mice, and thereby achieved considerably higher antitumor activity against C-26 in comparison with free Dox [38].

As mentioned above, in preparation of polymeric micelles for physical drug encapsulation, the affinity between inner core-forming blocks and drugs as well as the amount of drug loading should be taken into consideration to attain a high physicochemical stability of the micelles, high drug loading efficiency and high loading amount, and sustained drug release over hours or days. Kwon et al reported that amphotericin B (AmB) was efficiently encapsulated into block copolymer micelles possessing AmB compatible moieties, i.e., saturated fatty acid ester, in inner core-forming blocks [60, 61]. Also, Yokoyama et al reported efficient encapsulation of KRN5500 into the micelles comprising cetyl ester residue-indroduced PEG-PBLA derivatives (PEG-P(C_{16}, BLA)) [62]. Recently, our laboratory successfully incorporated a oligopeptide, [Arg^8]-vasopressin (AVP) which is an antidiuretic hormone comprising nine amino acids, into polymeric micelles through the hydrogen bonding with PEG-poly(L-aspartic acid) with a free acid form [63]. Hydrogen bonding also appears to be available for encapsulation of the drugs into polymeric micelles without a covalent polymer-drug linkage.

The drug release manner might be one of the most important factors for micellar drugs to exert the antitumor activity reasonably. The release of active form of drugs from the carriers may be needed at the tumor site following accumulation to solid tumors based on the EPR effect, while the drug release should be kept minimal during their blood circulating period. Even if enhanced tumor accumulation of drug carriers is accomplished, high antitumor efficacy can not be achieved without the reasonable drug release. For example, it was reported that the discrepancy between remarkably high tumor accumulation of Dox-encapsulated PEG-liposomes and their in vivo antitumor activity much lower than expectations from their in vitro cytotoxicity may be due to extremely slow drug release from the liposomes [64]. In general, effective accumulation of macromolecules in solid tumors based on the EPR effect occurs in a time-dependent manner over hours or days, and hence the drug release rate in the order of hours or days may be appropriate to attain both the effective tumor targeting and the local drug action at the tumor site. In this regard, an increasing number of polymeric micelles has been reported, which are designed to possess the controllable drug release rate in the order of hours or days. Indeed, polymeric micelles developed in our laboratory achieved the sustained drug release over hours or days as reviewed in this chapter. Optimization of structure matching between inner core-forming blocks and the drugs as well as the amount of drug loading may allow control of the drug release rate. Langer et al and Cho et al separately reported that a higher loading of hydrophobic drugs (lidocaine and clonazepam, respectively) caused drug crystallization inside the micellar core, leading to slower drug release (over 14 h and 5 days, respectively) [65, 66]. The crystalline formation of encapsulated drugs was confirmed by differential scanning calorimetry (DSC) measurement. In addition to aforementioned parameters, to attain efficient drug loading and sustained drug release, microviscosity and fluidity of the micellar core should be considered for some block copolymer micelle systems possessing a low glass transition temperature (T_g) of inner core-forming blocks such as PEG-PDLLA and PEG-poly(caprolacton) (PEG-PCL) block copolymers [67]. Furthermore, a new class of polymeric micelles has recently been reported, which are designed to achieve the site-specific drug release responsive to several types of stimuli such as temperature [15-17] and pH [19].

4.3 CDDP-Complexed Polymeric Micelles

Cisplatin (CDDP) is a well-known metal complex exhibiting a wide range of antitumor spectrum [68], but its clinical use is limited due to significant toxic side effects such as acute nephrotoxicity and chronic neurotoxicity [69]. CDDP is known to show rapid distribution to the whole body and high glomerular clearance within 15 min after i.v. administration [70, 71]. Therefore, great efforts have been devoted to the development of drug delivery systems which can increase the blood residence time of CDDP and deliver to solid tumors [72-78]. However, the unfavorable properties of CDDP have prevented from developing successful formulations. For instance, formulations with liposomes may result in rapid leakage of their contents during storage and within the bloodstream due to low compatibility between the lipid bilayer and the free drug. Hence, many current formulations have utilized a coordination bond between CDDP and polymers or lipids containing carboxylic groups [73-77], since two chloride ligands in the leaving group of Pt(II) atom in CDDP are known to be substituted with a variety of reactive groups depending on the concentration of chloride ion in the surroundings [79]. The coordination bond between Pt(II) and carboxylic ligands may be appropriate as a polymer-drug linkage because of its reversibility, while amine or thiol groups form too stable coordination bonds with Pt(II) to be re-substituted with chloride ion or other ligands for the recovery of its antitumor activity [79].

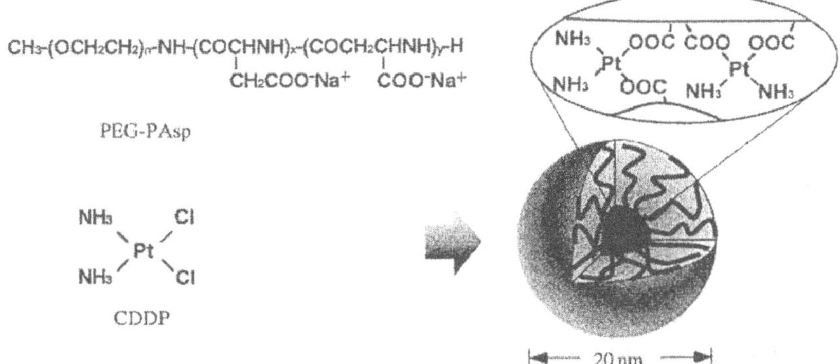

Figure 4. Chemical structure of CDDP-complexed PEG-PAsp (PEG-PAsp(CDDP)) block copolymers.

However, the solubility problem is often encountered in the polymer-CDDP conjugates at a high substitution ratio due to the increased cohesive force as well as inter-polymer cross-linking formation [80]. Then, we expected that such a solubility problem could advantageously turn into a driving force of block copolymer micelles. Indeed, the ligand substitution reaction between CDDP and PEG-PAsp block copolymer in aqueous media led to the spontaneous formation of polymeric micelles (PEG-PAsp(CDDP) micelles) having a diameter of approximately 20 nm with a considerably narrow distribution (Fig. 4) [81, 82].

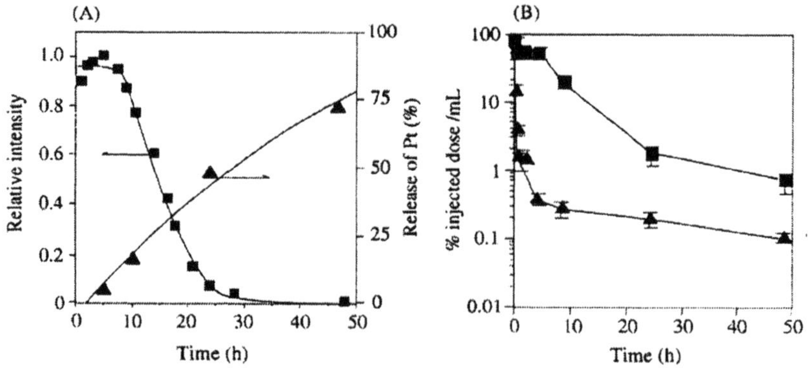

Figure 5. (A) Time change in the relative scattering light intensity (■) and CDDP release (▲) for PEG-PAsp(CDDP) micelles in physiological saline at 37°C (Reprinted with permission from Ref. [82]. Copyright 1999 American Chemical Society.). (B) Time profiles of free CDDP (▲) and PEG-PAsp(CDDP) micelles (■) in the plasma in LLC-bearing mice (n = 4). Free CDDP or PEG-PAsp(CDDP) micelles were administered intravenously at a dose of 4.7 mg/kg on a CDDP basis 10 days after the tumor inoculation (tumor weight: 0.13 ± 0.04 g). (Reprinted with permission from Ref. [9]. Copyright 2001 Kluwer Academic.).

It was found that such micelle formation occurred above a critical ligand substitution ratio (CDDP/Asp > 0.5), and thus formed micelles had remarkable stability upon dilution in distilled water [82]. In physiological saline (37 °C), PEG-PAsp(CDDP) micelles released CDDP in a sustained manner over 80 h due to the opposite ligand exchanging reaction of Pt(II) from carboxylates to chloride ions, and concomitantly dissociated slowly with an induction period of approximately 10 h (Fig. 5 A) [82]. This phenomenon suggests that PEG-PAsp(CDDP) micelles could be a new class of polymeric micelle (polymer-metal complex micelle) which exhibits the time-modulated decaying property accompanied with the sustained drug release. It should be noted that the Pt release rate depended on the concentration and species of the environmental nucleophiles (ligand ions) in the media, suggesting that the ligand exchanging reaction of Pt(II) would determine the drug release rate and micellar decaying profile (unpublished data). Importantly, in biodistribution assay using Lewis lung carcinoma (LLC)-bearing mice, PEG-PAsp(CDDP) micelles exhibited the time-dependent change in plasma Pt level consistent with their unique in vitro decaying profiles observed in physiological saline (Fig. 5 B) [9]. Namely, PEG-PAsp(CDDP) micelles kept a high plasma Pt level (~ 61 % of the injected dose) up to 4 -8 h followed by a gradual decrease in the plasma Pt level after that time, while free CDDP disappeared rapidly from the blood circulation after i.v. administration (Fig. 5 B). The tissue-to-plasma partitioning ratios (K_p values) suggested that PEG-PAsp(CDDP) micelles localize in the vascular space (~ 0.1 mL/g) in all tested organs (kidney, liver, spleen and tumor) up to 4 h, and the substantial tissue accumulation of the micellar drug may occur after 8 h. In the kidney where the dose-limiting side effect is observed in free CDDP treatment, PEG-PAsp(CDDP) micelles did not show such rapid and high Pt accumulation up to 15 min as observed for free CDDP. Consequently, PEG-PAsp(CDDP) micelles showed no increase in the blood urea nitrogen (BUN) value, a nephrotoxic marker, which was significantly increased by free CDDP treatment [9]. On the other hand, PEG-PAsp(CDDP) micelles showed 6-fold higher tumor accumulation than free CDDP at 8 h, resulting in slightly higher in vivo antitumor activity than free CDDP treatment at the same dose (6 mg/kg) [9].

To achieve more effective tumor accumulation, it may be needed to extend blood circulation time of CDDP-loaded micelles. In this regard, we more recently prepared polymer-metal complex micelles (PEG-PGlu(CDDP) micelles) having a diameter of approximately 30nm through the ligand substitution reaction between CDDP and poly(ethylene glycol)-poly(α-glutamic acid) (PEG-PGlu) block copolymers in aqueous media [83]. In physiological saline (37 °C), PEG-PGlu(CDDP) micelles showed a slower release rate (half-value period: > 95 h) than aforementioned PEG-PAsp(CDDP) micelles (half-value period: ca 30 h), and longer induction period (> 20 h) for the micellar decaying than PEG-PAsp(CDDP) micelles (ca 10 h). These results suggest that the control of the drug release as well as micellar stability in physiological saline can be achieved by optimizing the chemical structure of the metal complex-forming blocks. In biodistribution assay, PEG-PGlu(CDDP) micelles kept a high plasma Pt level longer (11 % of the injected dose at 24 h) than PEG-PAsp(CDDP) micelles (1.5 % at 24 h), and showed decreased liver and spleen accumulation [83]. As a result of prolonged blood circulation, the tumor accumulation of PEG-PGlu(CDDP) micelles was kept increasing over 24 h, and eventually reached a 20-fold higher level than free CDDP [83]. Due to enhanced tumor accumulation as well as decreased accumulation in normal tissues, PEG-PGlu(CDDP) micelles exhibited the tumor targeting efficiency (tumor AUC / normal tissue AUC) more than 1.0 for all tested organs, indicating the selective drug targeting to solid tumors. In pharmacological assay, PEG-PGlu(CDDP) micelles showed an expanded therapeutic window (in LLC-bearing mice). Furthermore, we recently observed that the treatment with PEG-PGlu(CDDP) micelles (five times (every 2 days) i.v. administration at 4mg/kg) showed complete tumor regression for 5 out of 10 mice with minimal body weight loss (within 5% of the initial body weight), whereas the treatment with CDDP at the same drug dose regimen showed tumor regression for only one mouse out of 10 with significant body weight loss (approximately 20% of the initial weight) (in C-26 bearing mice) [84].

4.4 Photodynamic Therapy (PDT)

In addition to the aforementioned hydrophobic drugs and metal complexes, the charged macromolecules can be encapsulated into the polymeric micelle carrier systems (polyion complex (PIC) micelles) via an electrostatic interaction with oppositely charged block copolymers [85, 86]. The charged macromolecules including plasmid DNA, antisense DNA, bioactive proteins and enzymes have a great potential as a therapeutic agent, and have recently received increasing attention. However, such bioactive macromolecules are generally unstable in the body due to the enzymatic degradation as well as unfavorable phramacokinetic properties, hampering their practical use in clinical study. Incorporation of these charged macromolecular therapeutics into the polymeric micelle carrier systems may allow protection from their enzymatic degradation, improvement in their bioavailability, and even their targeting to the diseased tissues or cells [87-92]. Thus, PIC micelles are expected as a useful carrier system for charged macromolecular therapeutics. This issue would be referred to our another reviews [2, 93].

In this chapter, we would like to introduce PIC micelles encapsulating ionic dendrimer porphyrins as a photosensitiser (PS) for photodynamic therapy (PDT). PDT is a topical therapeutic modality of malignant tumors, which treats tumor cells with cytotoxic singlet oxygen ($^1O_2$) produced by PS through photo-excitation at its characteristic wavelength [94]. A successful PDT may be completed by the development of potent PSs [94], their tumor-selective delivery [19, 95, 96], and selective and effective photoirradiation at the diseased sites [97]. Recently, Aida et al. have elaborated ionic dendrimer porphyrins (DPs) in which a Zn-porphyrin chromophore is spatially isolated by the 3rd generation aryl ether dendrimer framework and 32 positively- or negatively-charged groups ($CONH(CH_2)_2N^+(CH_3)_3$ or COO^-, respectively) are installed on their periphery (Fig. 6) [98, 99], intriguing us towards the development of a novel type of dendrimer-based PS. DPs are expected to show different biological effects from typical low molecular PSs used in clinical study due to their size (~ 5 nm), surface charge and water solubility. Indeed, positively- and negatively-charged DPs (32(+)DPZn and 32(-)DPZn, respectively) were internalized via adsorptive and fulid phase endocytosis, respectively, and localized in membrane-limited organelles in LLC cells, whereas protoporphyrin IX (PIX), a typical hydrophobic and low molecular PS, diffused through the cell except for the nucleus [100]. Consequently, 32(+)DPZn showed much higher photo-induced cytotoxicity than 32(-)DPZn, and it was superior even to PIX in photo-induced cytotoxicity in spite of the lower cellular association amount [100]. Nevertheless, both DPs had extremely low dark toxicity, whereas PIX showed significant non-specific toxicity in absence of photoirradiation. Further, worth noting is that the photodamage by PIX severely disrupted the characteristic structures of membrane organelles such as a plasma membrane, mitochondrion and lysosome, while the photodamage by DPs toward them was negligible[100]. From these observations, the efficient phtodynamic effect of 32(+)DPZn may be due to photo-inactivation of specific target molecules (e.g., transporters, ion channels, cytoskeletons or lipids) in the plasma and subcellular membranes, although such exact molecular targets for the efficient PDT are an issue to be clarified in future. Another important aspect of DPs is their applicability to drug delivery systems. Namely, the surface charges of DPs might provide an opportunity to be encapsulated into PIC micelles. Indeed, both 32(+)DPZn and 32(-)DPZn formed PIC micelles through an electrostatic interaction with PEG-PAsp and PEG-poly(L-lysine) (PEG-PLys) block copolymers, respectively, and those micelles were confirmed to be stable in physiological saline (37 °C) (Fig. 6) [101]. The research towards in vivo antitumor activity of DPs-incorporated PIC micelles is now ongoing in our laboratory.

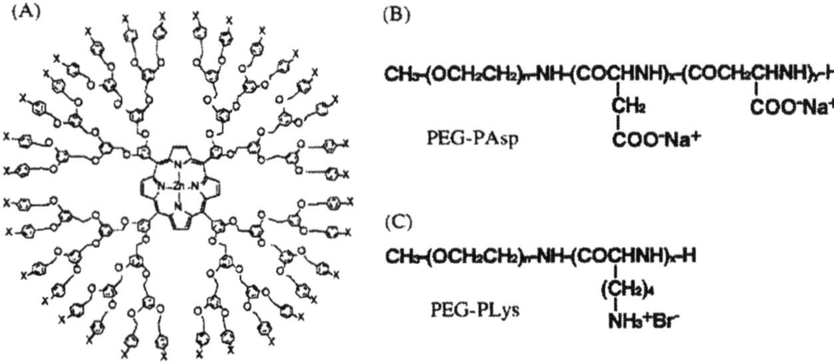

Figure 6. Schematic structures of (A) third-generation ionic dendrimer porphyrins, (B) PEG-PAsp, and (C) PEG-PLys block copolymers.

5. CONCLUSION

Polymeric micelles are a useful drug carrier system that can circulates stably in bloodstream and accumulates effectively in solid tumors. They can encapsulate a variety of drugs such as hydrophobic drugs, metal complexes and charged macromolecules. The micellar structure can be tailor-made on the purposes. More recently, great efforts are devoted for the development of mechanism-based drugs through an identification of molecular targets for the tumor treatment, accelerated by recent progress in synthetic combinatorial chemistry and high through-put screening technology. These drugs include inhibitors of growth factor receptor tyrosine kinases [102], farnesyltransferase [103], mitogen-activaed protein (MAP) kinases [104], cyclin-dependent kinases (CDKs) [105, 106] and so on. Basically, most of these drugs are cytostatic, so that continuous drug exposure would be required to achieve clinical efficacy. Therefore, controlled drug release from an appropriate drug carrier system may provide more practical and effective drug dose regime for these cytostatic drugs in clinical use. On the other hand, multi-hit drugs capable of affecting multiple molecular targets have recently received much attention, since hitting one target may be insufficient to eradicate tumor cells due to their heterogeneity as well as parallel and redundant signaling pathways supporting their survival. This class of drugs includes geldanamycin, and a heat shock protein-90 (Hsp90) inhibitor [107]. However, these drugs are known to cause serious toxic side effects due to a lack of selective access to the tumor cells. Hence, the use of tumor-targeted drug carrier systems may greatly increase the clinical efficacy of these drugs [108, 109]. Thus, successful clinical use of the newly developed drugs may be accompanied with the development of their appropriate carrier systems. In this regard, polymeric micelles is superior due to their encapsulating applicability to a variety of therapeutic agents without a covalent drug-carrier linkage. Further, the drug release rate can be controlled by optimization of structure matching between inner core-forming blocks and the drugs as well as the drug loading amount, lending polymeric micelles to have the great potential as a versatile drug carrier system in clinical use in the future.

REFERENCES

1. Kataoka, K., Kwon, G. S., Yokoyama, M., Okano, T., Sakurai, Y., 1993, Block copolymer micelles as vehicles for drug delivery. *J. Contr. Rel.* **24**: 119-132.
2. Kataoka, K., Harada, A., Nagasaki, Y., 2001, Block copolymer micelles for drug delivery: design, characterization and biological significance. *Adv. Drug Deliv. Rev.* **47**: 113-131.

3. Kabanov, A., Batrakova, E. V., Melik-Nubarov, N. S., Fedoseev, N. A., Dorodnich, T. Y., Alakhov, V. Y., Chekhonin, V. P., Nazarova, I. R., Kabanov, V. A., 1992, A new class of drug carriers: micelles of poly(oxyethylene)-poly(oxypropylene) block copolymers as microcontainers for drug targeting from blood in brain. *J. Contr. Rel.* **22**: 141-158.
4. Allen, C., Maysinger, D., Eisenberg, A., 1999, Nano-engineering block copolymer aggregates for drug delivery. *Colloids and Surfaces B: Biointerfaces* **16**: 3-27.
5. Lavasanifar, A., Sanuel, J., Kwon, G. S., 2002, Poly(ethylene oxide)-block-poly(L-amino acid) micelles for drug delivery. *Adv. Drug Deliv. Rev.* **54**: 169-190.
6. Torchilin, V. P., 2002, PEG-based micelles as carriers of contrast agents for different imaging modalities. *Adv. Drug Deliv. Rev.* **54**: 235-252.
7. Kwon, G. S., Kataoka, K., 1995, Block copolymer micelles as long-circulating drug vehicles. *Adv. Drug Deliv. Rev.* **16**: 295-309.
8. Yokoyama, M., Okano, T., Sakurai, Y., Fukushima, S., Okamoto, K., Kataoka, K., 1999, Selective delivery of adriamycin to a solid tumor using a polymeric micelle carrier system. *J. Drug Targeting* **7**: 171-186.
9. Nishiyama, N., Kato, Y., Sugiyama, Y., Kataoka, K., 2001, Cisplatin-loaded polymer-metal complex micelle with time-modulated decaying property as a novel drug delivery system. *Pharm. Res.* **18**: 1035-1041.
10. Weissig, V., Whiteman, K. R., Torchilin, V. P., 1998, Accumulation of protein-loaded long-circulating micelles and liposomes in subcutaneous Lewis Lung Carcinoma. *Pharm. Res.* **15**: 1552-1556.
11. Scholz, C., Iijima, M., Nagasaki, Y., Kataoka, K., 1995, A novel reactive polymeric micelle. Polymeric micelle with aldehyde groups on its surface. *Macromolecules* **28**: 7295-7297.
12. Nagasaki, Y., Okada, T., Scholz, C., Iijima, M., Kato, M., Kataoka, K., 1998, The reactive polymeric micelle based on an aldehyde-ended poly(ethylene glycol)-poly(lactide) block copolymer. *Macromolecules* **31**: 1473-1479.
13. Yasugi, K., Nakamura, T., Nagasaki, Y., Kato, M., Kataoka, K., 1999, Sugar-installed polymer micelles: synthesis and micellization of poly(ethylene glycol)-poly(D,L-lactide) block copolymers having sugar groups at the PEG chain end. *Macromolecules* **32**: 8024-8032.
14. Cammas, S. M., Okano, T., Kataoka, K., 1999, Functional and site-specific macromolecular micelles as high potential drug carriers. *Colloids and Surfaces B: Biointerfaces* **16**: 207-215.
15. Kohori, F., Sakai, K., Aoyagi, T., Yokoyama, M., Sakurai, Y., Okano, T., 1998, Preparation and characterization of thermally responsive block copolymer micelles comprising poly(N-isopropylacrylamide-b-DL-lactide). *J. Contr. Rel.* **55**: 87-98.
16. Chung J. E., Yokoyama, M., Okano, T., 2000, Inner core segment design for drug delivery control of thermo-responsive polymeric micelles. *J. Contr. Rel.* **65**: 93-103.
17. Cammas, S., Suzuki, K., Sone, C., Sakurai, Y., Kataoka,, K., Okano, T., 1997, Thermo-responsive polymer nanoparticles with a core-shell micelle structure as site-specific drug carriers. *J. Contr. Rel.* **48**: 157-164.
18. Kakizawa, Y., Harada, A., Kataoka, K., 1999, Environment-sensitive stabilization of core-shell structured polyion complex micelle by reversible cross-linking of the core through disulfide bond. *J. Am. Chem. Soc.* **121**: 11247-11248.
19. Taillefer, J., Brasseur, N., van Lier, J. E., Lenaerts, V., Le Garrec, D., Leroux, J.-C., 2001, In-vitro and in-vivo evaluation of pH-sensitive polymeric micelles in a photodynamic cancer therapy model. *J. Pharm. Pharmacol.* **53**: 155-156.
20. Kataoka, K., 1996, Targetable polymeric drugs, chapter 4 in "*Controlled drug delivery: the next generation* (K. Park, ed.), American Chemical Society, Washington D.C..

21. Matsumura, Y., Maeda, H., 1986, A new concept for macromolecular therapeutics in cancer chemotherapy: mechanism of tumoritropic accumulation of proteins and the antitumor agent Smancs. *Cancer Res.* **46**: 6387-6392.
22. Maeda, H., Matsumura, Y., 1989, Tumoritropic and lymphotropic principles of macromolecular drugs. *Critical Rev. in Ther. Drug Carrier Syst.* **6**: 193-210.
23. Noguchi, Y., Wu, J., Duncan, R., Steohalm, J., Ulbrich, K., Akaike, T., Maeda, H., 1998, Early phase tumor accumulation of macromolecules: a great difference in clearance rate between tumor and normal tissues. *Jpn. J. Cancer Res.* **89**: 307-314.
24. Seymour, L. W., Duncan, R., Strohalm, J., Kopecek, J., 1987, Effect of molecular weight (M_w) of N-(2-hydroxypropyl)methacrylamide copolymers on body distribution and rate of excretion after subcutaneous, intraperitoneal, and intravenous administration to rats. *J. Biomed. Mater. Res.* **21**: 1341-1358.
25. Stolnik, S., Illum, L., Davis, S. S., 1995, Long circulating microparticulate drug carriers. *Adv. Drug Del. Rev.* **16**: 195-214.
26. Mosqueria, V. C. F., Legrand, P., Gulik, A., Bourdon, O., Gref, R., Labarre, D., Barratt, G., 2001, Relationship between complement activation, cellular uptake and surface physicochemical aspects of novel PEG-modified nanoparticles. *Biomaterials* **22**: 2967-2979.
27. Harris, J. M., 1992, Introduction to biotechnical and biomedical applications for poly(ethylene glycol), in *Poly(ethylene glycol) chemistry* (J. M. Harris ed.), Plenum Press, New York.
28. Jeon, S. I., Lee, J. H., Andrade, J. D., De Gennes, P. G., 1991, Protein-surface interactions in the presence of polyethylene oxide. I. Simplified theory. *J. Colloid Interface Sci.* **142**: 149-158.
29. Maeda, H., Sawa, T., Konno, T., 2001, Mechanism of tumor-targeted delivery of macromolecular drugs, including the EPR effect in solid tumor and clinical overview of the prototype polymeric drug SMANCS. *J. Contr. Rel.* **74**: 47-61.
30. Dvorak, H. F., Brown, L. F., Detmar, M., Dvorak, A. M., 1995, Vascular permeability factor / vascular endothelial growth factor, microvascular hyperpermeability, and angiogenesis. *Am. J. Pathol.* **146**: 1029-1039.
31. Hobbs, S.K, Monsky, W. L., Yuan, F., Roberts, W. G., Griffith, L., Torchilin, V. P., Jain, R. K., 1998, Regulation of transport pathways in tumor vessels: role of tumor type and microenvironment. *Proc. Natl. Acad. Sci. USA* **95**: 4607-4612.
32. Jain, R. K., 2001, Delivery of molecular and cellular medicine to solid tumors. *Adv. Drug Deliv. Rev.* **46**: 149-168.
33. Maeda, H., 2001, The enhanced permeability and retention (EPR) effect in tumor vasculature: the key role of tumor-selective macromolecular drug targeting. *Adv. Enzyme Regul.* **41**: 189-207.
34. Maeda, H., Noguchi, Y., Sato, K., Akaike, T., 1994, Enhanced vascular permeability in solid tumor is mediated by nitric oxide and inhibited by both new nitric oxide scavenger and nitric oxide synthase inhibitor. *Jpn. J. Cancer Res.* **85**: 331-334.
35. Wu, J., Akaike, T., Maeda, H., 1998, Modulation of enhanced vascular permeability in tumors by a bradykinin antagonist, a cyclooxygenase inhibitor, and a nitric oxide scavenger. *Cancer Res.* **58**: 159-165.
36. Wu, J., Akaike, T., Hayashida, K., Okamoto, T., Okuyama, A., Maeda, H., 2001, Enhanced vascular permeability in solid tumor involving peroxynitrite and matrix metalloproteinases. *Jpn. J. Cnacer. Res.* **92**: 439-451.
37. Kwon, G. S., Naito, M., Yokoyama, M., Okano, T., Sakurai, Y., Kataoka, K., 1993, Micelles based on AB block copolymers of poly(ethylene oxide) and poly(β-benzyl L-aspartate). *Langmuir* **9**: 945-949.
38. Kataoka, K., Matsumoto, T., Yokoyama, M., Okano, T., Sakurai, Y., Fukushima, S., Okamoto, K., Kwon, G. S., 2000, Doxorubicin-loaded poly(ethylene oxide) and poly(β-

benzyl L-aspartate) copolymer micelles: their pharmaceutical characteristics and biological significance. *J. Contr. Rel.* **64**: 143-153.

39. Yamamoto, Y., Nagasaki, Y., Kato, Y., Sugiyama, Y., Kataoka, K., 2001, Long-circulating poly(ethylene glycol)-poly(D,L-lactide) block copolymer micelles with modulated surface charge. *J. Contr. Rel.* 77: 27-38.
40. Yamamoto, Y., Nagasaki, Y., Kato, M., Kataoka, K., 1999, Surface modification of poly(ethylene glycol)-poly(D,L-lactide) block copolymer micelles: conjugation of charged peptide. *Colloids and Surfaces B: Biointerfaces* **16**: 135-146
41. Verrechia, T., Spenlehauer, G., Bazile, D. V., Murry-Brelier, A., Archimbaud, Y., Veillard, M., 1995, Non-stealth (poly(lactic acid / albumin)) and stealth (poly(lactic acid-polyethylene glycol)) nanoparticles as injectable drug carriers. *J. Contr. Rel.* **36**: 49-61.
42. Bazile, D., Prudhomme, C., Bassoullet, M. T., Marlard, M., Spenlehauer, G., Veillard, M., 1995, Stealth Me-PEG-PLA nanoparticles avoid uptake by the mononuclear phagocytes system. *J. Pharm. Sci.* **84**: 493-498.
43. Nakada, Y., Tudomi, R., Sakurai, K., Takahashi, Y., 1998, Evaluation of long-circulating nanoparticles using biodegradable ABA triblock copolymers containing of poly(L-lactic acid) A-blocks attached to central poly(oxyethylene) B-blocks in vivo. *Int. J. Pharm.* **175**: 109-117.
44. Burt, H. M., Zhang, X., Toleikis, P., Embree, L., Hunter, W. L., 1999, Development of copolymers of poly(D,L-lactide) and methoxypolyethylene glycol as micellar carriers of paclitaxel. *Colloids and Surfaces B: Biointerfaces* **16**: 161-171.
45. Allen, T. M., Hansen, C., 1991, Pharmacokinetics of stealth versus conventional liposomes: effect of dose. *Biochim. Biophys. Acta* **1068**: 133-141.
46. Woodle, M. C., Matthay, K. K., Newman, M. S., Hidayat, J. E., Collins, L. R., Redemann, C., Martin, F. J., Papahadjopoulos, D., 1992, Versatility in lipid composition showing prolonged circulation with sterically stabilized liposome. *Biochim. Biophys. Acta* **1105**: 193-200.
47. Takakura, Y., Fujita, T., Hashida, M., Sezaki, H., 1990, Distribution characteristics of macromolecules in tumor-bearing mice. *Pharm. Res.* **7**: 339-346.
48. Y. Takakura, Hashida, M., 1996, Macromolecular carrier systems for targeted drug delivery: pharmacokinetic considerations on biodistribution. *Pharm. Res.* **13**: 820-831.
49. Nagasaki, Y., Yasugi, K., Yamamoto, Y., Harada, A., Kataoka, K., 2001, Sugar-installed block copolymer micelles: their preparation and specific interaction with lectin molecules. *Biomacromolecules* **2**: 1067-1070.
50. Yokoyama, M., Okano, T., Sakurai, Y., Ekimoto, H., Shibazaki, C., Kataoka, K., 1991, Toxicity and antitumor activity against solid tumors of micelle-forming polymeric anticancer drug and its extremely long circulation in blood. *Cancer Res.* **51**: 3229-3236.
51. Yokoyama, M., Okano, T., Sakurai, Y., Kataoka, K., 1994, Improved synthesis of adriamycin-conjugated poly(ethylene glycol)-poly(aspartic acid) block copolymer and formation of unimodal micellar structure with controlled amount of physically entrapped adriamycin. *J. Contr. Rel.* **32**: 269-277.
52. Fukushima, S., Machida, M., Akutsu, T., Shimizu, K., Tanaka, S., Okamoto, K., Machida, H., Yokoyama, M., Okano, T., Sakurai, Y., Kataoka, K., 1999, Roles of adriamycin and adriamycin dimer in antitumor activity of the polymeric micelle carrier system, *Colloids and Surfaces B: Biointerfaces* **16**: 227-236.
53. Yokoyama, M., Sugiyama, T., Okano, T., Sakurai, Y., Naito, M., Kataoka, K., 1993, Analysis of micelle formation of an adriamycin-conjugated poly(ethylene glycol)-poly(aspartic acid) block copolymer by gel permeation chromatography. *Pharm. Res.* **10**: 895-899.
54. Yokoyama, M., Sugiyama, T., Okano, T., Sakurai, Y., Naito, M., Kataoka, K., 1993, Analysis of micelle formation of an adriamycin-conjugated poly(ethylene glycol)-poly(aspartic acid) block copolymer by gel permeation chromatography. *Pharm. Res.* **10**: 895-899.

55. Kwon, G. S., Naito, M., Kataoka, K., Yokoyama, M., Sakurai, Y., Okano, T., 1994, Block copolymer micelles as vehicles for hydrophobic drugs. *Colloids and Surfaces B: Biointerfaces* **2**: 429-434.
56. Kwon, G. S., Naito, M., Yokoyama, M., Okano, T., Sakurai, Y., Kataoka, K., 1995, Physical entrapment of adriamycin in AB block copolymer micelles. *Pharm. Res.* **12**: 192-195.
57. Kwon, G. S., Naito, M., Yokoyama, M., Okano, T., Sakurai, Y., Kataoka, K., 1997, Block copolymer micelles for drug delivery: loading and release of doxorubicin. *J. Contr. Rel.* **48**: 195-201.
58. La, S. B., Okano, T., Kataoka, K., 1996, Preparation and characterization of the micelle-forming polymeric drug indomethacin-incorporated poly(ethylene oxide)-poly(β-benzyl L-aspartate) block copolymer micelles. *J. Pharm. Sci.* **85**: 85-90.
59. Liaw, J., Aoyagi, T., Kataoka, K., Sakurai, Y., Okano, T., 1998, Visualization of PEO-PBLA-pyrene polymeric micelles by atomic force microscopy. *Pharm. Res.* **15**: 1721-1726.
60. Lavasanifar, A., Samuel, J., Kwon, G. S., 2000, Micelles of poly(ethylene oxide)-block-poly(N-alkyl stearate L-aspartamide): synthetic analogues of lipoproteins for drug delivery. *J. Biomed. Mater. Res.* **52**: 831-835.
61. Lavasanifar, A., Samuel, J., Kwon, G. S., 2001, The effect of alkyl core structure on micellar properties of poly(ethylene glycol)-block-poly(L-aspartamide) derivatives. *Colloids and Surfaces B: Biointerfaces* **22**: 115-126.
62. Yokoyama, M., Satoh, A., Sakurai, Y., Okano, T., Matsumura, Y., Kakizoe, T., Kataoka, K., 1998, Incorporation of water-insoluble anticancer drug into polymeric micelles and control of their particle size. *J. Contr. Rel.* **55**: 219-229.
63. Aoyagi, T., Sugi, K., Sakurai, Y., Okano, T., Kataoka, K., 1999, Peptide drug carrier: studies on incorporation of vasopressin into nano-associates comprising poly(ethylene glycol)-poly(L-aspartic acid) block copolymer. *Colloids and Surface B: Biointerfaces* **16**: 237-242.
64. Parr, M. J., Masin, D., Cullis, P. R., Bally, M. B., 1997, Accumulation of liposomal lipid and encapsulated doxorubicin in murine Lewis lung carcinoma: The lack of beneficial effects by coating liposomes with poly(ethylene glycol). *J. Phamacol. Exp. Ther.* **280**: 1319-1327.
65. Gref, R., Minamitake, Y., Peracchia, M. T., Trubetskoy, V., Torchilin, V., Langer, R., 1994, Biodegradable long-circulating polymeric nanospheres. *Science* **263**: 1600-1603.
66. Jeong, Y.-I., Cheon, J.-B., Kim, S.-H., Nah, J.-W., Lee, Y.-M., Sung, Y.-K., Akaike, T., Cho, C.-S., 1998, Clonazepam release from core-shell type nanoparticles in vitro. *J. Contr. Rel.* **51**: 169-178.
67. Burt, H. M., Zhang, X., Toleikis, P., Embree, L., Hunter, W. L., 1999, Development of copolymers of poly(D,L-lactide) and methoxypolyethylele glycol as micellar carriers of paclitaxel. *Colloids and Surfaces B: Biointerfaces* **16**: 161-171.
68. Rosenberg, B., 1978, Platinum complexes for the treatment of cancer. *Interdisciplinary Science Reviews* **3**: 134-147.
69. Ponzani, V., Bressolle, F., Haug, I. J., Galtier, M., Blayac, J. P., 1994, Cisplatin-induced renal toxicity and toxicity-modulating strategies: review. *Cancer Chemother. Pharmacol.* **35**: 1-9.
70. Siddik, Z. H., Newell, D. R., Boxall, F. E., Harrap, K. R., 1987, The comparative pharmacokinetics of carboplatin and cisplatin in mice and rats. *Biochemical Pharmacology* **36**: 1925-1932.
71. Korst, A. C. E., Boven, E., van der Sterre, M. L. T., Fichtinger-Schepman, A. M. J., van der Vijgh, W. J. F., 1998, Pharmacokinetics of cisplatin with and without amifostine in tumour-bearing nude mice. *Eur. J. Cancer* **34**: 412-416.
72. Newman, M. S., Colbern, G. T., Working, P. K., Engbers, C., Amantea, M. A., 1999, Comparative pharmacokinetics, tissue distribution, and therapeutic effectiveness of

cisplatin encapsulated in long circulating, pegylated liposomes (SPI-077) in tumor-bearing mice. *Cancer Chemother. Pharmacol.* **43**:1-7.

73. Avichechter, D., Schechter, B., Arnon, R., 1998, Functional polymers in drug delivery: carrier-supported CDDP (cis-platin) complexes of polycarboxylates - effect on human ovarian carcinoma. *React. Funct. Polym.* **36**: 59-69.
74. Bogdanov Jr., A, Wright, S. C., Marecos, E. M., Bogdanova, A., Martin, C., Petherick, P., Weissleder, R., 1997, A long-circulating co-polymer in "passive targeting" to solid tumors. *J. Drug Targeting* **4**: 321-330.
75. Perez-Soler, R., Han, I., Al-Baker, S., Khokhar, A. R., 1994, Lipophilic platinum complexes entrapped in liposomes: improved stability and preserved antitumor activity with complexes containing linear alkyl carboxylate leaving groups. *Cancer Chemother. Pharmacol.* **33**: 378-384.
76. Ohya, Y., Masunaga, T., Baba, T., Ouchi, T., 1996, Synthesis and cytotoxic activity of dextran carrying cis-dichloro(cyclohexane-trans-l-1,2-diamine) platinum(II) complex. *J. Biomater. Sci. Polymer Edn.* **7**: 1085-1096.
77. Ferruti, P., Ranucci, E., Trotta, F., Gianasi, E., Evagorou, E. G., Wasil, M., Wilson, G., Duncan, R., 1999, Synthesis, characterization, and antitumor activity of platinum(II) complexes of novel functionalised poly(amido amine)s. *Macromol. Chem. Phys.* **200**:1644-1654.
78. Gianasi, E., Wasil, M., Evagarou, E. G., Keddle, A., Wilson, G., Duncan, R., 1999, HPMA copolymer platinates as novel antitumor agents: in vitro properties, pharmacokinetics and antitumor activity in vivo. *Eur. J. Cancer* **35**: 994-1002.
79. Howe-Grant, M. E.; Lippard, S. J., 1980, Aqueous platinum(II) chemistry: Binding to Biological Molecules (chapter 2 in *Metal Ions in Biological Systems*), Mercel Dekker, New York, NY, 11: 63-125.
80. Schechter, B., Newmann, A., Wilchek, M., Arnon, R., 1989, Soluble polymers as carriers of cis-platinum. *J. Contr. Rel.* **10**: 75-87.
81. Yokoyama, M., Okano, T., Sakurai, Y., Suwa, S., Kataoka, K., 1996, Introduction of cisplatin into polymeric micelle. *J. Contr. Rel.* **39**: 351-356.
82. Nishiyama, N., Yokoyama, M., Aoyagi, T., Okano, T., Sakurai, Y., Kataoka, K., 1999, Preparation and characterization of self-assembled polymer-metal complex micelle from cis-dichlorodiammineplatinum(II) and poly(ethylene glycol)-poly(aspartic acid) block copolymer in an aqueous medium. *Langmuir* **15**: 377-383.
83. Nishiyama, N., Kato, Y., Sugiyama, Y., Kataoka, K., 2001, Development of cisplatin-loaded polymeric micelles with a prolonged circulation in the bloodstream and an enhanced accumulation in the solid tumor. *Proceedings of the 20th International Symposium on Controlled Release of Bioactive Compounds* **28**: 5155-5156.
84. Okazaki, S., Nishiyama, N., Kato, Y., Sugiyama, Y., Miyamoto, M., Kataoka, K., 2002, Enhanced tumor accumulation and anticancer activity of cisplatin-loaded polymeric micelles. *Proceedings of the 2nd International Symposium on Tumor Targeted Delivery Systems*
85. Harada, A., Kataoka, K., 1995, Formation of polyion complex micelles in aqueous milieu from a pair of oppositely-charged block copolymers with poly(ethylene glycol) segments. *Macromolecules* **28**: 5294-5299.
86. Harada, A., Kataoka, K., 1999, Chain length recognition: core-shell supermolecular assembly from oppositely charged block copolymers. *Science* **283**: 65-67.
87. Wolfert, M. A., Schacht, E. H., Toncheva, V., Ulbrich, K., Nazarova, O., Seymour, L. W., 1996, Characterization of vectors for gene therapy formed by self-assembly of DNA with synthetic block co-polymers. *Hum. Gene Ther.* **7**: 2123-2133.
88. Katayose, S., Kataoka, K., 1997, Water-soluble polyion complex associates of DNA and poly(ethylene glycol)-poly(L-lysine) block copolymer. *Bioconj. Chem.* **8**: 702-707.

89. Kabanov, A. V., Vinogradov, S. V., Suzdaltseva, Y. G., Alakhov, V. Y., 1995, Water-soluble block polycations as carriers for oligonucleotide delivery. *Bioconj. Chem.* **6**: 639-643.
90. Kataoka, K., Togawa, H., Harada, A., Yasugi, K., Matsumoto, T., Katayose, S., 1996, Spontaneous formation of polyion complex micelles with narrow distribution from antisense oligonucleotide and cationic block copolymer in physiological saline. *Macromolecules* **29**: 8556-8557.
91. Harada, A., Kataoka, K., 1998, Novel polyion complex micelles entrapping enzyme molecules in the core: preparation of narrowly-distributed micelles from lysozyme and poly(ethylene glycol)-poly(aspartic acid) block copolymer in aqueous medium. *Macromolecules* **31**: 4208-4212.
92. Harada, A., Kataoka, K., 1999, On-off control of enzymatic activity synchronizing with reversible formation of supramolecular assembly from enzyme and charged block copolymers. *J. Am. Chem. Soc.* **121**: 9241-9242.
93. Kakizawa, Y., Kataoka, K., 2002, Block copolymer micelles for delivery of gene and related compounds. *Adv. Drug Deliv. Rev.* **54**: 203-222.
94. Macdonald, I. J., Dougherty, T. J., 2001, Basic principles of photodynamic thrapy. *J. Porphyrins Phthalocyanines* **5**: 105-129.
95. Shiah, J.-G., Sun, Y., Peterson. C. M., Kopecek, J., 1999, Biodistribution of free and N-(2-hydroxypropyl)methacrylamide copolymer-bound mesochlorin e_6 and adriamycin in nude mice bearing human ovarian carcinoma OVCAR-3 xenografts. *J. Contr. Rel.* **61**: 145-157.
96. Shiah, J.-G., Sun, Y., Kopeckova, P., Peterson, C. M., Straight, R. C., Kopecek, J., 2001, Combination therapy and photodynamic therapy of targetable N-(2-hydroxypropyl)methacrylamide copolymer-doxorubicin / mesochlorin e_6-OV-TL 16 antibody immunoconjugates. *J. Contr. Rel.* **74**: 249-253.
97. Fisher, A. M. R., Murphree, A. L., Gomer, C. J., 1995, Clinical and preclinical photodynamic therapy. *Lasers in Surgery and Medicine* **17**: 2-31.
98. Sadamoto, R., Tomioka, N., Aida, T., 1996, Photoinduced electron transfer reaction through dendrimer architecture. *J. Am. Chem. Soc.* **118**: 3978-3979.
99. Jiang D.-L., Aida, T., 1998, Morphology-dependent photochemical events in aryl ether dendrimer porphyrins: cooperation of dendron subunits for singlet energy transduction. *J. Am. Chem. Soc.* **120**: 10895-10901.
100. Nishiyama, N., Stapert, H. R., Zhang, G.-D., Takasu, D., Jiang, D.-L., Nagano, T., Aida, T., Kataoka, K., Light-harvesting dendrimer porphyrins as new photosensitizers for photodynamic therapy, *Bioconj. Chem.* In press.
101. Stapert, H. R., Nishiyama, N., Kataoka, K., Jiang, D.-L., Aida, T., 2000, Poly-ion complex micelles encapsulating light-harvesting dendrimer porphyrins. *Langmuir* **16**: 8182-8188.
102. Mendelsohn, J., Baselga, J., 2000, The EGF receptor family as targets for cancer therapy. *Oncogene* **19**: 6550-6565.
103. Sebti, S. M., Hamilton, A. D., 2000, Farnesyltransfetase and geranylgeranyltransferase I inhibitors and cancer therapy: Lessons from mechanism and bench-to-bedside translational studies. *Oncogene* **19**: 6584-6593.
104. Sebolt-Leopold, J. S., 2000, Development of anticancer drugs targeting the MAP kinase pathway. *Oncogene* **19**: 6594-6599.
105. Pestell, K. E., Ducruet, A. P., Wipf, P., Lazo, J. S., 2000, Small molecule inhibitors of dual specificity protein phosphatases. *Oncogene* **19**: 6607-6612.
106. Senderowicz, A. M., Small molecule modulators of cyclin-dependent kinases for cancer therapy. *Oncogene* **19**: 6600-6606.
107. Blagosklonny, M. V., 2002, Hsp-90-associated oncoproteins: multiple targets of geldanamycin and its analogs. *Leukemia* **16**: 455-462.

108. Kasuya, Y., Lu, Z.-R., Kopeckova, P., Tabibi, S. E., Kopecek, J., 2002, Influence of the structure of drug moieties on the in vitro efficacy of HPMA copolymer-geldanamycin derivative conjugates. *Pharm. Res.* **19**: 115-123.
109. Kasuya, Y., Lu, Z.-R., Kopeckova, P., Minko, T., Tabibi, S.-E., Kopecek, J., 2001, Synthesis and characterization of HPMA copolymer-geldanamycin derivative conjugates. *J. Contr. Rel.* **74**: 203-211.

An Interim Analysis of Phase I Clinical Trial of MCC-465, a Doxorubicin (DXR) Encapsulated in PEG-immunoliposome, in Patients with Metastatic Stomach Cancer

Y. MATSUMURA
Investigative Treatment Division, National Cancer Center Research Institute East, 6-5-1 Kashiwanoha, Kashiwa, Chiba 277-8577, Japan, E-mail: yhmatsum@east.ncc.go.jp

1. INTRODUCTION

A low-molecular-weight anticancer agent is distributed readily into almost all tissues and intracellular compartments. Such compound is rapidly cleared from blood by glomerular excretion, limiting its therapeutic availability. In order to raise its therapeutic concentration and AUC (area under the concentration curve), injection of the maximum tolerable amount of the low-molecular-weight drug often results in severe toxicity without significant antitumor efficacy. Therefore, several novel forms of drug delivery system (DDS) have been designed to obtain a selective tumor targeting of anticancer agents. There are two main concepts in the DDS, active targeting and passive targeting. The former involves monoclonal antibodies to tumor related molecules which can target the tumor by utilizing specific binding ability between the antibody and antigen. The latter system can be achieved by the so-called EPR effect (enhanced permeability and retention effect) (1-5). The EPR effect was named according to the pathophysiological characteristics of solid tumor tissue: hypervascularity, incomplete vascular architecture, secretion of vascular permeability factors stimulating extravasation within the cancer, and also the absence of effective lymphatic drainage of macromolecules and nano particulates. Macromolecules and nano particulates have long plasma half-lives because they are too large to extravasate through the normal vessel walls unless they are trapped by the reticuloendothelial system in various organs. Such macromolecules can diffuse out of tumor blood vessels, and reach to the solid tumor tissue effectively, but they are retained in the tumor tissue for a long period due to the EPR effect.

PEG-coated liposomes are stable, long-circulating drug carriers useful for delivering doxorubicin (DXR) to the sites of solid tumors. Compared with conventional liposomes, pegylated liposomes are less effectively taken up by the reticuloendothelial system (RES) and remains in circulation for a long time (6-8). The long circulating pegylated liposomes also extravasate through leaky tumor vasculartυre resulting in delivery of DXR to tumor tissue probably due to the EPR effect. In fact, in numbers of animal and human tumors, pegylated liposomal DXR produced higher intratumor drug concentrations and better therapeutic responses than equivalent doses of nonpegylated-liposome encapsulated DXR or free DXR (9,10).

MCC-465 is the newly formulated immunoliposome encapsulated DXR. This liposome is chemically conjugated with PEG and a monoclonal antibody, GAH which recognizes a cell surface molecule on various kinds of cancer cells (Fig.1) (11,12). Therefore this formulation should possess the ability of both active and passive targeting. The antibody bound to liposome is human antibody F(ab')$_2$. At present, the antigen recognized by the antibody has not been well identified, probably because the antibody may recognizes the conformation of the antigen(s) as the epitope. However at the time of the initiation of this phase I study, it was found that the antigen was on the cell surface, and 90% of stomach cancer tissue was positively stained while normal cells were always negative (11). Antitumor activity of MCC-465 against GAH-positive stomach cancer cells B37 was compared with GAH non-conjugated PEG liposomal DXR in vivo. The result clearly showed that MCC-465 was much more effective against B37 than GAH non-conjugated PEG liposomal DXR. The internalization study using immunoliposome containing fluorescence PKH-2 instead of DXR revealed that B37 internalized MCC-465 extensively but not GAH non-conjugated PEG liposomal DXR (11). In nude mice, MCC-465 exhibited higher antitumor activity against several GAH positive stomach cancers inoculated to the renal capsules of mice in comparison with free DXR or GAH non-conjugated PEG liposomal DXR (12). Taking all data together, we concluded that GAH-conjugated immunoliposome was highly potent antitumor drug with targeting device for human stomach cancer. Therefore, this phase I study was confined to pts with advanced gastric cancer.

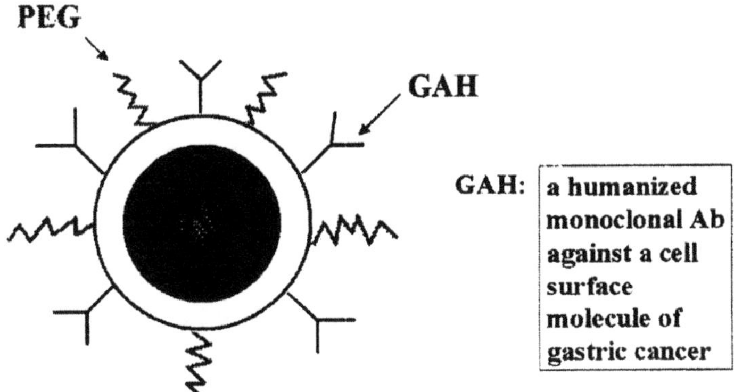

Figure 1. Structure of MCC-465

2. PATIENTS AND METHODS

2.1 Eligibility Criteria

Pts with a cytologically or histologically confirmed advanced or recurrent gastric cancer refractory to conventional therapy were candidates for this study. Pts with a serious infection including HBsAg, HCVab, syphilis, HIV positive, uncontrollable hypertension, brain metastasis showing symptoms, allergy against anthracycline-type drugs, cardiofunction disorders (e.g., pt with suspected congestive heart failure, pt with a treatment history of congestive heart failure, pt with a history of myocardial infarction, and pt with an electrocardiographic abnormality who requires pharmacotherapy.), vascular disorder including a history of pulmonary embolism, deep venous thrombosis, and peripheral artery occlusive disease were excluded. Pts were also excluded if they were pregnant or lactating, or showing gastrointestinal bleeding. Also, pts for whose principal investigator or investigators considered ineligible were excluded. Eligibility criteria also included the following: (1) World Health Organization performance status of ≡ 2; (2) age ≡ 20 years, < 75 years; (3) normal hematologic (WBC count ≡ 4,000/μL; platelet count ≡ 100,000/μL), hepatic (Total bilirubin level ≡ 1.5mg/dL; AST and ALT ≡ 2.5 times the upper limit of normal, unless the elevation was a result of hepatic metastasis, in which case elevations ≡ 3 times the upper normal limits were permitted), renal (serum creatinine = the upper limit of normal), cardiac (NYHA = 1), pulmonary function (PaO_2 = 60mHg); (4) no anticancer therapy in the previous 4 weeks for radiotherapy and chemotherapy (6 weeks for nitrosoureas and mitomycin) before administration of MCC-465, confirmation of history of anthracyclin treatment and doxorubicin dose = 100mg/m^2 or epi- or pira-rubicin dose = 200mg/m^2 ; (5) life expectancy of = 3 months: (6) no coexisting medical problems of sufficient severity; (7) full recovery from toxicity caused by other test drug previously administrated. The institutional review boards for each hospital approved the protocol and informed-consent brochures. All pts gave written informed consent at study entry.

2.2 Study drug and drug administration

MCC-465 was supplied by Mitsubishi Pharma Corporation (Osaka, JPN) in glass vials. Each vial contained lyophilized PEG-immunoliposome including 10 mg of doxorubicin hydrochloride (JP: converted to the DXR titer). Appropriate amounts of MCC-465 which was dissolved in cold sterile saline for injection were diluted with 250 mL or 500 mL (in case of administering eight or more vials) of sterile saline. MCC-465 was infused iv for 60 minutes or 120 mines (in case of 500ml volume) by electric-driven pump with fine filter F162 (Forte Grow Medical Co., Tochigi, JPN) monitoring vital signs including blood pressure, pulse, and respiratory rate during infusion. After infusion, the line was washed out by 50 ml of saline. For the first course, pts were hospitalized for monitoring clinical toxicity and blood sampling for pharmacokinetic analysis from one day before 1st administration to day 23, the next day of 2nd administration.

2.3 Dosage and Dose Escalation

The starting dose of MCC-465 was 6.5mg/m^2 which was equivalent to one tenth of the LD_{10} in rats. MCC-465 was administered once every three week and treatment was continued for up to 6 cycles unless either DLT, or progressive disease were observed. Dose escalation proceeded according to the accelerated titration method described by Simon R *et al* (13) up to Grade 2 or higher toxicity, which were evaluated by the criteria of Japan Clinical Oncology Group (JCOG) at each dose by Day 21. After observation of Grade 2 or higher toxicity the dose should be increased according to the modified Fibonacci method from the next level. Intrapatient dose escalation was not permitted. In the event of DLT, toxicity was confirmed in as many as six pts. MTD was defined as 1 level lower than level in that 3 of 6 pts expressed DLT. The recommended dose for phase II trial was defined by

Safety and Efficacy Assessment Committee concerning with the results of safety and efficacy of this trial. DLT was defined as: (1) Neutrophil less than 500/μL lasting longer than 5 days or associated with fever more over than 38.5 °C by infection; (2) platelets less than 25,000/μL; (3) non-hematologic toxicity ≥ grade 3 except for nausea, vomiting and alopecia.

2.4 Pretreatment Assessment and Follow-Up Studies

Medical histories, physical examinations, vital signs and routine laboratory studies were performed before treatment. On the 1st day of infusion, vital signs included temperature, blood pressure, pulse, respiratory rate ratio was evaluated before infusion, and monitored until the termination of infusion. Furthermore, vital signs were checked at 1,4,8 24 hour. At days 4, 8, 15, 21, 22, 23 (if possible) after the termination of infusion, and the day of every treatment (the time before, interval during and after infusion). ECG was performed before and during treatment. Ultrasonic cardiogram was performed before every odd administration to evaluate ejection fraction. Routine laboratory examination for serum electrolytes, chemistries, renal and liver function tests, a complete blood count with differential WBCs, urinalysis were obtained day 1,2,4,8,15 and 21. Human anti-human antibody (HAHA) was evaluated before every course to prevent hypersensitivity against the antibody conjugated to MCC-465 and decrease of anticancer effect. Also, tumor markers were measured at the same point as HAHA. Tumor response was evaluated and measured before treatment and every 4-6 weeks after treatment (x-ray or endoscopy for original lesions were performed every two courses). A complete response was defined as disappearance of cancerous lesions and partial response required greater than 50% reduction in the sum of the bidimentional length of tumors on two time points separated by at least 4 weeks. No change was defined as less than 25% reduction or less than 25% growth of lesions for at least continuous 4 weeks. To conduct this study properly, the Clinical Trial Coordinating Committee and the Efficacy and Safety Assessment Committee advised to investigators of the study involving three different institutions.

2.5 Sampling and storage

Measurement items were as follows: (1) Plasma concentrations of DXR (total DXR concentration); (2) concentrations of DXR after gel filtration (encapsulated-DXR); (3) concentration of DXR after ultrafiltration (free-DXR); (4) plasma concentrations of DXR metabolites; (5) urinary concentrations of DXR; (6) urinary concentrations of DXR metabolites. In the first course, measurement points were almost same as vital check except ones at days 3 and 6. In the third or subsequent administration, blood collection should be conducted before each administration. After the second course, only total DXR was measured. All samples were chilled on ice during preparation and processed appropriately according to the method described in "Assay condition." Urine samples were stored in refrigerator from the day before administration up to immediately before administration (Day-1 to Day1), thereafter every 24 hours after the first administration, Day 1-2, Day 2-3, and Day3-4 to measure urinary total DXR concentration and urinary DXR metabolites concentrations. Prepared plasma and urinary samples were stored –20 °C except encapsulated-DXR samples which were stored at –80 °C. All plasma and urinary samples should be subjected to each concentration collective measurement at Mitsubishi Pharma Corporation.

2.6 Assay conditions

The assay conditions were as follows. For the measurement of total-DXR and metabolites (doxorubicinol (Dxol) and 7-deoxydoxorubicinol aglycon (7H-Dxol)) in plasma, 200 μL of boric acid buffer (pH9.8) and 3 ml of chloroform/methanol (80:20 v/v) was added to 200 μL of human plasma and mixed. The separated organic phase was evaporated by dryness under nitrogen stream. Residue was re-dissolved with mobile phase and injected into high performance liquid chromatograph (HPLC). HPLC conditions were used "HPLC conditions 1" of Table 1. For the measurement of encapsulated-DXR with HPLC, plasma samples were prepared and filtrated as follows. Sixty μL of patient's plasma and 60 μL of marker solution containing sufficiently empty MCC-465 (no DXR), were mixed. The empty MCC-465 solution was used as the marker for UV detection. And 100 μL of the mixture was applied to gel-filtration. One hundred μL of sample which was collected from peak fraction of encapsulated-DXR through gel-filtration was mixed with 230 μL of methanol containing 0.15% TFA, and injected into HPLC. Gel-filtration conditions were as follows. Column was ECONO Column 5.0×200mm (Bio-Rad); Gel was Bio-Gel A-15m (Bio-Rad); Mobile phase was saline; Flow rate was 0.06 mL/min; Temperature of HPLC was at room temperature; Detection wavelength was UV280nm. HPLC conditions were used "HPLC conditions 2" of Table 1. For free-DXR measurement, 1ml of freshly prepared plasma at each point was centrifuged immediately at 2000xg at room temperature in Centrifree (Amicon Co., Ltd.) for 10 minutes and the filtrate was collected. One hundred μL of the collected sample was mixed with 250?μL of the mobile phase (Table 1) containing internal standard and stored.

DXR and the metabolites in urine were measured with the same method for plasma except for the urine volume (400 μL).

Table 1. HPLC conditions

	HPLC conditions 1	HPLC conditions 2	HPLC conditions 3
Column	CAPCELLPAK C18 UG120 (Shiseido)		
Column size	2.0×250mm	4.6×250mm	2.0×250mm
Column temperature	50°C		
Mobile phase	0.05M phosphoric acid : acetonitrile: THF : PIC B-7 = 75:23:2:1.5 v/v	0.05M phosphoric acid : acetonitrile (containing 7.5% THF) : PIC B-7 =75:23:2:1.5 v/v	0.05M phosphoric acid :acetonitrile : THF : PIC B-7 =70:28:2:2.5 v/v
Flow rate	0.2mL/min	1.2mL/min	0.18mL/min
Fluorescent detector wavelength	EX=475nm, Em=554nm		

2.7 Pharmacokinetic Analysis

Pharmacokinetic parameters of total-DXR, free-DXR and metabolites in human plasma were calculated by non-compartmental model using WinNonlin Ver.2.1 (Pharsight Corporation). The parameters calculated were as follows: peak plasma concentration (Cmax); time to reach the peak plasma concentration (Tmax); half-life of terminal phase (T1/2λz); area under the concentration-time curve (AUC); total clearance (CL); volume of distribution at steady state (Vdss); mean residence time (MRT). The parameters were calculated using scheduled sampling time. However, in case the actual infusion times was more than 15% of scheduled infusion time, pharmacokinetic parameters of the subject were calculated using actual sampling time. Mean and S.D. value of DXR and metabolites at each time point were expressed as N.D. when concentrations of half or more of the subjects were N.D. (which were below limit of quantification). But, when less than half of subjects were N.D., the mean was calculated by substituting 0 for N.D. The total urinary excretion rates of DXR and metabolites were calculated in each subject, and mean urinary excretion rates of DXR and metabolites were calculated at each level. "Microsoft Excel 97 software" was used for data management.

3. RESULTS

To date, 16 patients have been entered into the trial: The details of patients background was shown in Table 2. First pt, 1-101, experienced grade 3 toxicity in liver function with elevation of total bilirubin up to 4.4 mg/dL. This pt did not have liver metastasis, but was suspected to have bile duct obstruction, a tumor thrombosis of the bile duct by invasion of neoplasm was proven by autopsy. The Efficacy and Safety Assessment Committee suggested that the pt could not be a subject for pharmacokinetics and efficacy but safety, additional pt was recommended to enroll. Second pt, 1-102, revealed grade 3 hypertension with grade 2 fever and shivering during infusion. At this time, administration was stopped immediately and re-started cautiously after recovery of all symptoms by medication of antihypertensive drug. This reaction was thought to be infusion related reaction (IRR). Consequently, 6 pts had to be entered for level 1 and dose escalation was changed as modified Fibonacci method thereafter.

Table 2. Patient Characteristic

			Dose	(mg/m^2)		
		Level 1	Level 2	Level 3	Level 4	
		6.5	13.0	21.0	32.5	Total
No. of Patients		7	3	3	3	16
	(Male : Female)	(6 : 1)	(3 : 0)	(3 : 0)	(2 : 1)	(14 : 2)
Age	(Median)	58	57	54	68	56
	(Range)	(40-68)	(57-58)	(30-60)	(56-72)	(30-72)
PS	0	1	2	1	1	5
	1	5	1	2	2	10
	2	1	0	0	0	1
Original Lesion						
	Yes	3	1	1	0	5
	No	4	2	2	3	11
Metastatic Lesion						
	Lung	1	0	1	1	3
	Liver	3	1	0	2	6
	adrenal gland	1	0	0	0	1
	Bone	0	0	2	0	2
	peritonea	3	1	0	0	4
	esophagus	0	0	1	0	1
	Lymph node	3	2	3	1	9
Prior Therapy						
	1	5	1	1	2	9
	2	1	2	0	1	4
	≥3	1	0	2	0	3

Abbreviations: por, Poorly differentiated adenocarcinoma; tub1, Tubular adenocarcinoma, Well differentiated type; tub2, Tubular adenocarcinoma, Moderately differentiated type; pap, Papillary adenocarcinoma; sig, Signet-ring cell carcinoma; *both of por and sig

Table 3. Toxicity in Level 1-4

	$6.5 mg/m^2$		$13.0 mg/m^2$		$21.0 mg/m^2$		$32.5 mg/m^2$		Total No.
Hematologic	Grade 1-2	Grade 3-4	Grade 1-2	Grade 3-4	Grade 1-2	Grade 3-4	Grade 1-2	Grade 3-4	of Pts
Leukopenia					1		1	1	3
Neutropenia					1		1	1	3
Thrombocytophenia									0
Non-Hematologic									
General disorders									
Pyrexia	3		1		2		2		8
Rigors	2		1		2		2		7
Malaise							2		2
Shivering	2		1		1		1		5
Performance status decreased	1								1
Chest discomfort					1				1
Feeling hot									0
Gastrointestinal disorders									
Nausea	2		2				1		5
Anorexia			1		1				2
Vomiting					1		1		2
Stomatitis	1		1				2		4
Diarrhea	1								1
Skin and subcutaneous tissue disorders									
Urticaria NOS	1						1		2
Depilation									0
Others									
Blood pressure increased	1	1	1		1				4
Flushing	1						1		2
Back pain							1		1
Taste disturbance			1						1
Heart rate increased	1		1						2

3.1 Infusion related reaction and other non-hematologic toxicity

All pts who were enlisted in Table 2 were accessed for safety. Major non-hematologic toxicity was summarized in Table 3 with dose and number of pts. Reactions to infusion were observed on first exposure to the drug in 10 pts. Early reactions to infusion developed between 5 to 20 minutes after the start of infusion and were characterized by flushing, chest discomfort, lumbago or itching. All symptoms disappeared shortly with no treatment or after chlorpheniramine maleate infusion. Late reactions to infusion developed usually at the end of infusion of MCC-465 and were characterized by chills and shivering. All symptoms disappeared shortly with no treatment. However, in one instance of level 1, chills and shivering were accompanied by grade 3 hypertension. Some of 16 pts treated to date developed a grade 1 or grade 2 fever 30 min or 60 min after the termination of infusion, however all fevers were transient. Pts experienced such infusion related reactions were tried to treat repeatedly, and they had no or lesser reactions without pre-medications. No skin toxicity was observed. Only 2 patients experienced grade 1 nausea. There was no evidence of liver function or kidney function abnormalities related to treatment. Neither pain nor local toxicity in the area of injection was observed.

Anti-human antibody (HAHA) has not been detected yet throughout all treatment.

3.2 Hematologic toxicity

No significant myelosuppression has been seen up to level 3. Leucopenia and neutropenia were started from day 4 to 8 and a median time to nadir was 15 days.

3.3 Antitumor toxicity

Antitumor responses have not been observed yet at this stage. A slight decrease in serum tumor markers (CEA, CA19-9, CA125) was observed in 7 patients.

3.4 Pharmacokinetics

Pharmacokinetis were evaluated in 15 pts. Mean plasma concentrations of total-DXR, free-DXR, encapsulated-DXR at level 4 was shown in Fig 2. Table 4 shows the mean pharmacokinetic parameters of total-DXR, free-DXR–and metabolites in plasma at level 1 to level 4. The plasma concentration of total-DXR at each level reached Cmax at the end of infusion. The plasma concentration profiles of total-DXR at level 1 to 3 showed biphasic elimination pattern but showed monophasic elimination pattern at level 4, because one subject at level 4 showed monophasic elimination pattern with a long half-life. CL, Vdss, and MRT of total-DXR were almost the same among dose levels. $T1/2\lambda z$ of total-DXR was prolonged by dose escalation, because the concentration of terminal phase was detected as dose increased (Table 4). Most of total-DXR could exist in circulating blood as an encapsulated form, because plasma concentration of encapsulated-DXR was almost equal to that of total-DXR. There was no difference in terms of total-DXR concentration during the repeated administration (data not shown). It was suggested that the pharmacokinetic profile of total-DXR in plasma was not affected by the repeated administration of MCC-465 every 3 weeks.

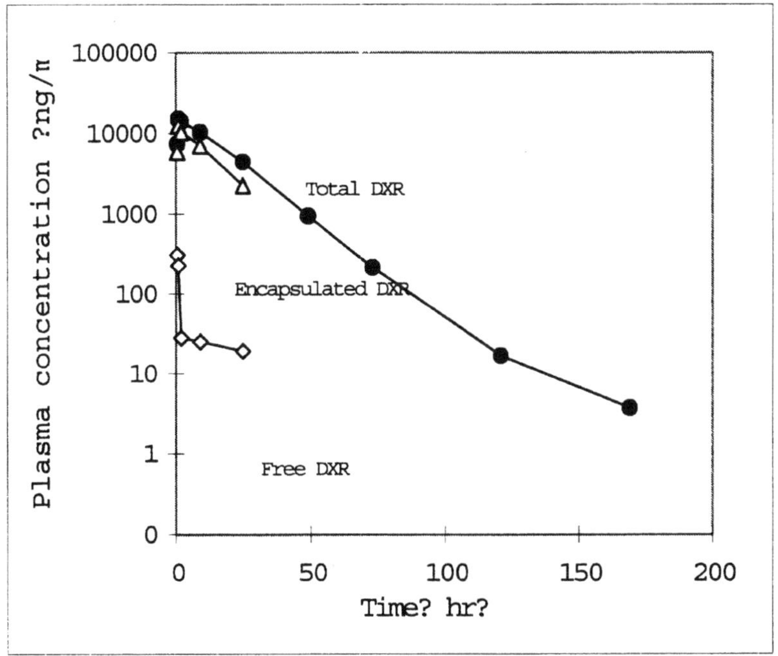

Figure 2. PK profile of MCC-465. Plasma concentrations of DXR in level 4 (mean, n=3). Time in the figures was expressed by scheduled time.

4. DISCUSSION

More than thirty years have passed since Bangham described a liposome for the first time (14). Liposomes had been considered to be a carrier for the delivery of drug because of non-toxic cell-like structure. However the original liposomes possessed a drawback as the liposomes injected intravenously into animals were rapidly cleared primarily by the RES. Consequently they disappear before reaching the tumor tissues and exerting their cell-killing effect. Thus requirements for liposomes with longer circulation times and improved avoidance of RES capture, became prerequisite, which was later accomplished by the development of stealth liposome for cytotoxic drug delivery (6-10). In the cases of stealth

Table 4. Mean PK parameters at each level in phase-I clinical study

Total and free DXR

	n	Dose	Cmax	Tmax	AUC_{0-8}	CL	Vdss	MRT	T1/2λz
		mg/m²	μg/mL	hr	μg•hr/mL	mL/hr/kg	(×10²) mL/kg	hr	hr
Level 1	6	6.5	2.49±1.45	1.01±0.01	31.5±23.7	(4.45±1.78)*3 20.4±25.4	(0.413±0.114)*3 2.61±3.43	10.9±2.53	9.09±4.30
Level 2	3	13.0	7.18±0.847	1.28±0.13	120±44.6	3.36±1.13	0.325±0.0499	10.3±3.11	7.66±1.68
Level 3	3	21.0	11.4±1.42	1.06±0.10	177±27.5	3.39±0.509	0.282±0.0190	8.39±0.761	21.7±12.0
Level 4	3	32.5	15.1±1.47	1.39±0.54	310±139	4.00±1.97	0.511±0.140	14.5±6.42	33.2±17.7
Free-DXR in Level 4	3	32.5	0.325±0.0990	0.67±0.29	3.07	504	210	73.5	54.5

Metabolites

	n	Dose	Cmax	Tmax	AUC_{0-t}	AUC_{0-8}	CL	Vdss	MRT	T1/2λz
		mg/m²	μg/mL	hr	μg•hr/mL	μg•hr/mL	(×10²) mL/hr/kg	(×10³) mL/kg	hr	hr
Dxol in Level 4	3	32.5	0.0049 ±0.0008	25.06 ±24.09	0.476 ±0.117	0.696 ±0.144	15.9±3.90	204±41.0	130±6.43	85.1±9.63
7H-Dxol in Level 4	3	32.5	0.0024	5.5	0.0291	-	-	-	-	-

- : Not calculated

Urinary excretion rate of DXR and metabolites from 0 to 72 hours (mean ± S.D.)

	Level 1	Level 2	Level 3	Level 4
n	6	3	3	3
Doxorubicin	8.3±3.1	5.0±0.8	6.1±1.3	7.3±3.8
Doxorubicinol	2.2±0.7	1.2±0.3	1.5±0.2	1.6±0.8
7-Deoxydoxorubicinol Aglycone	0.0	0.0	0.0	0.0
Total excretion rate	10.5±3.7	6.2±1.0	7.6±1.5	8.9±4.5

liposomal doxorubicin (doxil, Alza, Pharmaceuticals Inc., USA), the liposomes are small (about 100 nm diameter) and contain a small proportion of phospholipid derivative with the hydrophilic polymer, PEG. The linear PEG groups extend from the liposome surface to create a hydrophilic layer that reduces interactions between liposome and plasma components or immune responsive cells.

The plasma pharmacokinetics of Doxil are markedly different from conventional doxorubicin in human (8). Also, in pre-clinical studies, it was revealed that there was a correlation between increasing circulation half-life and the antitumor efficacy of the pegylated liposomal doxorubicin (8). This was presumably obtained by the selective accumulation of the pegylated liposonal doxorubicin utilizing previously described EPR effect (1-5).

Phase II and III studies of Doxil for Kaposi's sarcoma revealed that Doxil exhibits comparable effect to conventional regimens in terms of antitumor effect and over all survival but less toxic especially in cardiac toxicity (15-17).

A phase II study of doxil in ovarian cancer refractory to platinum and paclitaxel showed remarkable antitumor activity with minimal toxicity (18). A Phase III study of doxil against relapsed ovarian cancer revealed that there was no significant difference between doxil and topotecan in terms of progression-free survival and over all survival. Most interestingly, doxil was superior to topotecan in terms of over all survival in a platinum sensitive subset group (19). In addition, toxicity differences between the two agents suggested that doxil would be milder than topotecan (19). At a current status, doxil is approved for Kaposi's sarcoma and ovarian cancer by FDA. Given the comparable antitumor activity and mild myelosuppression in single agent studies, combinations with other agents are being actively pursued against several tumor types. In any event, the stealth liposomes represent an impc tant milestone in the history of the development of liposome technology.

MCC-465 is a pegylated-liposomal doxorubicin tagged with a newly developed monoclonal human antibody, named GAH (11,12). At the present, the antigen recognized by GAH antibody is not well characterized; one reason for this is that the western blot analysis with GAH is not applicable probably because the antibody may recognizes the complex conformational integrity of the antigenic epitope.

Goren D. *et al.* prepared immunoliposome conjugated with whole monoclonal antibody against Her-2 and studied tumor targeting efficacy of the immunoliposome in vitro and in vivo in comparison with plain liposome. They suggested that antitumor efficacy of the liposomal drug was dependent on drug delivery to tumor and hence the rate-limiting step of tumor accumulation of liposome was extravasation process, regardless with liposome affinity or targeting to tumor cells (20). Maruyama *et al.* reported that immunoliposomes conjugated with whole IgG showed shorter plasma half life because of the entrapment of liposomes by RES. In order to overcome this problem, they prepared $F(ab')_2$ conjugated immunoliposome and succeeded in reducing the entrapment of the immunoliposome by RES (21). Based on this finding, $F(ab')_2$ of GAH was conjugated to MCC-465.

Pre-clinical studies showed selective accumulation of DXR in stealth PEG-liposome within gastric cancer tissue following iv injection of MCC-

465, to the nude mice xenograft model with high GAH positive with human gastric cancer tissue, led us to initiate this phase I study (11,12).

The present clinical data indicate that the pharmacokinetics of MCC-465 differ from those of the free doxorubicin but are very similar to doxil in humans. Also, MCC-465 shows peak plasma levels and AUCs similar to the doxil. The increased AUCs result from the increased plasma levels. The volume of distribution at steady state (Vdss) of MCC-465 is also similar to that reported for doxil (8). These pharmacokinetics data indicate that the stability in blood circulation of MCC-465 is similar to doxil. These results suggest that the conjugation of the F(ab')2 of GAH did not interfere with the stealth effect of the pegylated liposomes. Until now, we have not reached MTD yet.

The infusion related reaction was the most common adverse effect. Ten of evaluable 15 pts showed variety of symptoms during the infusion. Major symptoms were fever, rigors, shivering, flushing, chest discomfort, back pain, red eye, itching, feeling hot, numbness and hypertension, were observed. Some pts showed two or more symptoms at the same time. But these symptoms were transient and mild. Other non-hematological toxicities were mild and no malfunctioning of organ such as that of the liver and the kidney occurred. No pt with cardiac toxicity was seen symptomatically as well as functionally in terms of left ventricular ejection fraction. This phase I study is still on going.

ACKNOWLEDGMENTS

I thank the members of MCC-465 phase I study group, as follows: Drs. M. Goto, K. Muro, Y. Yamada, K. Shimada, M. Okuwa, S. Matsumoto, Y. Miyata, H. Okura, S. Baba, K. Chin, T. Yamao, A. Kannami, Y. Takamatsu, K. Ito, and K. Takahashi.

I am also grateful to Misses Michiru Okano and Hiromi Orita for their secretarial assistance.

REFERENCES

1) Matsumura Y, Maeda H: A new concept for macro-molecular therapeutics in cancer chemotherapy: mechanism of tumoritropic accumulation of proteins and the antitumor agent smancs. Cancer Res 46:6387-6392, 1986
2) Maeda H, Matsumura Y: Tumoritropic and lymphotropic principles of macromolecular drugs. Crit Rev Ther Drug Carrier Syst 6: 193-210, 1989
3) Matusmura Y, Maruo K, Kimura M, *et al*: Kinin-generating cascade in advanced cancer patients and *in vitro* study. Jpn J Cancer Res 82: 732-741, 1991
4) Maeda H, Sawa T, and Konno T: Mechanism of tumor-targeted delivery of macro

molecular drugs, including the EPR effect in solid tumor and clinical overview of the prototype polymeric drug SMANCS. J Controlled Release 74: 47-61, 2001

5) Maeda H.: The enhanced permeability and retention (EPR) effect in tumor vasculature: the key role of tumor-selective macromolecular drug targeting. Advan. Enzyme Regul. 41: 189-207, 2001
6) Allen TM, Hansen C, Martin F, *et al*: Liposome containing synthetic lipid derivertives of poly (ethyleneglycol) show prolonged circulation half-lives in vivo. Biochem Biophys Acta 1066: 29-36, 1991.
7) Klibanov AL, Maruyama K, Torchilin VP, *et al*: Amphipathic polyethyleneglycols effectively prolong the circulation time of liposomes. FEBS Lett 268: 235-237, 1990
8) Gabizon A, Catane R, Uziely B, *et al*: Prolonged circulation time and enhanced accumulation in malignant exudates of doxorubicin encapsulated in polyethylene-glycol coated liposomes. Cancer Res 54: 987-992, 1994
9) Gabizon A, Chemla M, Tzemach D, *et al*: Liposome longevity and stability in circulation: effects on the in vivo delivery to tumors and therapeutic efficacy of encapsulated anthracyclines. J Drug Target 3: 391-398, 1996
10) Unezaki S, Maruyama K, Ishida O, *et al*: Enhanced tumor targeting and improved antitumor activity of doxorubicin by long-circulating liposomes containing amphipathic poly (ethylene glycol) Int J Pharm 126: 41-48, 1995
11) Hosokawa, S, Hirakawa, Y, Niki, H, *et al*: Establishment of a human monoclonal antibody (hu-McAb) GAH, exhibiting a specific reactivity to viable cancer cells from fresh tissues and evaluation of the use of the antibody GAH in targeting cancer therapy. Presented at 92nd Annual Meeting of the American Association for Cancer Research, New Orleans, LA, March 24- 28, 2001
12) Nagaike, K, Tagawa, T, Niki, H, *et al*: Anti-Tumor Activity of imunoliposomes conjugated with Human monoclonal antibody-GAH and modified with a branched-PEG derivative in gastric cancers. Presented at 92nd Annual Meeting of the American Association for Cancer Research, New Orleans, LA, March 24- 28, 2001
13) Simon R, Freidlin B, Rubinstein L, *et al.*: Accelerated titration designs for phase I clinical trials in oncology. J Natl Cancer Inst 89: 1138-1147, 1997
14) Bangham AD, Standish MM, Watkins JC: Diffusion on univalent inos across the lamellae of swollen phospholipids J Mol Biol 13: 238-252, 1965
15) Northfelt DW, Dezube BJ, Thommes JA, *et al*: Efficacy of pegylated-liposomal doxorubicin in the treatment of AIDS-related Kaposi's sarcoma after failure of standard chemotherapy J Clin Oncol 15: 653-659, 1997
16) Harrison M, Tomlinson D, Stewart S, *et al*: Loposomal-entrapped doxorubicin: an active agent in AIDS-related Kaposi's sarcoma J Clin Oncol 13: 914-920, 1995
17) Northfelt DW, Dezube BJ, Thommes JA, *et al*: Pegylated-Liposomal Doxorubicin Versus Doxorubicin, Bleomycin, and Vincristine in the Treatment of AIDS-Related Kaposi's Sarcoma: Results of a Randomized Phase III Clinical Trial J Clin Oncol 16: 2445-2451, 1998
18) Muggia FM, Hainsworth JD, Jeffers S, *et al*: Phase II study of liposomal doxorubicin in refractory ovarian cancer: antitumor activity and toxicity modification by liposomal encapsulation J Clin Oncol 15: 987-993, 1997
19) Gordon AN, Fleagle JT, Guthrie D, *et al*: Recurrent epithelial ovarian carcinoma: a randomized phase III study of pegylated liposomal doxorubicin versus topotecan J Clin Oncol 19: 3312-3322, 2001
20) Goren D, Horowitz AT, Zalipsky S, *et al*: Targeting of stealth liposomes to erbB-2 (Her/2) receptor: in vitro and in vivo studies BR J Cancer 74: 1749-1756, 1996
21) Maruyama K, Takahashi N, Tagawa T, *et al.* Immunoliposomes bearing poloethylenglycol-coupled Fab' fragment show prolonged circulation time and high ectravasation into targeted solid tumors in vivo. FEBS Lett 413: 177-180, 1997

Polymer Conjugates for Imaging

ALAN C. PERKINS
Academic Medical Physics, University of Nottingham, Medical School, Queen's Medical Centre. Nottingham, NG7 2UH, UK

1. INTRODUCTION

Medical imaging provides anatomical and physiological information from within the human body without the need for invasive surgical procedures. Clinical imaging procedures are regarded as an essential component of modern clinical care. The information obtained from imaging investigations is of value in the initial diagnosis and staging of disease, in monitoring the effectiveness of treatment and the in the follow up of patient wellbeing. More recently imaging techniques have developed to the extent that they can depict physiological processes rather than structural detail. In particular, certain techniques now have the capacity to image at the molecular level. Such imaging modalities include nuclear medicine (positron emission tomography (PET) and single photon emission computed tomography (SPECT)) and magnetic resonance imaging (MRI). Progress in these areas is partly due to a combination of advances in instrumentation, electronics and computing, however a significant contribution to the increased capabilities of imaging investigations has resulted from the introductions of new image contrast agents and radiopharmaceuticals.

The administration of pharmaceutical grade formulation incorporating a "reporter" moiety that gives rise to the imaging signal and a "targeting" moiety that controls the *in vivo* biodistribution provides additional information on the nature of pathological diseases. Furthermore an important branch of pharmaceutical science originally aimed at utilising polymers and polymeric conjugates as carriers for targeted drug delivery is proving to be

Polymer Drugs in the Clinical Stage, Edited by Maeda et al.
Kluwer Academic/Plenum Publishers, New York, 2003

of increasing importance in medical imaging[1]. A number of polymer conjugates have potential as imaging agents and some have now been evaluated in both experimental systems and patients[2]. This chapter reviews some of the advances in polymeric imaging agents with particular reference to tumour targeting.

2. PHARMACEUTICAL IMAGING AGENTS

In many respects the requirements for imaging are the same as those for drug targeting i.e. the desire to maximise the uptake of an administered agent in pathological tissues in comparison to that in normal tissues. The main difference between the two applications is in the kinetics of uptake in the lesion. Imaging procedures should be quick to minimise patient discomfort and maximise throughput, whereas chemotherapy involves sustained delivery of drug over long periods of time. The majority of anticancer drugs are low molecular weight compounds, which on entering the blood stream extravasate and cross the cell membrane, hopefully resulting in increased uptake in tumour tissue compared with that in normal organs. In drug delivery the biological basis of the design of macromolecular polymer conjugates is the addition of a polymer backbone to control the clearance from the blood pool, minimising the uptake in non-target tissues and hence increase the therapeutic ratio. Clinically this strategy has demonstrated reduced toxicity during cancer chemotherapy[3]. The mechanism involved is considered to be a passive accumulation of drug in the tumour, due to the enhanced permeability and retention (EPR)[4] of the drug. For imaging applications it is essential to control the biodistribution and uptake of the pharmaceutical agent to suit the required application. In some cases this may be a simple vascular agent for intravenous injection, or a non-absorbable agent administered orally, however, for site specific targeting it is necessary to add an additional vector molecule such as an antibody, hormone or receptor binding peptide to the polymer conjugate in order to promote uptake in the lesion or tumour.

2.1 X-ray Contrast Agents

Contrast agents have been widely used in radiological imaging. The majority of the traditional X-ray contrast agents are inert non-specific materials. These generally rely on the use of dense materials (capable of attenuating the X-ray photons) such as barium for oral administration and iodine for intravenous use. The potentially long clearance time of polymer formulations in the circulation makes these agents attractive for use as vascular contrast agents in X-ray procedures. Amphiphilic polymers and polychelating agents have been used for a variety of image contrast applications. The use of polymer based iodine complexes was reported by Bogdanov *et. al.*, in 1995[5]. It was shown that these had attractive properties for clinical diagnostic use including long survival times in the circulation. Other workers have used a block-copolymer of methoxy-polyethylene glycol (MPEG) with iodine as a long-circulating blood pool contrast agent for CT imaging. This copolymer formed a stable micelle that could be heavily loaded with iodine (up to 30% by weight)[6].

The site specific targeting of X-ray contrast agents has not proven to be of any clinical value, mainly because the reporter moieties (barium and iodine) have to be delivered in such large amounts that it is not considered to be a viable possibility. Most work on the development of pharmaceutical agents with specific biological characteristics for tumour targeting has been aimed at other imaging modalities. These are described subsequently.

3. POLYMERIC RADIOPHARMACEUTICALS

Although polymeric imaging agents have been developed for X-ray, magnetic resonance and ultrasound imaging it is probably in the field of nuclear medicine that the imaging of polymer conjugates has been of greatest significance. The use of the gamma camera to image *invivo* drug biodistribution is a powerful technique in its own right[7]. Experimental studies can be undertaken at the pre-clinical stage in an appropriate experimental model and subsequently as non-invasive techniques for clinical Phase I/II evaluation. The production of a stable radiolabelled conjugate is a prerequisite for experimental and clinical investigation. It is interesting to note that the addition of a polymer to a conventional cytotoxic drug can provide means for radiolabelling which would not be possible for the drug alone. A range of polymers and polymeric drug conjugates have been successfully radiolabelled with radionuclides such as ^{131}I, ^{123}I, ^{111}In and ^{99m}Tc which are suitable for gamma camera imaging[8-12]. Many of the methods originally used for radiolabelling peptides and proteins have been used for radiolabelling polymer conjugates[13]. Labelling with radioiodine involves either the direct oxidative incorporation of the iodine atom into tyrosine amino acids using chloramine-T or iodogen, or the indirect attachment of chemical groups such as Boulton and Hunter reagent. The radionuclides ^{123}I or ^{131}I can be used for imaging with the gamma camera whereas ^{124}I may be used for PET imaging. Radiolabelling with metals such as ^{111}In and ^{99m}Tc is usually achieved by the pre-conjugation of a chelating agent such as the bicyclic anhydride of DTPA.

Using the gamma camera, scintigraphic imaging in normal and tumour-bearing experimental models has provided information on the tumour targeting properties of polymer conjugates. Such studies have been extremely valuable in the development and understanding of the tumour targeting and biodistribution of polymeric materials prior to clinical therapeutic trails. A pioneering example of the use of imaging in the clinical development of polymeric drug carriers can be seen in the studies undertaken with the HPMA-doxorubicin copolymer conjugates. These conjugates were initially radiolabelled with ^{131}I and subsequently with ^{123}I by Pimm et al[11,14,15]. The choice of radionuclide will affect the quality of the images obtained, with ^{123}I being preferable to ^{131}I since its lower gamma energy provides superior image resolution when using the gamma camera. These studies not only demonstrated that it was feasible to radiolabel and image copolymer conjugates, but that it was possible to demonstrate tumour uptake by imaging mice with transplanted tumours. Furthermore specific targeting to the liver was achieved by the addition of galactosamine.

Using the same methodology these radiolabelled conjugates were then used clinically in Phase I studies. Julian et. al.[16] used whole body imaging

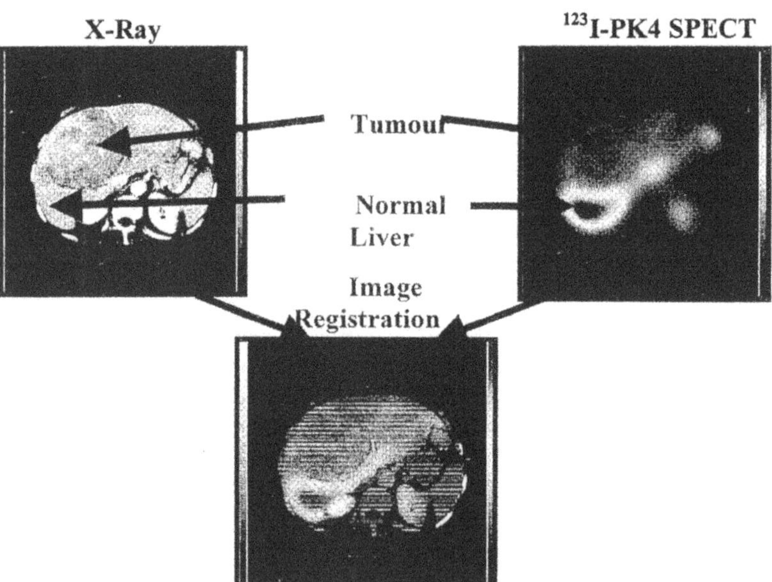

Figure 1. Images of a patient with hepatoma taken from the Birmingham clinical studies, courtesy of P J Julyan[16]. Top left: X-ray CT image through the upper abdomen. Top right: SPECT image of ^{123}I-HPMA-doxorubicin-galactosamine conjugate taken at the same level as the CT image. Bottom: Fused anatomical and functional images.

and single photon emission tomography (SPECT imaging) to show *invivo* biodistribution in patients with malignant disease. An example of targeting the liver of a patient with hepatoma using the ^{123}I-HPMA-doxorubicin-galactosamine conjugate is shown in Fig. 1. The relative uptake between tumour and normal liver tissue can be seen.

Detailed imaging and collection of blood, urine and faeces following the administration of the conjugate has provided critical information on biodistribution and organ uptake in addition to valuable data on pharmacokinetics and mass balance.

The ability to design molecular forms with specific targeting abilities is an important and exciting aspect of polymeric formulation development. The addition of a suitable polymer to a drug or ligand can change simple passive characteristics, such as molecular weight or charge. For example, it has been shown in imaging studies in mice with tumour xenografts that modification of the molecular charge will affect the biodistribution of a branched chain polypeptide[17,18]. Similar properties have been exploited using synthetic polymers to negatively charge-modify monoclonal antibodies, thus altering their *in vivo* biodistribution[19].

It is becoming increasingly evident that polymers in their own right are an important source of materials for the production of radiopharmaceuticals. Some important pharmaceutical products currently in regular clinical use are manufactured from materials obtained from pooled human blood. There remain serious concerns regarding the viral contamination of human blood products. The increased incidence of HIV in the population had serious implications for patients receiving the blood clotting Factor 8. Despite careful screening of donors and appropriate treatment of products problems still remain. In November 1997 and March 1998 the U.K. Department of Health withdrew a number of pharmaceuticals based on blood products from clinical use because of concern over contamination with new variant CJD. In nuclear medicine two routine diagnostic procedures are still undertaken throughout the world using products manufactured from pooled donor human serum albumin[20]. The first is lung perfusion imaging using ^{99m}Tc-macro aggregated albumin (MAA) and the second is sentinel node imaging using ^{99m}Tc-nanocolloid. Whilst the use of recombinant albumin offers one alternative source of material, the use of polymers as potential synthetic radiopharmaceuticals would seem a logical alternative to some of the current radiopharmaceuticals which rely on pooled human blood products for their production[21]. Ultimately these products could be formulated as a radiopharmaceutical kit for use in routine clinical practice[22].

A common clinical problem is the detection of infection and inflammation, especially in the patient with pyrexia of unknown origin. There are a number of radiopharmaceuticals for the clinical investigation of such patients, however, non are ideal. Recently there has been interest in the use of liposomes for this application. These phospholipid vesicles have been extensively investigated as drug carriers and as radiopharmaceuticals. However, rapid removal from the circulation by the mononuclear phagocyte system (MPS) compromises their targeting ability. Surface modification with polyethylene glygol has been shown to reduce recognition by the MPS and hence increase blood residence time. Clinical studies have demonstrated the potential of ^{99m}Tc-PEG liposomes in patients with conditions such as soft tissue infection, septic arthritis, autoimmune polyarthritis, colitis, abdominal abscess and pheumonia[23]. It is interesting to observe however, that the same group later carried out experimental studies using avidin clearance of biotin-PEG liposomes to reduce blood pool activity at the time of imaging[24].

Examples of some polymeric radiopharmaceuticals are given below.

Radiopharmaceutical	***application***	***Reference***
^{99m}Tc-DTPA-BCP	blood pool imaging	Perkins *et. al.*[12]
^{99m} Tc-DTPA-PL-MPEG	blood pool imaging	Bogdanov *et. al.*[22]
^{99m} Tc-PEG liposomes	infection imaging	Dams *et. al.*[23]
^{99m} Tc-DTPA-mannosyl-dextran	sentinel node detection	Vera *et. al.*[25]

In 2001 Vera *et. al.* reported the use of a promising formulation of Tc-99m-DTPA-mannosyl-dextran for sentinel node detection[25]. The identification and biopsy of the sentinel node (the first node in the lymph node chain draining from a tumour) has had a dramatic prognostic implications for patients with malignant tumours such as those of breast and melanoma. The technique for identification of the sentinel node has involved the parenchymal injection of a nanocolloidal human serum albumin particulate originally formulated for lymph node imaging. The production of a radiotracer specifically designed for sentinel node detection is an exciting new development. Potentially these formulations would be capable of providing more specific diagnostic information and will therefore become of increased importance in patient management.

4. MRI CONTRAST AGENTS

In magnetic resonance imaging the image is formed by measuring and mapping out the T_1 and T_2 relaxation times of protons in tissues. MRI contrast agents are based on injectable forms of paramagnetic metals that produce a high intensity signal in the computer generated image. Gadolinium chelates such as gadolinium-DTPA have been routinely used in the clinic, however superparamagnetic ferrite and magnetite formulation are under development. One attractive aspect of polymer formulations is their ability to bind a high density of reporter groups (in this case gadolinium) which will produce high contrast in the final image. An extraordinary range of polymer based formulations have been used for magnetic resonance angiography, tumour imaging, myocardial and pulmonary perfusion and lymphography[26,27,28,29,30]. An elegant example of such a formulation is the synthesis of the dendritic contrast agent GADOMER 17 (Shering AG, Berlin) which contains up to 24 gadolinium complexes trapped in the branched dendrimer structure[31].

The phenominal development of MRI as a major medical imaging modality over the past 10 years will ensure the production and utilisation of paramagnetic contrast agents. Polymers will undoubtedly be an important source of materials for diagnostic MR contrast formulations. Some examples of MR contrast agents are given below.

MRI contrast agent	***Application***	***Reference***
Gd-DTPA-cascade polymer	angiography	Schwickert *et. al.*[26]
Dendrimer Gd chelates	angiography	Wiener *et. al.*[27]
	angiography	Schmitt-Willich *et. al.*[31]
CMD Gd-DTPA carboxymethyl dextran	tumour imaging	Siauve *et. al.*[28]
Polylysine Gd-DTPA	lung perfusion	Berthezène *et. al.*[29]
Gd-DTPA-PGM polyglucose complex	lymphography	Harika *et. al.*[30]

5. ULTRASOUND CONTRAST AGENTS

The clinical application of injectable contrast media in medical ultrasound imaging has been slower to develop than in the other main imaging modalities. The physical basis of ultrasound imaging is the production of a backscattered echo within the frequency range between 1 and 20MHz. Echogenic contrast agents have been based on the use of injectable formulations of stable gas filled microbubbles that produce a strong reflection of the incident sound beam[32]. The bubbles must be less than 10 μm in diameter if they are to pass though the blood vessels of the lungs. Any greater in size and they will be trapped in the pulmonary capillaries. Once injected small gas bubbles dissolve rapidly in the blood. They will be subject to high pressure during transpulmonary and intracardiac passage. It is therefore necessary to stabalise the microbubbles so that they remain intact over a period of time sufficiently long to perform the clinical ultrasound investigation. This has been achieved by encapulating the gas within a thin film made from a suitable material. Biodegradable polymers are attractive materials for the encapsulation of gas microbubbles and a range of echo contrast have been developed based on such materials[33,34]. One promising formulation SH U 563 produced by Shering AG, uses a biodegradable shell of polybutyl-2 cyanoacrylate with a wall thickness of 100nm[35] This is stable enough to protect an enclosed gas bubble from dissolution in the blood stream and is of sufficient elasticity to oscillate in the ultrasonic field. Experimental studies have demonstrated that these particles are ultimately phagocytosed by the reticuloendothelial system. with most of the microcapsules ultimately residing in the liver.

One approach to prolong the survival of these microcapsules in the circulation and hence extend the period of ultrasound contrast enhancement has been to prevent opsonization by covering the surface of the microparticles with polyethylene gylcol. Clinical applications of these agents are in cardiovascular investigation, tumour imaging and in the determination of fallopian tube patency in patients with infertility. The application of these agents is expected to increase as targeting strategies are employed to direct microcapsules to pathological sites such as tumour or thrombus. It is also envisaged that at high acoustic intensities the ultrasound beam could be used to burst the microcapsule which could be loaded with an appropriate drug, thus increasing local availability of drug at the target site.

The comparative low cost of ultrasound equipment has resulted in its widespread clinical use. This will ensure a strong developing market for ultrasound contrast agents in the future.

6. CONCLUSION

The capabilities of modern medical imaging techniques can be greatly enhanced by the use of injectable imaging pharmaceuticals. These take a number of forms, from passive vascular contrast agents to highly specific agents targeted to specific receptors. One problem encountered with formulations based on biological materials has created a need for alternative sources of material for incorporation into imaging formulations. Synthetic polymers are expected to meet that need and are now established as a new generation of image contrast agents with the potential for clinical application in all medical imaging modalities.

REFERENCES

1. Maeda, H., 1994, Polymer conjugated macromolecular drugs for tumor-specific targeting. In *Polymeric Site-Specific Pharmacotherapy* (A.J. Domb, ed), J Wiley & Sons New York pp.96-116.

2. Perkins, A. C., 1998, Polymer Diagnostics: The next generation of image contrast agents. *J. Drug. Targeting* 6:79-84.
3. Duncan, R., Dimitrijevic, S., Evagorou, E. G., 1996, The role of polymer conjugates in the diagnosis and treatment of cancer. *STP Pharma Sciences* 6:237-263.
4. Maeda, H., 2001, The enhanced permeability and retention (EPR) effect in tumor vasculature: The key role of tumor-selective macromoleucluar drug targeting. *Advanced Enzyme Regul.* 41:189-207.
5. Bogdanov, A. A., Weissleder, R., Brady, T.J. (1995) Long circulating blood pool imaging agents. *Advanced Drug Delivery Rev.* 16, 335-348.
6. Torchilin, V. P., 2000. Polymeric contrast agents for medical imaging. *Current Pharmaceutical biotechnology* 1:183-215.
7. Perkins, A.C., and Frier, M., eds. 1999, *Nuclear Medicine in Pharmaceutical Research.* Taylor and Francis, London.
8. Pimm, M. V, Clegg, J. A., Hudecz F, Baldwin RW, 1991, ^{111}In labelling of a branched polypeptide drug carrier with a poly(L-lysine) backbone. *Int. J. Pharmaceutics* 79:77-80.
9. Pimm, M. V., Perkins, A. C., Hudecz, F., 1992, Scinitigraphic evaluation of the pharmacokinetics of a soluble polymeric drug carrier. *Eur. J. Nucl, Med.* 19:449-452.
10. Pimm, M. V., Perkins, A. C., Gribben, S. J., Hudecz, F., 1994, J. Scintigraphic determination of the biodistribution of an ^{111}In labelled poly(L-lysine) backbone branched polypeptide drug carrier in tumour-bearing mice. *Nucl. Biol. Med.* 38 (Suppl):104-108.
11. Pimm, M., V., Perkins, A.,C., Duncan, R., Ulbrich, K., 1993, Targeting of N-(2-Hydroxypropyl) methacrylamide copolymer-doxorubicin conjugate to the hepatocyte galactose-receptor in mice: visualisation and quantification by gamma scinitgraphy as a basis for clinical targeting studies. *J. Drug. Targeting* 1:125-131.
12. Perkins, A. C., Frier, M., Pimm, M. V., Hudecz, F., 1998, ^{99m}Tc-branched-chain-polypeptide (BCP): A potential synthetic radiopharmaceutical. J. Labelled Comp. Radiopharm XLI:631-638.
13. Pimm, M. V., 1999, Scintigraphic study of drug carriers and conjugates. In *Nuclear Medicine in Pharmaceutical Research.* A. C. Perkins and M. Frier, eds. Taylor and Francis London, pp133-169.
14. Pimm, M. V., Perkins, A. C., Strohalm, J., Ulbrich, K., Duncan, R., 1996, Gamma Scintigraphy of a ^{123}I-Labelled N-(2-Hydroxypropyl) Methacrylamide Copolymer-Doxorubicin Conjugate Containing Galactosamine Following Intravenous Administration to Nude Mice Bearing Hepatic Human Colon Carcinoma. *J. Drug Targeting* 3:385-390.
15. Pimm, M. V., Perkins, A. C., Strohalm, J., Ulbrich, K., Duncan, R., 1996, Gamma Scintigraphy of the Biodistribution of ^{123}I-Labelled N-(2-Hydroxypropyl) Methacryllamide Copolymer-Doxorubicin Conjugates in Mice with Transplanted Melanoma and Mammary Carcinoma. *J. Drug Targeting* 3:375-383.
16. Julyan P, J., Seymore, L. W., Ferry, D. R., Daryani, S., Boivin, C. M., Doran, J., David, M., Anderson, D., Christodoulou, C., Young, A. M., Hesselwood, S., Kerr, D. J., 1999, Preliminary clinical study of the distribution of HPMA copolymers bearing doxorubicin and galactosamine. *J. Controlled Release* 57: 281-290.
17. Pimm, M. V., Perkins, A.C., Gribben, S. J., Mezo, G., Gaal D and Hudecz, F. 1995 Gamma scintigraphy of ^{111}In-labelled branched chain polypeptides (BCP) with a poly(L-lysine) backbone in mice with mammary carcinoma: Effect of charge on biodistribution and tumour imaging potential. *Annals. Nucl. Med.*, 9:247-251.
18. Pimm, M. V., Gribben, S. J., Bogdán, K., Hudecz, F., 1995, The effect of charge on the biodistribution in mice of branched chain polypeptides with a poly(L-lysine) backbone labelled with ^{123}I, ^{111}In and ^{51}Cr. *J. Controlled Release* 37:161-172.

19. Khaw, B-A., Kilbanov, A., O'Donnell, S. M., Saito, T., Nossiff, N., Slinkin, M. A., Newell, J. B., Strauss, W., Torchilin, V. P. 1991, Gamma imaging with negatively charge-modified monoclonal antibody: modification with synthetic polymers. *J. Nucl. Med.* 32:1742-1751.
20. Perkins, A.C. and Frier, M., 1999, Bad blood and biologicals: the need for new radiopharmaceutical source materials. *Nucl. Med. Commun.* 20:1-3
21. Verbeke, K., Ons, S., De Roo, M., Verbruggen, A. (1994) Labelling of poly-l-lysine with 99mTc and evaluation as a possible tracer agent for ventriculography. *J. Nucl. Biol. Med.* 38, (Suppl 1 to No 4) 75-78.
22. Bogdanov, A. A., Callahan R.J., Wilkinson, R.A., Martin, C., Cameron, J.A., Fisschman, A. J., Brady, T. J., Weissledr, R., 1994 Synthetic copolymer kit for radionuclide blood-pool imaging. *J. Nucl. Med.*, 35:1880-1886.
23. Dams, E. T. M., Oyen, W. J. G., Boerman, O. C., Storm, G., Laverman P., Kok, P. J. M., Buijs, W. C. A. M., Bakker, H., van der Meer, J. W. M., Corstens, F. H. M., 2000, ^{99m}Tc-PEG liposomes for the scintigraphic detection of infection and inflammation:clinical evaluation. *J. Nucl. Med.* 41:622-630.
24. Laverman, P., Zalipsky, S., Oyen, W. J. G., Dams, E. T. M., Storm, G., Mullah, N., Corstens F. H. M., Boerman, O. C., 2000, Improved imaging of infections by avidin-induced clearance of ^{99m}Tc-biotin-PEG liposomes. *J. Nucl. Med.* 41:912-918.
25. Vera D R, Wallace A M, Hoh C K, Mattrey R F, 2001, A Synthetic Macromolecule for Sentinel Node Detection: ^{99m}Tc-DTPA-Mannosyl-Dextran. *J. Nucl. Med.* 42:951-959.
26. Schwickert, H. C., Roberts, T. P. L., Mühler, A,. Stiskal, M., Demsar, F., Brasch, R. C. 1995, Angiographic properties of Gd-DTPA-24-cascade-polymer - a new macromolecular MR contrast agent. *Eur. J. Radiol.* 20, 144-150.
27. Wiener, E. C., Brechbiel, M. W., Brothers, H., Magin, R. L., Gansow, O. A., Tomalia, D. A., Lauterbur, P. C., 1994, Dendrimer-based metal chelates: a new class of magnetic resonance image contrast agents. *Magn. Reson. Med.* 13:1-8.
28. Siauve, N., Clément, O., Cuénod, C-A., Benderbous, S., Frija, G., 1996, Capillary leakage of a macromolecular MRI agent, carboxymethyldextran-Gd-DTPA, in the liver: pharmacokinetics and imaging implications. *Magn. Reson. Imaging.*, 14, 381-390.
29. Berthezène, Y., Vexler, V., Price, D. C, Wisner-Dupon, J., Mosely, M. E., Aicher, K. P., Brasch R.C., 1992, Magnetic resonance imaging detection of an experimental pulmonary perfusion deficit using a macromolecular contrast agent. *Invest. Radiol.* 27, 346-351.
30. Harika, L., Weissleder, R., Poss, K., Zimmer, C., Papisov, M. I., Brady, T. J., M. R., 1995, Lymphography with a lymphotropic T1-type MR contrast agent Gd-DTPA-PGM. *Magn. Reson. Med.*, 33, 88-92.
31. Schmitt-Willich, H., Ebert, W., Frenzel, T., Misselwitz, B., Platzek, J., Radüchel, B., Weinmann H-J., 1997, Synthesis and preclinical evaluation of a 24-mer dendrimer as a new contrast agent in MR imaging of the vascular system. Proceedings of the second International Symposium on Polymer Therapeutics: From laboratory to the clinic. Kumamoto, Japan (P-19), 40.
32. Hindle, A. J. and Perkins, A. C., 1995, History and basic principles of echo-contrast media. *Brit. Med. Ultrasound Bulletin,* 3 (No 1): 17-23.
33. Schneider, M., Bussat, P., Barrau, M-B., Arditi, M., Yan, F., Hybl, E. (1992) Polymeric microballoons as ultrasound contrast agents: Physical and Ultrasonic properties compared with sonicated albumin. *Invest. Radiol.*, 27, 134-139.
34. Schneider, M., Broillet, A., Bussat, P., Ventrone, R., 1994, The use of polymeric microballoons as ultrasound contrast agents for liver imaging. *Invest. Radiol.*, 29:S149-S151.

35. Fritzsch, T., Heldman, D., and Reinhardt, M., 1997, The potential of a novel ultrasound contrast medium. In *Ultrasound Contrast Agents* (B. B. Goldberg, ed.), Martin Dunitz, London. pp.169-176.

S-Nitrosylated Polyethylene Glycol-conjugated Hemoglobin Derivative as a Candidate Material for Oxygen Therapeutics

KUNIHIKO NAKAI*, ICHIRO SAKUMA#, HIROKO TOGASHI†, MITSUHIRO YOSHIOKA†, TAKESHI SUGAWARA#, HIROSHI SATOH*, and AKIRA KITABATAKE#

**Environmental Health Sciences, Tohoku University Graduate School of Medicine, Aoba, Sendai; Departments of #Cardiovascular Medicine and †Pharmacology, Hokkaido University Graduate School of Medicine, Kita-15 Nishi-7, Sapporo Japan.*

1. INTRODUCTION

Several hemoglobin (Hb)-based derivatives have been studied for use as artificial oxygen carriers. However, they have several limitations[1]. The major side effects include vasoconstriction, abnormal gastrointestinal constriction and platelet stimulation. The most plausible mechanism for these side effects is the nitric oxide (NO) scavenging by acellular Hb itself, since the heme of Hb has a high affinity to NO. A universal problem among all Hb derivatives is their short plasma residence time. The half life time of Hb derivatives in the circulation ranges from 6 to 24 h in animals, and these values are very much shorter than the mean residence time of 120 days for human red blood cells. The hope, therefore, is that the new products will have better applicability in clinical situations where the short-term use of an oxygen carrier is essential.

Recently, it was proposed that the Cysβ93 of Hb is covalently bound with NO, and that this *S*-nitrosylated Hb (SNO-Hb) retains EDRF/NO-like bioactivity[2,3]. Since *S*-nitrosothiols do not react with heme of Hb, SNO-Hb can provide a protected way of delivery of bioactive NO to the tissues. Indeed, SNO-Hb induces relaxation of pre-capillary vessels and inhibits platelet aggregation[3,4]. These insights suggest that SNO-Hb can release NO preferentially where pO_2 is low, dilating small vessels, thus providing more blood to the ischemic tissues. In the circulation, SNO-Hb may still have vasoconstrictive activity because Fe(II)-Hb, which binds oxygen, also has an affinity to NO, though SNO-Hb can compensate for this vasoconstricting effect by releasing NO. These dual functions as both a scavenger and donor of NO not only contribute to avoidance of Hb-induced vasoconstriction, but increase the therapeutic potential of SNO-Hb for use in the area of oxygen therapeutics.

2. S-NITROSOHEMOGLOBIN

Hb is a tetramer composed of two α- and two β-subunits. In human Hb, the β-subunit contains one highly reactive sulfhydryl group (Cysβ93). This sulfhydryl residue has been reported to be *S*-nitrosylated to form SNO-Hb within red blood cells[2]. The authors showed a dynamic cycle in which the binding of oxygen to heme iron promotes the binding of NO to the sulfhydryl residues, and deoxygenation is accompanied by an allosteric conformational change that releases the NO group. In this context, Hb is *S*-nitrosylated in the lung when red blood cells are oxygenated, and the NO group is released during arterial-venous transit dependent on the oxygen gradient in the tissues[3]. SNO-Hb, therefore, can release an NO-group to induce vasorelaxation and increase regional blood flow, and then deliver oxygen more efficiently to the tissues with oxygen requirements.

2.1 Preparation of SNO-PEG-Hb

To utilize SNO-Hb as an oxygen carrier, we have developed a pyridoxalated and pegylated SNO-Hb derivative having low oxygen affinity and an optimum plasma residence time. The preparation steps are schematically illustrated in Figure 1. The detailed preparation method is described elsewhere[5]. Briefly, human Hb purified from outdated hman red cell products was mixed with pyridoxal-5' phosphate and pyridoxalation was started by the addition of sodium borohydrate under anaerobic conditions. For the pegylation of pyridoxalated Hb, the activated ester of PEG-bis(succinimidyl succinate) was added very slowly with stirring. *S*-nitrosylation of PEG-Hb was then performed with addition of *S*-nitrosoglutathione. The yield of *S*-nitrosylation was estimated by using a high-performance liquid chromatography (HPLC) coupled with flow reactors of metal and Griess reagent (Fig. 2)[6]. In human Hb, Cysβ93 is

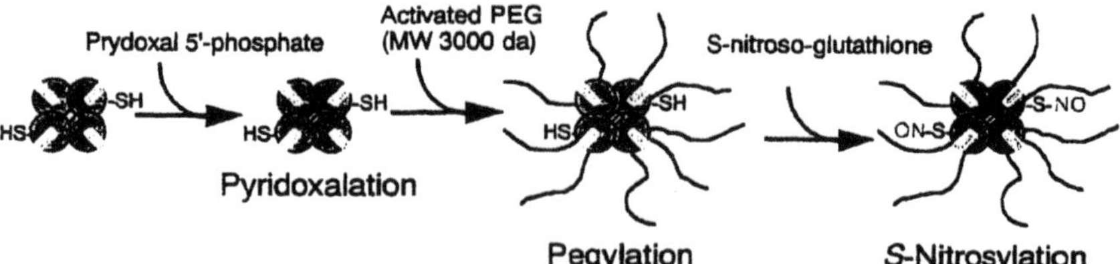

Figure 1. SNO-PEG-Hb preparation. Hb was pyridoxalated, pegylated and then *S*-nitrosylated.

highly reactive and the prefered target for *S*-nitrosylation. The content of NO in SNO-Hb reported in the text was, therefore, expressed on the basis that a fully s-nitrosylated Hb (100% SNO-Hb) contains two NOs because one tetramic Hb is constituted from two β-subunits. The yield of *S*-nitrosylation was usually set to 30-37%.

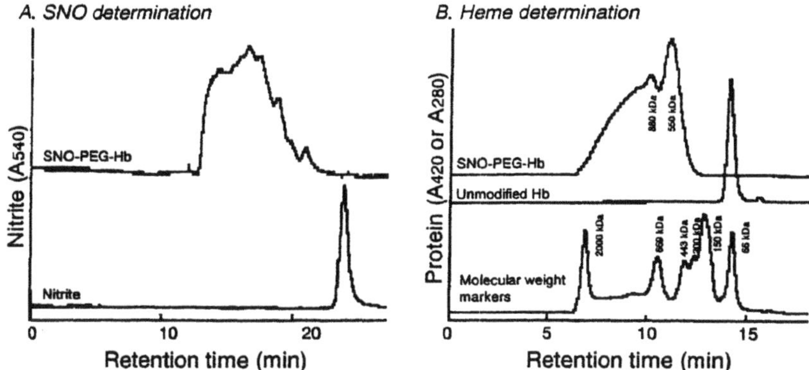

Figure 2 HPLC characterization of (A) Hb-bound NO and (B) heme of SNO-PEG-Hb. (A) Samples were separated on a gel-filtration column (8 x 300 mm, GFC-200, Eicom, Kyoto, Japan) eluted with 10 mM acetate buffer, 0.1 mM EDTA, 100 mM sodium chloride, pH 5.5, at the flow rate of 0.55 mL/min. The eluate was mixed with 1.75 mM mercury chloride at the flow rate of 0.20 mL/min to decompose S-nitrosylated protein, and further mixed with Griess reagent at the flow rate of 0.22 mL/min. The red azo-dye formed was determined by the absorption at 540 nm. (B) For the characterization of molecular weight distribution, proteins were separated on a gel-filtration column (7.6 x 300 mm, TSK G3000SW, Toyo Soda Co. Ltd, Tokyo, Japan) in 10 mM sodium phosphate buffer, 100 mM sodium chloride, pH 6.9, at the flow rate of 0.9 mL/min. Proteins were monitored at 420 nm for heme and at 280 nm for molecular weight markers.

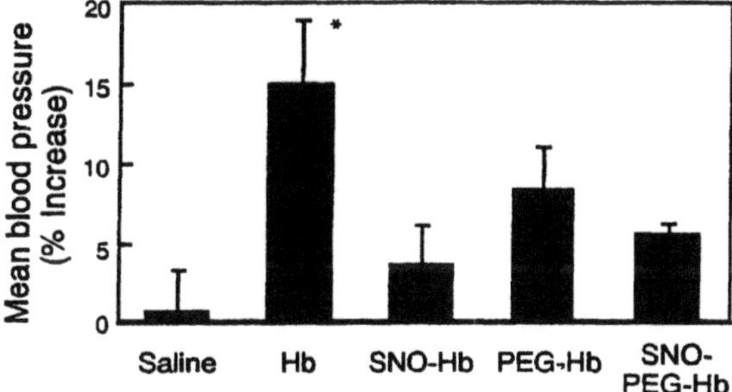

Figure 3 Changes in mean arterial blood pressure 5 min after a bolus injection of Hb materials (125 mg Hb/kg, Hb 10% solution) into male Wistar rats. Relative increase was calculated from the data before and after the injection. Each value represents the mean±SEM of 6-9 animals. *$p<0.05$ vs saline control by ANOVA followed by Scheffe's test.

3. EFFICACY AND SAFETY OF SNO-PEG-HB

3.1 Vasoactivity of SNO-PEG-Hb

Systemic administration of unmodified Hb resulted in a hypertensive reaction, which result is in agreement with previous reports[7,8]. In contrast, SNO-Hb did not raise blood pressure, suggesting that NO released from SNO-Hb may have compensated for NO scavenging by the heme in SNO-Hb. Since PEG-Hb also caused no significant increase of blood pressure, PEG-modification itself may also contribute to avoidance of Hb-induced hypertension, probably because the extravasation of Hb molecules and the resultant NO scavenging in the vessel walls is critical for Hb-induced vasoconstriction[9]. Pegylation effectively prevents the extravasation of Hb molecules. SNO-PEG-Hb showed reduced hypertensive activity like that of SNO-Hb (Fig. 3).

The release of NO from SNO-Hb was reported to be accelerated in the presence of low molecular weight thiols such as glutathione and a trace amount of copper ions[6]. Since both components should be present in blood plasma, we assumed that the half-life of NO bound to PEG-Hb in the plasma might be very short. We measured the half-life of Hb-bound NO as shown in Figure 4. The present data indicated that the plasma residence time was not so short. One possible reason for this might be the very low concentration of free copper ion in plasma. Finally, these findings suggested that SNO-PEG-Hb was a slow-releasing agent for NO.

3.2 Oxygen Transporting Capacity

The oxygen transporting capacity of SNO-PEG-Hb was evaluated using a hemorrhagic shock model in rats by monitoring the redox state of cytochrome oxidase reduction of cerebral tissues, in which a near-infrared spectroscopy

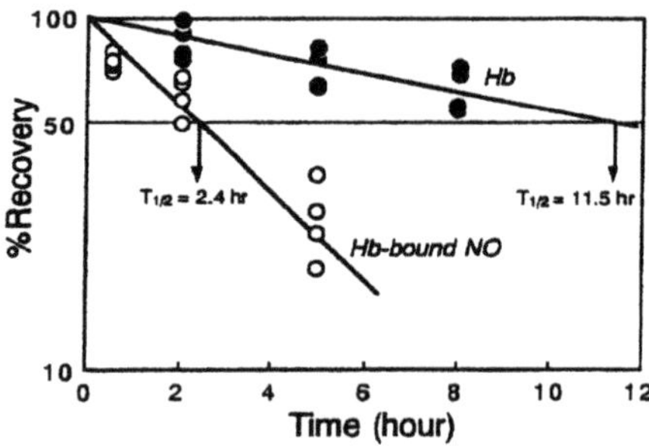

Figure 4 Plasma retention of NO (open circles) and heme (closed circles) of SNO-PEG-Hb in the circulation of rats after a bolus injection at 125 mg/kg.

was used[10]. After blood was removed (up to 30%) from anesthetized male Wistar rats under 21% O_2 ventilation, saline, PEG-Hb or SNO-PEG-Hb (5% Hb solution) was isovolumetrically infused. The pO_2 in the cervical vein and arterial blood pressure were monitored throughout the experiments. The intravenous infusion of SNO-PEG-Hb and PEG-Hb restored oxy-Hb, total-Hb, and cytochrome oxidase reduction levels of cerebral tissues (Fig. 5). This suggested that SNO-PEG-Hb could supply enough oxygen to the brain, like PEG-Hb. During the Hb infusion, PEG-Hb could quickly restore blood pressure, while this recovery was slower after the infusion of SNO-PEG-Hb. This suggested that SNO-PEG-Hb causes vasodilation as an NO donor.

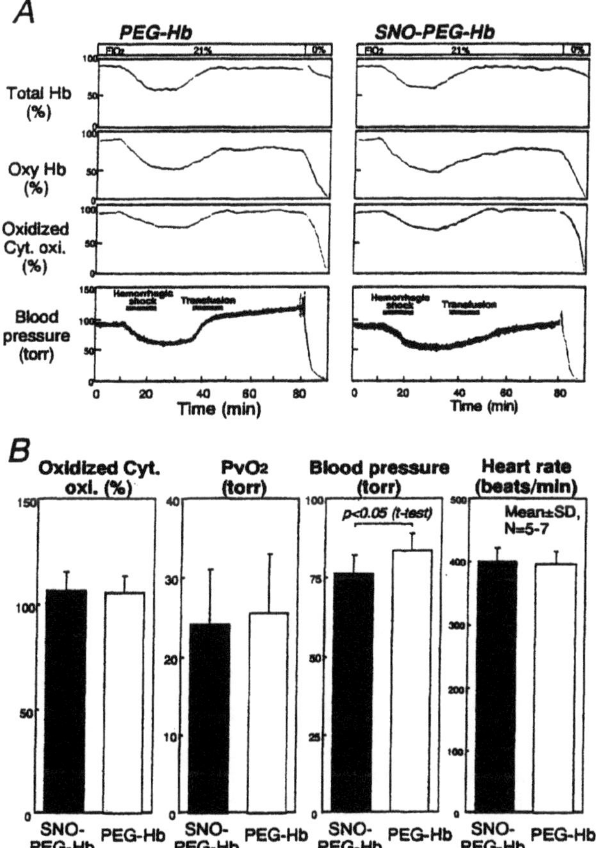

Figure 5 **The redox status of cytochrome oxidase in the rat brain after hemorrhagic shock and Hb infusion. (A) Typical tracings; (B) Comparison at the end of Hb infusion. The duration of hemorrhage and transfusion was indicated by bars. The relative change against the value obtained during the resting period is indicated in some figures.**

3.3. Safety Characteristics

Safety evaluation of SNO-PEG-Hb was performed in a volume overload experimental model using rats. Unmodified Hb, PEG-Hb and SNO-PEG-Hb were infused into male Wistar rats at 1.15 g/kg body weight (5% Hb solution). Bovine serum albumin was used as the control. Blood samples were obtained 1, 3, 7 and 14 days after administration. Plasma aspartate aminotransferase (AST), alanine aminotransferase (ALT), blood urea nitrigen (BUN) and creatinine were assayed, and the liver and kidney were removed, fixed with

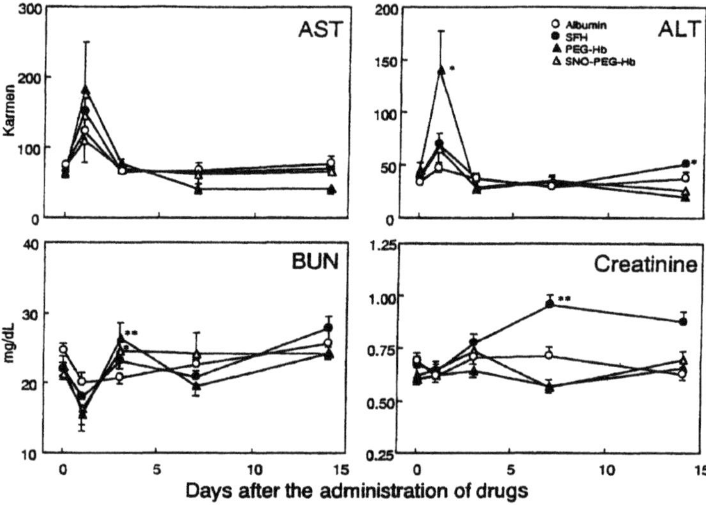

Figure 6 Changes in AST, ALT, BUN and creatinine after the administration of Hb solutions (1.15 g/kg, Hb 5% solution) into male Wistar rats. Each value represents the mean ± SEM of 7-13 animals. *$p<0.05$ and **$p<0.01$ vs albumin control by ANOVA followed by the Fisher PLSD test.

Table 1. Histopathological observation of the liver and kidney 7 days after the Hb administration into rats

Drugs Number of animals observed	Albumin 8	Hb 8	PEG-Hb 8	SPEG-Hb 9
Liver				
Focal capsulitis	4	3	5	3
Focal fibrous thickening of the capsule	3	3	5	4
Granuloma in the capsule	0	0	1	0
Focal necrosis	0	0	0	0
Fatty droplets in the hepatocytes	0	0	1	0
Kidney				
Vacuolization of the proximal tubular epithelium	0	0	8	8
Red (hemoglobinogenous) casts	0	2	0	0
Focal basophilic changes and atrophy of the renal tubules	1	2	1	1
Cellular infiltration in the interstitium	0	0	1	0
Pyelitis	0	0	1	0

formaline and stained for histopathological examination. All protein solutions induced transient increases in AST and ALT, and a decrease in BUN (Fig. 6). The most remarkable increase in ALT was observed with PEG-Hb, while SNO-PEG-Hb showed the smallest increase. These changes in AST and ALT returned to the baseline at 3 days postinfusion. Histological examinations of the liver supported these biochemical observations (Table 1). In kidneys, unmodified Hb caused red casts immediately after the administration and increased the plasma creatinine level at 7 days postinfusion, suggesting that unmodified Hb was nephrotoxic. PEG-Hb and SNO-PEG-Hb caused vacuole formation in the proximal tubular epithelium. Cellular infiltration in the interstitium was observed in the PEG-Hb group, while this change was rare in the SNO-PEG-Hb group. Renal function, as evaluated by BUN and creatinine, was, however, normal in both Hb groups. These findings suggested that two pegylated Hb derivatives induced some transient stress with regard to hepatic and renal functions, but it seemed to be well tolerated.

The most remarkable observation in the histology was the vacuolization in the proximal tubular epithelium of the kidneys in the animals transfused with the two pegylated Hb products (Fig. 7 for histology of rats treated with SNO-PEG-Hb). A similar phenomenon has been reported by Matsushita et al.[11], who showed that a PEG-Hb product caused vacuole formation in the epithelium of the canine kidney, without any pathological features of renal ischemic changes and the regeneration of the tubules. They demonstrated that these

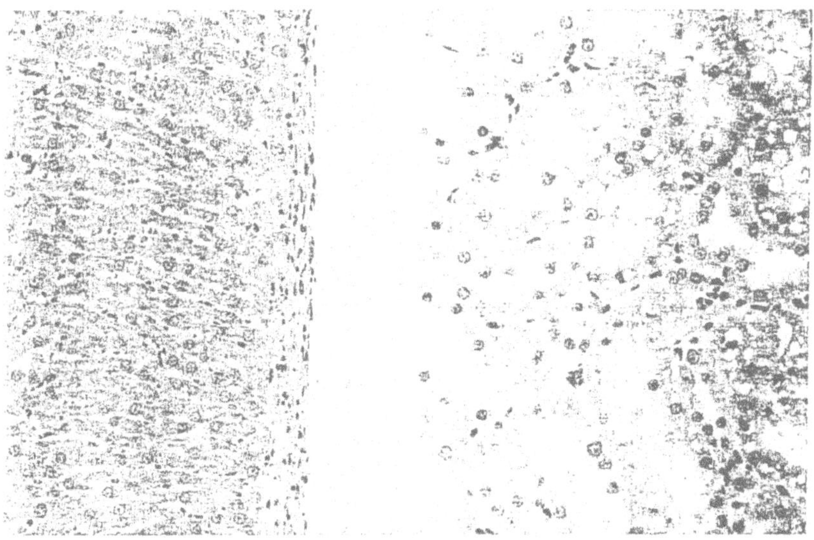

Figure 7 **Light microscopic examination of liver (left, x 66) and kidney (right, x 100) of rats treated with SNO-PEG-Hb at 7 days postinfusion. Hematoxylin and eosin stain.**

vacuoles included iron, possibly derived from the Hb product, based on the data of elemental X-ray microanalysis and ferric iron staining. Other substances such as dextran, hydroxyethyl starch, sucrose and mannitol have been also shown to cause vacuolization without any disturbance in renal functions. These reports suggest that the vacuolization reflects the degradation process of artificial materials in the proximal tubule cells.

4. IMPLICATION OF S-NITROSOTHIOLS

There is increased interest in NO in the body as a result of its formation by a variety of cell types as endothelial cells, platelets, neutrophils, and smooth muscle cells. The redox and chemical states of NO are critical in the diverse physiological and pathophysiological events induced by NO. One mechanism by which NO alters the biological function is through formation of S-nitrosothiols; there is increasing evidence that s-nitrosylation plays a large role in regulation of key enzymes and transcription factors. For example, the cardiac calcium release channel (ryanodine receptor) has been shown to be reversibly regulated by *S*-nitrosylation[12]. *S*-nitrosylation of α1-protease inhibitor (αPI), a major serine protease inhibitor protein in human plasma, gives a novel function to the protein; SNO-αPI exhibits remarkable cytoprotective effects in ischemia-reperfusion injury[13]. NF-kB is one of several transcription factors that display redox-sensitive DNA binding, and *S*-nitrosylation of its redox-sensitive cysteine-62 residue has been shown to inhibit NF-kB-dependent transcription[14]. Recently, several active transporting systems of RNSO-bound NO into live cells beyond the cell membrane have been reported[15,16]. The specific enzyme for GSNO degradation has been also identified as glutathione-dependent formaldehyde dehydrogenase, and this enzyme is evolutionally conserved from bacteria to humans[17]. Even though the total picture of the biology of RSNO is still unknown, these findings suggest the presence of an active regulatory system for RSNO metabolism, and that RSNO-bound NO may play essential roles in NO biology in health and disease. SNO-PEG-Hb can deliver not only oxygen but also NO to the tissues with oxygen requirements. Such delivered NO may contribute to regulate the above key enzymes and transcription factors. Considering that SNO-PEG-Hb will be applied to physiopathological situations such as ischemic disease and inflammation, further characterization of SNO-PEG-Hb as a tool for oxygen therapeutics should be encouraged.

5. CONCLUSION

We have developed a new Hb derivative that can deliver and release oxygen and NO-group molecules in the periphery. This product might be a valuable oxygen carrier as a tool for oxygen therapeutics.

ACKNOWLEDGMENTS

This work was supported in part by grants from the Ministry of Education, Science and Culture (No. 09557125,11694229, 11557112), and the Ministry of Health, Labour and Welfare of Japan for Research on Advanced Medical Technology. We thank J. Sakanoue for his assistance in measuring the oxygen supply in the rat brain, and A. Aida and Y. Shimahara for their experimental assistance.

REFERENCES

1. Nakai K, Sakuma I, Satoh H, Kitabatake A. Vascular activities of hemoglobin-based oxygen carriers: relationship between vasoconstrictive activity and endothelial permeability. In: Kitabatake A, Sakuma I. (eds). Recent Advances in Nitric Oxide Research. Tokyo: Springer-Verlag Tokyo; 1998. p. 33-45.
2. Jia L, Bonaventura C, Bonaventura J, Stamler J. *S*-nitrosohaemoglobin: a dynamic activity of blood involved in vascular control. Nature 1996; 380:221-226.
3. Stamler JS, Jia L, Eu JP, McMahon TJ, Demchenko IT, Bonaventura J, et al. Blood flow regulation by *S*-nitrosohemoglobin in the physiological oxygen gradient. Science 1997; 276:2034-3037.
4. Pawloski JR, Swaminathan RV, Stamler JS. Cell-free and erythrocytic *S*-nitrosohemoglobin inhibits human platelet aggregation. Circulation 1998; 97:263-267.
5. Nakai K, Hiroko T, Yasukohchi T, Sakuma I, Fujii S, Yoshioka M, et al. Preparation and characterization of SNO-PEG-hemoglobin as a candidate for oxygen transporting material. Int J Artif Organs 2001; 24:322-328.
6. Akaike T, Inoue K, Okamoto T, Nishino H, Otagiri M, Fujii S, et al. Nanomolar quantification and identification of various nitrosothiols by high performance liquid chromatography coupled with flow reactors of metals and Griess reagent. J Biochem 1997; 122:459-466.
7. Keipert PE, Gonzales A, Gomez CL, MacDonald VW, Hess JR, Winslow RM. Acute changes in systemic blood pressure and urine output of conscious rats following exchange transfusion with diaspirin-crosslinked hemoglobin solution. Transfusion 1993; 33:701-708.
8. Rioux F, Petitclerc E, Audet R, Drapeau G, Fielding RM, Marceau F. Recombinant human hemoglobin inhibits both constitutive and cytokine-induced nitric oxide-mediated relaxation of rabbit isolated aortic rings. J Cardiovasc Pharmacol 1994; 24:229-237.
9. Nakai K, Ohta T, Sakuma I, Akama K, Kobayashi Y, Tokuyama S, et al. Inhibition of endothelium-dependent relaxation by hemoglobin in rabbit aortic strips: Comparison between acellular hemoglobin derivatives and cellular hemoglobins. J Cardiovasc Pharmacol 1996; 28:115-123.
10. Hoshi Y, Hazeki O, Kakihana Y, Tamura M. Redox behavior of cytochrome oxidase in the rat brain measured by near-infrared spectroscopy. J Appl Physiol 1997; 83:1842-8.
11. Matsushita M, Yabuki A, Chen J, Takahashi T, Harasaki H, Malchesky PS, et al. Renal effects of a pyridoxalated-hemoglobin-polyoxyethylene conjugate solution as a blood substitute in exchange transfusions. Trans. Am. Soc. Artif. Intern. Organs 1988; 34:280-283.
12. Xu L, Eu JP, Meissner G, Stamler JS. Activation of the cardiac calcium release channel

(ryanodine receptor) by poly-*S*-nitrosylation. Science 1998; 279:234-237.
13. Ikebe N, Akaike T, Miyamoto Y, Hayashida K, Yoshitake J, Ogawa M, et al. Protective effect of *S*-nitrosylated α1-protease inhibitor on hepatic ischemia-reperfusion injury. J Pharamacol Exp Ther 2000; 295:904-911.
14. Marshall HE, Stamler JS. Inhibition of NF-kB by *S*-nitrosylation. Biochemistry 2001; 40:1688-1693.
15. Li X, Rose G, Dongre N, Pan H-L, Tobin JR, Eisenach JC. *S*-nitroso-l-cysteine releases norepinephrine in rat spinal synaptosomes. Brain Res 2000; 872:301-307.
16. Ramachandran N, Root P, Jiang XM, Hogg PJ, Mutus B. Mechanism of transfer of NO from extracellular *S*-nitrosothiols into the cytosol by cell-surface protein disulfide isomerase. Proc Natl Acad Sci USA 2001; 97:9539-9544.
17. Liu L, Hausladen A, Zeng M, Que L, Heitman J, Stamler JS. A metabolic enzyme for *S*-nitrosothiol conserved from bacteria to humans. Nature 2001; 410:490-494.

Index

www.ingramcontent.com/pod-product-compliance
Ingram Content Group UK Ltd.
Pitfield, Milton Keynes, MK11 3LW, UK
UKHW021333070726
13610UKWH00011B/59

* 9 7 8 1 4 7 5 7 7 8 3 9 7 *